Health Meale

T0092202

Health Measurement Scales
A practical guide to their development and use

SIXTH EDITION

David L. Streiner
Department of Psychiatry and Behavioural Neurosciences,
Department of Clinical Epidemiology and Biostatistics,
McMaster University, Hamilton, Ontario, Canada
Department of Psychiatry, University of Toronto, Toronto,
Ontario, Canada

Geoffrey R. Norman
Department of Clinical Epidemiology and Biostatistics,
McMaster University, Hamilton, Ontario, Canada

and

John Cairney
School of Human Movement and Nutrition Sciences,
University of Queensland, St Lucia, Australia

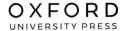
OXFORD
UNIVERSITY PRESS

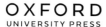

OXFORD
UNIVERSITY PRESS

Great Clarendon Street, Oxford, OX2 6DP,
United Kingdom

Oxford University Press is a department of the University of Oxford.
It furthers the University's objective of excellence in research, scholarship,
and education by publishing worldwide. Oxford is a registered trade mark of
Oxford University Press in the UK and in certain other countries

© Oxford University Press 2024

The moral rights of the authors have been asserted

First edition published in 1989
Second edition published in 1995
Third edition published in 2003
Reprinted 2004
Fourth edition published in 2008
Fifth edition published in 2015
Sixth edition published in 2024

All rights reserved. No part of this publication may be reproduced, stored in
a retrieval system, or transmitted, in any form or by any means, without the
prior permission in writing of Oxford University Press, or as expressly permitted
by law, by licence or under terms agreed with the appropriate reprographics
rights organization. Enquiries concerning reproduction outside the scope of the
above should be sent to the Rights Department, Oxford University Press, at the
address above

You must not circulate this work in any other form
and you must impose this same condition on any acquirer

Published in the United States of America by Oxford University Press
198 Madison Avenue, New York, NY 10016, United States of America

British Library Cataloguing in Publication Data
Data available

Library of Congress Control Number: 2023940289

ISBN 978–0–19–286948–7

DOI: 10.1093/med/9780192869487.001.0001

Printed in the UK by
Bell & Bain Ltd., Glasgow

Oxford University Press makes no representation, express or implied, that the
drug dosages in this book are correct. Readers must therefore always check
the product information and clinical procedures with the most up-to-date
published product information and data sheets provided by the manufacturers
and the most recent codes of conduct and safety regulations. The authors and
the publishers do not accept responsibility or legal liability for any errors in the
text or for the misuse or misapplication of material in this work. Except where
otherwise stated, drug dosages and recommendations are for the non-pregnant
adult who is not breast-feeding

Links to third party websites are provided by Oxford in good faith and
for information only. Oxford disclaims any responsibility for the materials
contained in any third party website referenced in this work.

MIX
Paper | Supporting
responsible forestry
FSC
www.fsc.org   FSC® C007785

Preface to the sixth edition

It has been said that the half-life of information in medicine is very short; that every 10 years or so, half of what we now believe to be true will have been shown to be wrong, replaced by new truths which will have their brief time in the sun before being replaced. Fortunately or not, the same is not the case for psychometrics or statistics. The formulae we use to define reliability, or to calculate the intra class correlation coefficient, or which underlie item response theory are the same as when they were first developed 50 to 100 years ago. So what has changed to justify a new edition of this book?

As a matter of fact, a lot has changed. When the previous editions were written, for example, coefficient alpha (α) was the undisputed index of the reliability of a scale. Granted that there was recognition that it was a flawed measure, but there wasn't much that could take its place. In recent years, though, the steady stream of articles criticizing α has become a torrent, and new (and free) computer programs have become available that do the necessary calculations. This also led us to completely rewrite the section on 'types' of scales, pointing out where α may be useful (tau-equivalent and parallel scales) and where it should be avoided (congeneric scales which, unfortunately, is what most scales are).

Changes in technology have also meant that the chapter on administration had to be extensively revised. The previous two editions extolled the virtues of personal data assistants (PDAs) as a method of delivering scales, and especially for measuring phenomena in real time, such as pain or depression. Now, perhaps the only place one can find PDAs is on the shelves of museums devoted to archaic technologies, such as eight-track tapes and dictation machines. By the same token, it has never been easier to enrol participants to fill out questionnaires. Between social media and Web-based services that cater to people willing to complete them, either for free or for a fee, it is now possible to achieve sample sizes in the hundreds or thousands in a very short time, albeit at the possible cost of reduced generalizability. We debated whether to delete the section on mailed questionnaires but, in the end, decided to retain it. Many parts of the world still do not have access to high-speed internet connections, and this applies to rural and remote areas of the developed world, so mail still remains a viable alternative. In addition, certain demographic groups, particularly those who grew up in a time when writing using pen and paper were standard fare, prefer this mode to digital options. Furthermore, many of the techniques used with mailed questionnaires to improve the return rate apply equally well to Web-based methods.

At the same time, what is old is new again. When we wrote the first edition of the book, we included a chapter on generalizability (G) theory, not because people were using it much, but rather we thought it provided a useful intellectual framework to better understand reliability and the factors, outside of the usual suspects, that can affect it. A quick Medline search showed about 5 to 10 articles a year were published using G-theory until last year, when the number jumped to nearly 25. Although we shouldn't generalize from such a small number of points, we will, and think that there may be revised interest in this technique. This has led to a complete rewrite of the chapter, relegating the equations (which not even we could remember) to an appendix, and focussing more on how to use a dedicated (and free) computer program to do the work for us.

Because of the new material we were adding, this version was threatening to equal *War and Peace* in length. To compensate, we eliminated some sections that we felt were addressing relatively obscure topics. So, if you want information about goal attainment scaling or (rarely used) alternatives to the standard error of the mean, you'll have to look at earlier versions.

Along the way, we updated most of the other chapters, highlighting the relevant literature. This version, as the previous ones, has benefitted greatly from comments readers have sent us. We don't know if we can promise a seventh edition, but keep the emails coming. Write to us at:

streiner@mcmaster.ca

norman@mcmaster.ca

j.cairney@uq.edu.au

D.L.S.

G.R.N.

J.C.

Contents

Dedication

According to the Talmud, Rabbi Chanina said, 'I have learned much from my teachers, more from my colleagues, and most from my students'. That is most definitely the case with this book. It has benefited greatly from feedback from our students, from their theses and dissertations, and from our interactions with them. In thanks, we dedicate this book to our students—past, present, and future.

Chapter 1

Introduction to health measurement scales

Introduction to measurement

Measure what is measurable, and make measurable what is not so. Galileo Galilei

Not everything that counts can be counted. Attributed (incorrectly) to Albert Einstein

The act of measurement is an essential component of scientific research, whether in the natural, social, or health sciences. Until the last couple of decades, however, discussions regarding issues of measurement were noticeably absent in the deliberations of clinical researchers. Certainly, measurement played as essential a role in research in the health sciences as that in other scientific disciplines. However, measurement in the laboratory disciplines presented no inherent difficulty. Like other natural sciences, measurement was a fundamental part of the discipline and was approached through the development of appropriate instrumentation. Subjective judgement played a minor role in the measurement process; therefore, any issue of reproducibility or validity was amenable to a technological solution. It should be mentioned, however, that expensive equipment does not, of itself, eliminate measurement errors. As Cicchetti et al. (2006, p. 560) have said:

> the fact that data derive from automated methods does not per se make them more reliable than data deriving from the evaluation of well-trained observers. Each type of assessment instrument has its own sources of variability that can serve to attenuate the level of reliability.

What can be more automated than measuring various blood parameters with a haemoglobinometer? Yet there is variability among successive drops of fingerprick blood (Bond and Richards-Kortum 2015) or between haemoglobin concentrations collected simultaneously from the right and left hand (Morris et al. 1999). Indeed, even if the measurement instrument were completely error free, measurement of such quantities as blood pressure, heart rate, or myriad other physiological variables is subject to variation, often large, between successive samples.

Conversely, clinical researchers were acutely aware of the fallibility of human judgement, as evidenced by the errors involved in processes such as radiological diagnosis (Garland 1959; Yerushalmy 1955). Fortunately, the research problems approached by many clinical researchers—cardiologists, epidemiologists, and the like—frequently did not depend on subjective assessment. Trials of therapeutic regimens focused on the prolongation of life and the prevention or management of such life-threatening conditions as heart disease, stroke, or cancer. In these circumstances, the measurement is reasonably straightforward. 'Objective' criteria, based on laboratory or tissue diagnosis where possible, can be used to decide whether a patient has the disease and warrants inclusion in the study. The investigator then waits an appropriate period of time and counts those who did or did not survive—and the criteria for death are reasonably well established, even though the exact cause of death may be a little more difficult.

In the past few decades, the situation in clinical research has become more complex. The effects of new drugs or surgical procedures on *quantity* of life are likely to be marginal indeed. Conversely, there is an increased awareness of the impact of health and healthcare on the *quality* of human life. Therapeutic efforts in many disciplines of medicine (e.g. psychiatry, respirology, rheumatology, and oncology) and other health professions, such as nursing, physiotherapy, and occupational therapy, are directed equally if not primarily to the improvement of quality, not quantity of life. If the efforts of these disciplines are to be placed on a sound scientific basis, methods must be devised to measure what was previously thought to be unmeasurable and to assess in a reproducible and valid fashion those subjective states that cannot be converted into the position of a needle on a dial.

The need for reliable and valid measures was clearly demonstrated by Marshall et al. (2000). After examining 300 randomized controlled trials in schizophrenia, they found that the studies were nearly 40 per cent more likely to report that treatment was effective when they used unpublished scales rather than ones with peer-reviewed evidence of validity; and in non-drug studies, one-third of the claims of treatment superiority would not have been made if the studies had used published scales.

The challenge is not as formidable as it may seem. Psychologists and educators have been grappling with the issue for many years, dating back to the European attempts at the turn of the twentieth century to assess individual differences in intelligence (Galton, cited in Allen and Yen 1979). Since that time, particularly since the 1930s, much has been accomplished so that a sound methodology for the development and application of tools to assess subjective states now exists. Unfortunately, much of this literature is virtually unknown to most clinical researchers. Health science libraries do not routinely catalogue *Psychometrica* or the *British Journal of Statistical Psychology*. Nor should they—the language would be incomprehensible to most readers, and the problems of seemingly little relevance.

Similarly, the textbooks on the subject are directed at educational or psychological audiences. The former is concerned with measures of achievement applicable to classroom situations, and the latter is focused primarily on personality or aptitude measures, again with no apparent direct relevance. In general, textbooks in these disciplines are directed to the development of achievement, intelligence, or personality tests.

By contrast, researchers in health sciences are frequently faced with the desire to measure something that has not been approached previously—arthritic pain, return to function of post-myocardial infarction patients, speech difficulties of aphasic stroke patients, or clinical competence of junior medical students. The difficulties and questions that arose in developing such instruments range from straightforward (e.g. How many boxes do I put on the response?) to complex (e.g. How do I establish whether the instrument is measuring what I intend to measure?). Nevertheless, to a large degree, the answers are known, although they are frequently difficult to access.

The intent of this book is to introduce researchers in health sciences to these concepts of measurement. It is not an introductory textbook, in that we do not confine ourselves to a discussion of introductory principles and methods; rather, we attempt to make the book as current and comprehensive as possible. The book does not delve as heavily into mathematics as many books in the field; such side trips may provide some intellectual rewards for those who are inclined, but frequently at the expense of losing the majority of readers. Similarly, we emphasize applications, rather than theory, so that some theoretical subjects (such as Thurstone's law of comparative judgement), which are of historical interest but little practical importance, are omitted. Nevertheless, we spend considerable time in the explanation of the concepts underlying the current approaches to measurement. One other departure from current books is that our focus is on those attributes of interest to researchers in health sciences—subjective states, attitudes, response to illness, etc.—rather than the topics such as personality or achievement familiar to readers in education and psychology. As a result, our examples are drawn from the literature in health sciences.

Finally, some understanding of certain selected topics in statistics is necessary to learn many essential concepts of measurement. In particular, the *correlation coefficient* is used in many empirical studies of measurement instruments. The discussion of reliability is based on the methods of *repeated measures analysis of variance*. Item analysis and certain approaches to test validity use the methods of *factor analysis*. It is not by any means necessary to have detailed knowledge of these methods to understand the concepts of measurement discussed in this book. Still, it would be useful to have some conceptual understanding of these techniques. If the reader requires some review of statistical topics, we have suggested a few appropriate resources at the end of this chapter.

A roadmap to the book

In the last edition of this book, we provided a roadmap or guide to summarize the process of scale construction and evaluation. While individual aspects of this are detailed in the chapters, the overall process can easily be lost in the detail. Of course in doing so, we run the risk that some readers will jump to the relevant chapters and conclude there is not much to this measurement business. That would be a gross misconception. The roadmap is an oversimplification of a complex process. However, we do feel it is a valuable heuristic device, which while necessarily lacking in detail, may nevertheless help to shed some light on the process of measurement—a process which, to those who are new to the field, can often seem like the darkest of black boxes (see Fig. 1.1).

Our roadmap begins the same way all research begins—with a question. It may be derived from the literature or, as is sometimes the case in health research, from clinical observation. Our question in this case, however, is explicitly connected to a measurement problem: do we have a measure or scale that can be used in pursuit of answering our research question? As we will discuss in Chapter 2, there are two important considerations here: are there really no existing measures that we can use? This of course

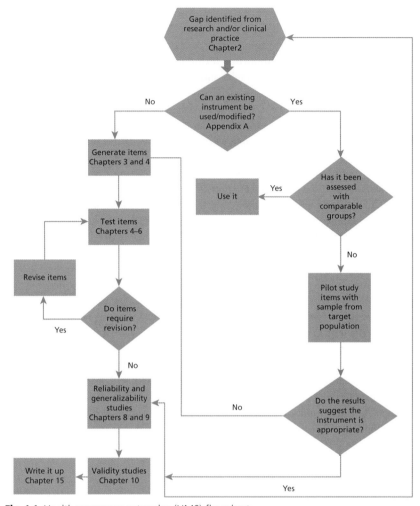

Fig. 1.1 Health measurement scales (HMS) flowchart.

can arise when the research question involves measuring a novel concept (or an old one) for which a measure does not currently exist. *Our position, always, is not to bring a new scale into the world unless it is absolutely necessary.* However, in situations where one is truly faced with no other option but to create a new scale, we begin the process of construction and testing—item generation, item testing, and retesting in Fig. 1.1. This is reviewed in detail in Chapters 3 to 6. Chapter 7 covers the transformation of items to scale. While not explicitly included in this diagram, we assume that once the items are devised and tested, then a scale will be created by combining items and further tested. It is here we concern ourselves with dimensionality of the scale (whether our new scale is measuring one thing or many). We discuss one common test of dimensionality, factor analysis, in Appendix B.

A far more common occurrence, however, is that we have a scale (or many scales) that can potentially be used for our research project. Following the top right side of the roadmap in Fig. 1.1, the important question now is whether we have a scale that has already been used in similar populations (and for similar purposes) to the one we will be sampling in our study. Appendix A lists many resources for finding existing scales. For example, there are many scales that measure depression. The selection of a particular scale will be in part based upon whether there is evidence concerning its measurement properties specifically in the context of our target population (e.g. a depression measure for children under the age of 12). Review of the literature is how we determine this. It is not uncommon at this stage to find that we have 'near' hits (e.g. a scale to measure depression in adolescents, but one that has not been used to measure depression in children). Here we must exercise judgement. If we believe that only minor modifications are required, then we can usually proceed without entering into a process of item testing. An example here comes from studies of pain. Pain scales can often be readily adapted for specific pain sites of clinical importance (hands, feet, knees, etc.). Absence of a specific scale measuring thumb pain on the right hand for adults aged 60–65 years, however, is not justification for the creation of a new scale. There are instances though where we cannot assume that a scale that has been tested in one population can necessarily be used in a different population without first testing this assumption. Here we may enter the process of item generation and testing if our pilot results reveal that important domains have been missed, or if items need to be substantially modified to be of use with our study population (on our diagram, this is the link between the right and left sides, or the pathway connecting 'No' regarding group to the item testing loop).

Once we have created a new scale (or revised an existing one for our population) we are ready to test reliability (Chapters 8 and 9) and validity (Chapter 10). Of course, if the purpose of the study is not the design and evaluation of a scale, researchers typically proceed directly to designing a study to answer a research question or test a hypothesis of association. Following this path, reporting of psychometric properties of the new or revised scale will likely be limited to internal consistency only, which is an easy, but extremely limited, psychometric property to assess (see the section entitled 'Kuder–Richardson 20 and coefficient alpha' in Chapter 5). However, study findings, while not explicitly stated as such, can nevertheless provide important information on validity. One researcher's cross-sectional study is another's construct validation study: it all depends on how you frame the question. From our earlier example, if the results of a study using our new scale to measure depression in children shows that girls have higher levels of depression than boys, or that children who have been bullied are more likely to be depressed than children who have not, this is evidence of construct validity (both findings show the scale is producing results in an expected way, given what we know about depression in children). On the other hand, simply finding a difference between two groups will not strengthen the case for construct validity if there is no theoretical rationale for the difference (e.g. finding a difference in quality of life scores between males and females). If the study in question is a measurement study, then we would be more intentional in our design to measure different aspects of both reliability and validity. The complexity of the design will depend on the scale (and the research question). If, for example, we are using a scale that requires multiple raters to assess a single object of measurement (e.g. raters evaluating play behaviour in children, tutors rating students), and we are interested in assessing whether raters agree or whether ratings are stable over time, we can devise quite complex factorial designs, as we discuss in Chapter 9, and use generalizability (G) theory to simultaneously assess different aspects of reliability. As another example, we may want to look at various aspects of reliability—inter-rater, test–retest, internal consistency; it then makes sense to do it with a single G study so we can look at the error resulting from the various factors. In some cases, a cross-sectional survey, where we compare our new (or revised) measure to a standard measure by correlating it with other measures hypothesized to be associated with the construct we are trying to measure, may be all that is needed. Of course, much has been written on the topic of research design already (e.g. Streiner and Norman 2009) and an extended discussion is beyond the scope of this chapter. We do, however, discuss different ways to administer scales (Chapter 13). Choice of administration method will be determined both by the nature of the scale and by what aspects of reliability and validity we are interested in assessing. But before any study is begun, be aware of ethical issues that may arise; these are discussed in Chapter 14.

Of course, as with all research, our roadmap is iterative. Most of the scales that have stood the test of time (much like this book) have been revised, retested, and tested again. In pursuit of our evaluation of reliability and validity, we often find that our scale needs to be tweaked. Sometimes, the required changes are more dramatic. As our understanding of the construct we are measuring evolves, we often need to revise scales accordingly. At any rate, it is important to dispel the notion that once a scale is created, it is good for all eternity. As with the research process in general, the act of research often generates more questions than answers (thereby also ensuring our continued employment). When you are ready to write up what you have found, check Chapter 15 regarding reporting guidelines for studies of reliability and validity.

A cautionary note—the 'jingle-jangle' fallacies

Earlier in the chapter, we admonished readers that they should seek out existing scales before embarking on the arduous journey of developing a new one. This could start by using some of the resources listed in Appendix A to locate tools that may be appropriate. There are two dangers lurking in the blind acceptance of a scale because its name makes it sound as if it's a likely candidate or, conversely, makes it sound irrelevant. These are known as the *jingle-jangle fallacies*.

The *jingle* fallacy, first identified by Thorndike (1904), is the assumption that two or more tests measure the same construct because they have the same name. Fried (2017), for example, looked at the seven most widely used scales of depressive symptomatology. Across the instruments, there were 52 disparate symptoms. Of these, 40 per cent appeared in only one scale; and only 12 per cent appeared in all. In one instrument (the Center for Epidemiological Studies—Depression (CES-D); Radloff 1977), one-third of the items appeared in no other scale. Similarly, there are many scales that purport to measure social support. Some do this by counting the number of people in one's social network, whereas others include only people considered to be friends. Some scales measure emotional support, while others tap instrumental support (e.g. financial assistance or other tangible, direct ways), and still others include informational support. The scales also differ among themselves regarding whether they measure support that has actually been given or the person's perception of the availability of support. These reflect differences not only in how social support is measured, but more importantly, in the conceptualization of what social support means. Needless to say, the correlations among the various measures are low, and the relationship between social support and other constructs, such as health, varies widely from one study to the next (Barrera 1986).

In contrast, the *jangle* fallacy (Kelly 1927) refers to constructs or scales with different names that are actually measuring the same thing. Sometimes, this arises from imprecise terminology in the field, but in psychology, a common problem concerns differences between how researchers or clinicians define (and measure) a phenomenon, and more colloquial understandings of the same concept (Block 2000). For example, 'sensation-seeking', 'disinhibition', and 'novelty-seeking' each have their own scales, but they are all highly correlated, suggesting that they are simply different names for the same phenomenon (Block 2000). Unfortunately, many other examples abound, such as the interrelationships among 'subjective well-being', 'quality of life', and 'happiness'; and the fact that aptitude and achievement tests not only are highly correlated but also often contain the same items.

These fallacies highlight that you must go beyond the name of the scale and examine how the construct was conceptualized, the individual items in the instrument, and the results of studies that have used the scales.

Further reading

Boateng, G.O., Neilands, T.B., Frongillo, E.A., Melgar-Quiñonez, H.R., and Young, S.L. (2018). Best practices for developing and validating scales for health, social, and behavioral research: A primer. *Frontiers of Public Health*, **6**, Article 149.

Freund, J.E. and Perles, B.M. (2005). *Modern elementary statistics* (12th edn). Pearson, Upper Saddle River, NJ.

Huff, D. (1954). *How to lie with statistics*. W.W. Norton, New York.

Norman, G.R. and Streiner, D.L. (2003). *PDQ statistics* (3rd edn). PMPH USA, Shelton, CT.

Norman, G.R. and Streiner, D.L. (2014). *Biostatistics: The bare essentials* (4th edn). PMPH USA, Shelton, CT.

References

Allen, M.J. and Yen, W.M. (1979). *Introduction to measurement theory*. Brooks Cole, Monterey, CA.

Barrera, M. (1986). Distinctions between social support concepts, measures, and models. *American Journal of Community Psychology*, **14**, 413–45.

Block, J. (2000). Three tasks for personality psychology. In *Developmental science and the holistic approach* (eds. L.R. Bergman, R.B. Cairns, L.G. Nilsson, and L. Nystedt), pp. 155–64. Erlbaum, Mahwah, NJ.

Bond, M.M. and Richards-Kortum, R.R. (2015). Drop-to-drop variation in the cellular components of fingerprick blood: Implications for point-of-care diagnostic development. *American Journal of Clinical Pathology*, **144**, 885–94.

Cicchetti, D., Bronen, R., Spencer, S., Haut, S., Berg, A., Oliver, P., *et al.* (2006). Rating scales, scales of measurement, issues of reliability: Resolving some critical issues for clinicians and researchers. *Journal of Nervous and Mental Disease*, **194**, 557–64.

Fried, E.I. (2017). The 52 symptoms of major depression: Lack of content overlap among seven common depression scales. *Journal of Affective Disorders*, **208**, 191–7.

Garland, L.H. (1959). Studies on the accuracy of diagnostic procedures. *American Journal of Roentgenology*, **82**, 25–38.

Kelley, E.L. (1927). *Interpretation of educational measurements*. World Book Company, Yonkers, NY.

Marshall, M., Lockwood, A., Bradley, C., Adams, C., Joy, C., and Fenton, M. (2000). Unpublished rating scales: A major source of bias in randomised controlled trials of treatments for schizophrenia. *British Journal of Psychiatry*, **176**, 249–52.

Morris, S.S., Ruel, M.T., Cohen, R.J., Dewey, K.G., de la Brière, B., and Hassan, M.N. (1999). Precision, accuracy, and reliability of hemoglobin assessment with use of capillary blood. *American Journal of Clinical Nutrition*, **69**, 1243–8.

Radloff, L.S. (1977). The CES-D scale: A self-report depression scale for research in the general population. *Applied Psychological Measurement*, **1**, 385–401.

Streiner, D.L. and Norman, G.R. (2009). *PDQ epidemiology* (3rd edn). PMPH USA, Shelton, CT.

Thorndike, E.L. (1904). *An introduction to the theory of mental and social measurements*. Teachers College, Columbia University, New York.

Yerushalmy, J. (1955). Reliability of chest radiography in diagnosis of pulmonary lesions. *American Journal of Surgery*, **89**, 231–40.

Chapter 2

Basic concepts

Introduction to basic concepts

One feature of the health sciences literature devoted to measuring subjective states is the daunting array of available scales. Whether one wishes to measure depression, pain, or patient satisfaction, it seems that every article published in the field has used a different approach to the measurement problem. This proliferation impedes research, since there are significant problems in generalizing from one set of findings to another.

Paradoxically, if you proceed a little further in the search for existing instruments to assess a particular concept, you may conclude that none of the existing scales is quite right, so it is appropriate to embark on the development of one more scale to add to the confusion in the literature. Most researchers tend to magnify the deficiencies of existing measures and underestimate the time and effort required to develop an adequate new measure. Of course, scales do not exist for all applications; if this were so, there would be little justification for writing this book. Nevertheless, perhaps the most common error committed by clinical researchers is to dismiss existing scales too lightly, and embark on the development of a new instrument with an unjustifiably optimistic and naive expectation that they can do better in a relatively short period. As will become evident, the development of scales to assess subjective attributes is not easy and requires considerable investment of both mental and fiscal resources. Therefore, a useful first step is to be aware of any existing scales that might suit the purpose. The next step is to understand and apply criteria for judging the usefulness of a particular scale. In subsequent chapters, these will be described in much greater detail for use in developing a scale; however, the next few pages will serve as an introduction to the topic and a guideline for a critical literature review.

The discussion that follows is necessarily brief. A much more comprehensive set of standards, which is widely used for the assessment of standardized tests used in psychology and education, is the manual called *Standards for Educational and Psychological Tests* that is published jointly by the American Educational Research Association, the American Psychological Association, and the National Council on Measurement in Education (AERA/APA/NCME 2014). Chapter 15 of this book summarizes what scale developers should report about a scale they have developed, and what users of these scales should look for (e.g. for reporting in meta-analyses). Here, again, the problem is a plethora of reporting guidelines. If you want to just jump in, the two most widely used ones are probably STARD (Bossuyt et al. 2015) and COSMIN (Mokkink et al. 2010), although both are biased toward diagnostic tests used in medical contexts that yield a dichotomous decision. For one more oriented to continuous measures (the type we discuss in this book), there is a modification of the STARD criteria (Streiner et al. 2016).

Searching the literature

An initial search of the literature to locate scales for measurement of particular variables might begin with the standard bibliographic sources, particularly Medline. However, depending on the application, one might wish to consider bibliographic reference systems in other disciplines, particularly *PsycINFO* for psychological scales; CINAHL (Cumulative Index to Nursing and Allied Health Literature) for nursing and rehabilitation (<https://www.ebsco.com/products/research-databases/cinahl-datab ase>); and ERIC (which stands for Educational Resource Information Center: <http://eric.ed.gov/>) for instruments designed for educational purposes.

In addition to these standard sources, there are a number of compendia of measurement scales, both in book form and as searchable, online resources. These are described in Appendix A. We might particularly highlight the volume entitled *Measuring Health: A Guide to Rating Scales and Questionnaires* (McDowell 2006), which is a critical review of scales designed to measure a number of characteristics of interest to researchers in the health sciences, such as pain, illness behaviour, and social support. However, as the most recent edition is now more than 1 7 years old, any new (or modified) scales developed since the early 2000s will obviously not be included; we could not locate a more recent, and similarly comprehensive, volume.

Critical review

Having located one or more scales of potential interest, it remains to choose whether to use one of these existing scales or to proceed to development of a new instrument. In part, this decision can be guided by a judgement of the appropriateness of the items on the scale, but this should always be supplemented by a critical review of the evidence in support of the instrument. The particular dimensions of this review are described in the following sections.

Face and content validity

The terms *face validity* and *content validity* are technical descriptions of the judgement that a scale looks reasonable—whether, on the face of it, the instrument appears to be assessing the desired qualities. The criterion represents a subjective judgement based on a review of the measure itself by one or more experts, and rarely are any empirical approaches used. Content validity is a closely related concept, consisting of a judgement whether the instrument samples all the relevant or important content or domains and does not include irrelevant content or domains. These two forms of validity consist of a judgement by experts whether the scale appears appropriate for the intended purpose. Guilford (1954) calls this approach to validation 'validity by assumption', meaning the instrument measures such-and-such because an expert says it does. However, an explicit statement regarding face and content validity, based on some form of review by an expert panel or alternative methods described later, should be a minimum prerequisite for acceptance of a measure.

In some instances, however, content validity may be more than this. Licensing bodies, such as the National Board of Medical Examiners, go to extreme lengths to ensure that their licensing examinations reflect the relevant content of medicine by, for example, recruiting expert clinicians to identify key concepts in their domain and to create test questions reflecting these domains.

Having said this, there are situations where face and content validity may not be desirable, and may be consciously avoided. For example, in assessing behaviour such as child abuse or excessive alcohol consumption, questions like 'Have you ever hit your child with a blunt object?' or 'Do you frequently drink to excess?' may have face validity, but are unlikely to elicit an honest response. Questions designed to effectively assess sensitive areas are likely to be less obviously related to the underlying attitude or behaviour and may appear to have poor face validity. In the end, it is rare for scales not to satisfy minimal standards of face and content validity, unless there has been a deliberate attempt from the outset to avoid straightforward questions.

Nevertheless, all too frequently, researchers dismiss existing measures on the basis of their own judgements of face validity—they did not like some of the questions, or the scale was too long, or the responses were not in a preferred format. As we have indicated, this judgement should comprise only one of several used in arriving at an overall judgement of usefulness, and should be balanced against the time and cost of developing a replacement.

Reliability

The concept of *reliability* is, on the surface, deceptively simple. Before one can obtain evidence that an instrument is measuring what is intended, it is first necessary to gather evidence that the scale is measuring *something* in a reproducible fashion. That is, a first step in providing evidence of the value of an instrument is to demonstrate that measurements of individuals on different occasions, or by different observers, or by similar or parallel tests produce the same or similar results.

That is the basic idea behind the concept—an index of the extent to which measurements of individuals obtained under different circumstances yield similar results. However, the concept is refined a bit further in measurement theory. If we were considering the reliability of, for example, a set of bathroom scales, it might be sufficient to indicate that the scales are accurate to ±1 kg. From this information, we can easily judge whether the scales will be adequate to distinguish among adult males (probably yes) or to assess weight gain of premature infants (probably no), since we have prior knowledge of the average weight and variation in weight of adults and premature infants.

Such information is rarely available in the development of subjective scales. Each scale produces a different measurement from every other. Therefore, to indicate that a particular scale is accurate to ±3.4 units provides no indication of its value in measuring individuals unless we have some idea about the likely range of scores on the scale. To circumvent this problem, reliability is usually computed as a ratio of the variability between individuals to the total variability in the scores; in other words, the reliability is a measure of the proportion of the variability in scores which was due to true differences between individuals. Thus, the reliability is expressed as a number between 0 and 1, with 0 indicating no reliability and 1 indicating perfect reliability.

An important issue in examining the reliability of an instrument is the manner in which the data were obtained that provided the basis for the calculation of a reliability coefficient. First of all, since the reliability involves the ratio of variability between subjects to total variability, one way to ensure that a test will look good is to conduct the study on an extremely heterogeneous sample : for example, to measure knowledge of clinical medicine using samples of first-year, third-year, and fifth-year medical students. However, this will be an overestimate of the scale's reliability if its ultimate use is to assess students in a single year. This further emphasizes the fact that reliability is not a fixed, immutable property of a scale that, once established, defines its properties. Rather, reliability depends on the scale, the characteristics of the group being assessed, and the circumstances of the assessment. It is imperative therefore to examine the sampling procedures carefully, and assure yourself that the sample used in the reliability study is approximately the same as the population you wish to study. If it is not, you will have to establish the reliability yourself using a more appropriate sample.

This discussion raises another important distinction in the concept—reliability refers both to agreement among raters and the degree to which a scale can differentiate among people who have different amounts of the attribute. If all raters label all students as 'above average', then the scale's reliability is zero, even if there is complete agreement among all of the raters, and total reproducibility over time. Thus, the only synonym for 'reliability' is 'reliability', and terms like 'reproducibility', 'stability', or 'agreement' are inadequate and only add to the confusion (Streiner and Norman 2006).

There are any number of ways in which reliability measures can be obtained depending on the particular source of error you are examining (e.g. observers, items, occasions), and the magnitude of the reliability coefficient will be a direct reflection of the particular approach used. Some broad definitions are described as follows:

1. *Internal consistency.* Measures of internal consistency are a reflection of the variability arising from different items, based on a single administration of the measure. If the measure has a relatively large number of items addressing the same underlying dimension, e.g. 'Are you able to dress yourself?', 'Are you able to shop for groceries?', 'Can you do the sewing?', as measures of physical function, then it is reasonable to expect that scores on each item would be correlated with scores on all other items. This is the idea behind measures of internal consistency—essentially they represent the average of the correlations among all the items in the measure. There are a number of ways to calculate these correlations, called *Cronbach's alpha*, *Kuder–Richardson*, or *split halves*, but all yield similar results. Since the method involves only a single administration of the test, such coefficients are easy to obtain. However, they do not take into account any variation from day to day or from observer to observer, and thus lead to an optimistic interpretation of the true reliability of the test. On the other hand, the use of these indices is dependent on strict criteria regarding properties of the individual items, and may underestimate the

overall reliability for scales that do not meet them (which is most scales). We will discuss this in greater depth in Chapter 8.

2. *Other measures of reliability.* There are various ways of examining the reproducibility of a measure derived from multiple administrations. For example, one might ask about the degree of agreement between different observers (inter-observer reliability); the agreement between observations made by the same rater on two different occasions (intra-observer reliability); observations on the patient on two occasions separated by some interval of time (test–retest reliability), and so forth. As a minimum, any decision regarding the value of a measure should be based on some information regarding stability of the instrument. Internal consistency, in its many guises, is not a sufficient basis upon which to make a reasoned judgement. (As we shall see in Chapter 9, one strategy to deal with this proliferation of reliabilities is 'generalizability theory', which deals simultaneously with multiple sources of error variance.)

One difficulty with the reliability coefficient is that it is simply a number between 0 and 1, and does not lend itself to common-sense interpretations. Various authors have made different recommendations regarding the minimum accepted level of reliability. Certainly, internal consistency should exceed 0.8 for narrowly focused scales (e.g. self-efficacy regarding sports) and 0.6 for measuring broader constructs (self-efficacy in general). On the other hand, values above 0.9 may indicate that the scale is too narrowly focused. Insofar as test –retest and inter-rater reliability are concerned, it might be reasonable to demand values greater than 0.7. Depending on the use of the test and the cost of misinterpretation, higher values might be required; for example, if the results will be used to make a decision about an individual patient or student, even a reliability of 0.9 may be too low.

Finally, although there is a natural concern that many instruments in the literature seem to have too many items to be practical, the reason for the length should be borne in mind. If we assume that every response has some associated error of measurement, then by averaging or summing responses over a series of questions, we can reduce this error. For example, if the original test has a reliability of 0.5, doubling the test will increase the reliability to 0.67, and quadrupling it will result in a reliability of 0.8. As a result, we must recognize that there is a very good reason for long tests; brevity is not necessarily a desirable attribute of a test, and is achieved at some cost (in Chapter 12, however, we will discuss item response theory, which is a direct a challenge to the idea that longer tests are necessary to maximize reliability).

Empirical forms of validity

Reliability simply assesses that a test is measuring something in a reproducible fashion; it says nothing about *what* is being measured. To determine that the test is measuring what was intended requires some evidence of 'validity'. To demonstrate validity requires more than peer judgements; empirical evidence must be produced to show that we can draw meaningful conclusions based on the tool's results. How is this achieved?

Although there are many approaches to assessing validity, and myriad terms used to describe these approaches, eventually the situation reduces to two circumstances:

1. *Other scales of the same or similar attributes are available.* In the situation where measures already exist, then an obvious approach is to administer the experimental instrument and one of the existing instruments to a sample of people and see whether there is a strong correlation between the two. As an example, there are many scales to measure depression. In developing a new scale, it is straightforward to administer the new and old instruments to the same sample. This approach is described by several terms in the literature, including *convergent validation, criterion validation,* and *concurrent validation.* The distinction among the terms (and why we should replace all of them with simply *construct validation*) will be made clear in Chapter 10.

   Although this method is straightforward, it has two severe limitations. First, if other measures of the same property already exist, then it is difficult to justify developing yet another unless it is cheaper or simpler. Of course, many researchers believe that the new instrument that they are developing is better than the old, which provides an interesting bit of circular logic. If the new method is better than the old, why compare it to the old method? And if the relationship between the new method and the old is less than perfect, which one is at fault?

   In fact, the nature of the measurement challenges we are discussing in this book usually precludes the existence of any conventional 'gold standard'. Although there are often measures which have, through history or longevity, acquired criterion status, a close review usually suggests that they have less than ideal reliability and validity (sometimes, these measures are better described as 'fool's gold' standards). Any measurement we are likely to make will have some associated error; as a result, we should expect that correlations among measures of the same attribute should fall in the mid-range of 0.4–0.8. Any lower correlation suggests that either the reliability of one or the other measure is likely unacceptably low, or they are measuring different phenomena.

2. *No other measure exists.* This situation is more likely, since it is usually the justification for developing a scale in the first instance. At first glance, though, we seem to be confronting an impossible situation. After all, if no measure exists, how can one possibly acquire data to show that the new measure is indeed measuring what is intended?

   The solution lies in a broad set of approaches labelled *construct validity.* We begin by linking the attribute we are measuring to some other attribute by a hypothesis, theory, or *construct.* Usually, this hypothesis will explore the difference between two or more populations that would be expected to have differing amounts of the property assessed by our instrument; or people at two time points, during which they are expected to change. We then test this hypothetical construct by applying our instrument to the appropriate samples. If the expected relationship is found, then the hypothesis and the measure are sound; conversely, if no relationship is found, the fault may lie with either the measure or the hypothesis.

Let us clarify this with an example. Suppose that the year is 1920, and a biochemical test of blood sugar has just been devised. Enough is known to hypothesize that diabetics have higher blood sugar values than normal subjects; but no other test of blood sugar exists. Here are some likely hypotheses, which could be tested empirically:

1. Individuals diagnosed as diabetic on clinical criteria will have higher blood sugar on the new test than comparable controls.

2. Dogs whose pancreases are removed will show increasing levels of blood sugar in the days from surgery until death.

3. Individuals who have sweet-tasting urine will have higher blood sugar than those who do not.

4. Diabetics injected with insulin extract will show a decrease in blood sugar levels following the injection.

These hypotheses certainly do not exhaust the number of possibilities, but each can be tested empirically. Further, it is evident that we should not demand a perfect relationship between blood sugar and the other variable, or even that each and all relationships are significant. But the weight of the evidence should be in favour of a positive relationship.

Similar hypotheses can be developed for almost any instrument, and in the absence of a concurrent test, some evidence of construct validity should be available. However, the approach is non-specific and is unlikely to result in very strong relationships. Therefore, the burden of evidence in testing construct validity arises not from a single powerful experiment, but from a series of converging experiments.

Nevertheless, a strong caveat is warranted. As we have said regarding reliability, validity is not a fixed, immutable property of scale that, once established, pertains to the scale in all situations. Rather, it is a function of the scale, the group to which it is administered, and the circumstances under which it was given. That means that a scale that may appear reliable and valid when, for example, it is completed by outpatients in a community clinic, may be useless for inpatients involved in a forensic assessment. Potential users of a scale must assure themselves that reliability and validity have been determined in groups similar to the ones with which they want to use it.

Feasibility

For the person wanting to adopt an existing scale for research or clinical purposes, or someone with masochistic tendencies who wants to develop a new instrument, there is one final consideration: feasibility. There are a number of aspects of feasibility that need to be considered: time, cost, scoring, method of administration, intrusiveness, the consequences of false-positive and false-negative decisions, and so forth.

Time is an issue for both developing a scale and using it. As will become evident as you read through this book, you cannot sit down one Friday evening and hope that by Monday morning you will have a fully developed instrument (although all too many do seem to have been constructed within this time frame). The process of writing items, seeing if they work, checking various forms of reliability, and carrying out even preliminary studies of validity is extremely time-consuming . It can take up to a year to do a decent job, and some people have devoted their entire careers to developing a single scale (we will forego any judgement whether this reflects a laudable sense of commitment or a pathological degree of obsessiveness).

Even when an existing scale has been adopted by a researcher, it must be realized that time is involved on the part of both the researcher and, more importantly, the respondent. It takes time to score the scale and enter the results into a database. Although computer-based administration can lessen this load, it means that time must be spent preparing the scale to be used in this way. For the respondent, the time involvement is naturally what is required to complete the instrument. Time may not be an issue for a person lying in a hospital bed recuperating from an operation; he or she may in fact welcome the distraction. However, it can be an issue for outpatients or non-patients; they may simply want to go home and get on with their lives. Having to complete an instrument, especially a long one, may result in anger and frustration, and lead them to answer in a haphazard manner—a point we will discuss in Chapter 6 when we look at biases in responding.

Cost can also be a problem. If the scale has been copyrighted, it cannot simply be used without appropriate permissions (although, to quote Hamlet, 'it is a custom more honor'd in the breach than the observance'). Similarly, *scoring* may or may not be an issue. Some scales are scored by simply counting the number of items that have been endorsed. Others may add a bit of complexity, such as having different weights for various items or response options, or requiring the user to reverse score some items (i.e. giving Strongly Agree a weight of 1 and Strongly Disagree a weight of 5 for some items and reversing this for others). If scoring is done by hand, this can introduce errors (and if there's a possibility of mistakes, it's guaranteed they will occur). Some commercially available scales require computerized scoring, which adds to both complexity and cost; fortunately, these aren't used too often for research purposes.

There are a number of different ways to *administer* a scale, and each has its own advantages and disadvantages. The easiest way is through direct administration to the respondents. However, this assumes they are able to read the items (raising issues of literacy level and vision) and answer, either by hand writing, typing by computer, or tapping or clicking on a screen. In some instances, such as a patient in a hospital ward with limited ability to move, these modes may be wholly impractical. There is also less control regarding the order in which the questions are read or ensuring that all of the items have been completed. If the scale is administered by a research assistant, costs are again involved for training and salary; and it precludes giving it to large groups at once. Computer-based methods or administration through tablets or even smartphones are becoming increasingly more feasible. This has the advantage of obviating the need for humans to score the responses and enter them into a database, but cost and the ability to test many people at once are still considerations (see Chapter 13 for an extended discussion of administration).

You may feel it is important to know the respondents' income level in order to describe the socioeconomic level of your sample; or to ask about their sex lives when you're looking at quality of life. Bear in mind, though, that some people, especially those from more conservative cultures, may view these questions as unduly *intrusive*. At best, they may simply refuse to answer, or if they are particularly offended, withdraw completely from the study. It is usually best to err on the side of propriety, and to emphasize to the respondents that they are free to omit any item they deem offensive.

This is more difficult, though, if an entire scale probes areas that some people may find offensive.

A scale that places a 'normal' person in the abnormal range (a *false-positive* result) or misses someone who actually does have some disorder (*false-negative* result) is not too much of an issue when the scale is being used solely within the context of research. It will lead to errors in the findings, but that is not an issue for the individual completing the scale. It is a major consideration, though, if the results of the scale are used to make a decision regarding that person—a diagnosis or admission into a programme. In these circumstances, the issue of erroneous results is a major one, and should be one of the top criteria determining whether or not a scale should be used.

The two traditions of assessment

Not surprisingly, medicine on the one hand and psychology and education on the other have developed different ways of evaluating people—ways that have influenced how and why assessment tools are constructed in the first place, and the manner in which they are interpreted. This has led each camp to ignore the potential contribution of the other: the physicians contending that the psychometricians do not appreciate how the results must be used to abet clinical decision-making, and the psychologists and educators accusing the physicians of ignoring many of the basic principles of test construction, such as reliability and validity. It has only been within the last three decades that some rapprochement has been reached—a mutual recognition that we feel is resulting in clinical instruments that are both psychometrically sound and clinically useful. In this section, we will explore two of these different starting points—categorical versus dimensional conceptualization and the reduction of measurement error—and see how they are being merged.

Categorical versus dimensional conceptualization

Medicine traditionally has thought in terms of diagnoses and treatments. In the most simplistic terms, a patient either has a disorder or does not, and is either prescribed some form of treatment or is not. Thus, blood pressure (DBP), which is measured on a continuum of millimetres of mercury, is often broken down into just two categories: normotensive (under 130 mmHg systolic or 80 mmHg diastolic in North America), in which case nothing needs to be done; and hypertensive (above these limits), which calls for some form of intervention.

Test constructors who come from the realm of psychology and education, though, look to the writings of S. Smith Stevens (1951) as received wisdom. He introduced the concept of 'levels of measurement', which categorizes variables as *nominal*, *ordinal*, *interval*, or *ratio*—a concept we will return to in greater depth in Chapter 4. The basic idea is that the more finely we can measure something, the better; rating an attribute on a scale in which each point is equally spaced from its neighbours is vastly superior to dividing the attribute into rougher categories with fewer divisions. Thus, psychometricians tend to think of attributes as continua, with people falling along the dimension in terms of how much of the attribute they have.

The implications of these two different ways of thinking have been summarized by Devins (1993) and are presented in modified form in Table 2.1. In the categorical mode, the diagnosis of, for example, major depression in the fifth edition of the *Diagnostic and Statistical Manual of Mental Disorders* (DSM-5; American Psychiatric Association 2013) requires that the person exhibit at least five of nine symptoms (one of which, depressed mood or loss of interest/pleasure, must be among the five) and that none of four exclusion criteria be present. In turn, each of the symptoms, such as weight change or sleep disturbance, has its own minimum criterion for being judged to be demonstrated (the threshold value). A continuous measure of depression, such as the Center for Epidemiological Studies Depression scale (CES-D; Radloff 1977), uses a completely different approach. There are 20 items, each scored 1 through 4, and a total score over 16 is indicative of depression. No specific item must be endorsed, and there are numerous ways that a score of 16 can be achieved—a person can have four items rated 4, or 16 items rated 1, or any combination in between. Thus, for diagnostic purposes, having many mild symptoms is equivalent to having a few severe ones.

Second, DSM-5 differentiates among various types of depression according to their severity and course. A bipolar depression is qualitatively and quantitatively different from a dysthymic disorder; different sets of criteria must be met to reflect that the former is not only more severe than the latter, but also cyclical in its time course, whereas dysthymia is not. On the other hand, the CES-D quantifies depressive symptomatology, but does not differentiate among the various types. Consequently, it would reflect that one person's symptoms may be more extensive than another's, irrespective of category.

One implication of this difference is that there is a clear distinction between cases and non-cases with the categorical approach, but not with the dimensional. In the former, either one meets the criteria and is a case, or the criteria are not satisfied and

Table 2.1 Categorical and dimensional conceptualization

Categorical model	Dimensional model
1. Diagnosis requires that multiple criteria, each with its threshold value, be satisfied	Occurrence of some features at high intensities can compensate for non-occurrence of others
2. Phenomenon differs qualitatively and quantitatively at different severities	Phenomenon differs only quantitatively at different severities
3. Differences between cases and non-cases are implicit in the definition	Differences between cases and non-cases are less clearly delineated
4. Severity is lowest in instances that minimally satisfy diagnostic criteria	Severity is lowest among non-disturbed individuals
5. One diagnosis often precludes others	A person can have varying amounts of different disorders

Source: data from Devins, G., *Psychiatric rating scales*, Paper presented at the Clarke Institute of Psychiatry, Toronto, Ontario, Copyright © 1993.

one is not a case. With the latter, 'caseness' is a matter of degree, and there is no clear dividing line. The use of a cut point on the CES-D is simply a strategy so that it can be used as a diagnostic tool. The value of 16 was chosen only because, based on empirical findings, using this score maximized agreement between the CES-D and clinical diagnosis; the number is not based on any theoretical argument. Furthermore, there would be less difference seen between two people, one of whom has a score of 15 and the other 17, than between two other people with scores of 30 and 40, although one is a 'case' and the other not in the first instance, and both would be 'cases' in the second.

Another implication is that, since people who do not meet the criteria are said to be free of the disorder with the categorical approach, differences in severity are seen only among those who are diagnosed (point 4 in Table 2.1). Quantification of severity is implicit, with the assumption that those who meet more of the criteria have a more severe depression than people who satisfy only the minimum number. With the dimensional approach, even 'normal' people may have measurable levels of depressive symptomatology; a non-depressed person whose sleep is restless would score higher on the CES-D than a non-depressed person without sleep difficulties.

Last, using the categorical approach, it is difficult (at least within psychiatry) for a person to have more than one disorder. A diagnosis of major depression, for example, cannot be made if the patient has a psychotic condition, or shows evidence of delusions or hallucinations. The dimensional approach does permit this; some traits may be present, albeit in a mild form, even when others coexist.

The limitations of adhering strictly to one or the other of these ways of thinking are becoming more evident. The categorical mode of thinking is starting to change, in part due to the expansion of the armamentarium of treatment options. Returning to the example of hypertension, now patients can be started on diets, followed by diuretics at higher levels of the DBP, and finally placed on ACE inhibitors. Consequently, it makes more sense to measure blood pressure on a continuum, and to titrate the type and amount of treatment to smaller differences than to simply dichotomize the reading. On the other hand, there are different treatment implications, depending on whether one has a bipolar or a non-cyclical form of depression. Simply measuring the severity of symptomatology does not allow for this. One resolution, which will be discussed in Chapter 4, called multidimensional scaling is an attempt to bridge these two traditions. It permits a variety of attributes to be measured dimensionally in such a way that the results can be used to both categorize and determine the extent to which these categories are present.

It should be noted that, at least in psychiatry, the reliability and validity of measures of pathology are significantly improved when measured on a continuum. Paradoxically, this holds true even when applied to discrete diagnostic conditions (Markon et al. 2011). Although, to the best of our knowledge, this has not been demonstrated in other areas of health care, we strongly suspect it is true for other conditions, such as irritable bowel syndrome, migraine headache, Alzheimer's disease, and a host of others where there is no definitive, objective diagnostic test.

The reduction of measurement error

Whenever definitive laboratory tests do not exist, physicians rely primarily on the clinical interview to provide differential diagnoses. The clinician is the person who both elicits the information and interprets its significance as a sign or symptom (Dohrenwend and Dohrenwend 1982). Measurement error is reduced through training, development, refinement and practice of interviewing skills, and especially clinical experience. Thus, older physicians are often regarded as 'gold standards' since they presumably have more experience and therefore would make fewer errors. (In a different context, though, Caputo (1980, p. 370) wrote, 'They haven't got seventeen years' experience, just one year's experience repeated seventeen times'.)

In contrast, the psychometric tradition relies on self-reports of patients to usually close-ended questions. It is assumed that the response to any one question is subject to error: the person may misinterpret the item, respond in a biased manner, or make a mistake in transcribing their reply to the answer sheet. The effect of these errors is minimized in a variety of ways. First, each item is screened to determine if it meets certain criteria. Second, the focus is on the consistency of the answers across many items, and for the most part, disregarding the responses to the individual questions. Last, the scale as a whole is checked to see if it meets another set of criteria.

The 'medical' approach is often criticized as placing unwarranted faith in the clinical skills of the interviewer. Indeed, as was mentioned briefly in Chapter 1, the reliability (and hence the validity) of the clinical interview leaves much to be desired. Conversely, psychometrically sound tests may provide reliable and valid data, but do not yield the rich clinical information and the ways in which patients differ from one another, which come from talking to them in a conversational manner. These two 'solitudes' are starting to merge, especially in psychiatry, as is seen in some of the structured interviews such as the Diagnostic Interview Schedule (DIS; Robins et al. 1981), and it s more recent iteration, the World Health Organization Composite International Diagnostic Interview (WHO-CIDI; https://www.cdc.gov/nchs/data/nhanes/cidi_quex.pdf), both of which are derived from the clinical examination used to diagnose psychiatric patients, but constructed in such a way to be administered by trained lay people, not just psychiatrists. It also relies on the necessity of answering a number of questions before an attribute is judged to be present. Thus, elements of both traditions guided its construction, although purists from both camps will be dissatisfied with the compromises.

Summary

The criteria we have described are intended as guidelines for reviewing the literature and as an introduction to the remainder of this book. We must emphasize that the research enterprise involved in development of a new method of measurement requires time and patience. Effort expended to locate an existing measure is justified, because of the savings if one can be located and the additional insights provided in the development of a new instrument if none proves satisfactory.

Further reading

American Educational Research Association, American Psychological Association, and National Council on Measurement in Education (2014). *Standards for educational and psychological testing*. American Educational Research Association, Washington, DC.

Boateng, G.O., Neilands, T.B., Frongillo, E.A., Melgar-Quiñonez, H.R., and Young, S.L. (2018). Best practices for developing and validating scales for health, social, and behavioral research: A primer. *Frontiers of Public Health*, **6**, Article 149.

Markon, K.E., Chmielewski, M., and Miller, C.J. (2011). The reliability and validity of discrete and continuous measures of psychopathology: A quantitative review. *Psychological Bulletin*, **137**, 856–78.

Stevens, S.S. (1946). On the theory of scales of measurement. *Science*, **10**, 677–80.

References

American Educational Research Association, American Psychological Association, and National Council on Measurement in Education (2014). *Standards for educational and psychological testing*. American Psychological Association, Washington, DC.

American Psychiatric Association (2013). *Diagnostic and statistical manual of mental disorders* (5th edn). American Psychiatric Publishing, Arlington, VA.

Bossuyt, P.M., Reitsma, J.B., Bruns, D.E., Gatsonis, C.A., Glasziou, P.P., Irwig, L., *et al.* (2015). STARD 2015: An updated list of essential items for reporting diagnostic accuracy studies. *BMJ*, **351**, h5527.

Caputo, P. (1980). *Horn of Africa*. Holt, Rinehart and Winston, New York.

Devins, G. (1993). *Psychiatric rating scales*. Paper presented at the Clarke Institute of Psychiatry, Toronto, Ontario.

Dohrenwend, B.P. and Dohrenwend, B.S. (1982). Perspectives on the past and future of psychiatric epidemiology. *American Journal of Public Health*, **72**, 1271–9.

Guilford, J.P. (1954). *Psychometric methods*. McGraw-Hill, New York.

Markon, K.E., Chmielewski, M., and Miller, C.J. (2011). The reliability and validity of discrete and continuous measures of psychopathology: A quantitative review. *Psychological Bulletin*, **137**, 856–78.

McDowell, I. (2006). *Measuring health* (3rd edn). Oxford University Press, Oxford.

Mokkink, L.B., Terwee, C.B., Patrick, D.L., Alonso, J., Stratford, P.W., Knol, D.L., *et al.* (2010). The COSMIN study reached international consensus on taxonomy, terminology, and definitions of measurement properties for health-related patient-reported outcomes. *Journal of Clinical Epidemiology*, **63**, 737–44.

Radloff, L.S. (1977). The CES-D scale: A self-report depression scale for research in the general population. *Applied Psychological Measurement*, **1**, 385–401.

Robins, L.N., Helzer, J.E., Crougham, R., and Ratcliff, K.S. (1981). National Institute of Mental Health Diagnostic Interview Schedule: Its history, characteristics, and validity. *Archives of General Psychiatry*, **38**, 381–9.

Stevens, S.S. (1951). Mathematics, measurement, and psychophysics. In *Handbook of experimental psychology* (ed. S.S. Stevens), pp. 1–49. Wiley, New York.

Streiner, D.L. and Norman, G.R. (2006). "Precision" and "accuracy": Two terms that are neither. *Journal of Clinical Epidemiology*, **59**, 327–30.

Streiner, D.L., Sass, D.A., Meijer, R.R., and Furr, M. (2016). STARDing again: Revised guidelines for reporting information in studies of diagnostic test accuracy. *Journal of Personality Assessment*, **98**, 559–62.

Chapter 3

Devising the items

Introduction to devising items

The first step in writing a scale or questionnaire is, naturally, devising the items themselves. This is far from a trivial task, since no amount of statistical manipulation after the fact can compensate for poorly chosen questions: those that are badly worded, ambiguous, irrelevant, or—even worse—not present. In this chapter, we explore various sources of items and the strengths and weaknesses of each of them.

The first step is to look at what others have done in the past. Instruments rarely spring fully grown from the brows of their developers. Rather, they are usually based on what other people have deemed to be relevant, important, or discriminating. Wechsler (1958), for example, quite openly discussed the patrimony of the subtests that were later incorporated into his various IQ tests. Of the 11 subtests that comprise the original adult version, at least nine were derived from other widely used indices. Moreover, the specific items that make up the individual subtests are themselves based on older tests. Both the items and the subtests were modified and new ones added to meet his requirements, but in many cases the changes were relatively minor. Similarly, the *Manifest Anxiety Scale* (Taylor 1953) is based in large measure on one scale from the *Minnesota Multiphasic Personality Inventory* (MMPI; Hathaway and McKinley 1951). Lest you think this practice is only historical (based on the dates of these publications), one of the most widely used, contemporary psychological distress scales, the Kessler 10, was developed using a statistical approach (item response theory; see Chapter 12) to identify the most discriminating items from a larger pool, all of which came from existing depression and anxiety scales (Slade et al. 2011).

The long, and sometimes tortuous, path by which items from one test end up in others is beautifully described by Goldberg (1971). He wrote that (p. 335):

> Items devised around the turn of the century may have worked their way via Woodworth's Personal Data Sheet, to Thurstone and Thurstone's Personality Schedule, hence to Bernreuter's Personality Inventory, and later to the Minnesota Multiphasic Personality Inventory, where they were borrowed for the California Personality Inventory and then injected into the Omnibus Personality Inventory—only to serve as a source of items for the new Academic Behavior Inventory.

Angleitner et al. (1986) expanded this to 'and, we may add, only to be translated and included in some new German personality inventories' (p. 66).

There are a number of reasons that items are repeated from previous inventories. First, it saves work involved in constructing new ones. Second, the items have usually gone through repeated processes of testing so that they have proven themselves to be useful and psychometrically sound. Third, there are only a limited number of ways to ask about a specific problem. If we were trying to tap into a depressed mood, for instance, it is difficult to ask about sleep loss in a way that has not been used previously.

Hoary as this tradition may be, there are (at least) four problems in adopting it uncritically. First, it may result in items that use outdated terminology. For example, the original version of the MMPI (in use until 1987) contained such quaint terms as 'deportment', 'cutting up', and 'drop the handkerchief'. Endorsement of these items most likely told more about the person's age than about any aspect of their personality. Perhaps, more importantly, the motivation for developing a new tool is the investigator's belief that the previous scales are inadequate for one reason or another, or do not completely cover the domain under study. We would add further that in an era where researchers are increasingly under pressure to produce products that generate revenue, the practice of lifting items from existing scales, especially those that are in the public domain or otherwise not protected by current patent or copyright protection, for use in the creation of scales that will be only available for cost, seems at best a dubious ethical and legal practice. The fourth problem is that, when using items from tests that have been copyrighted, there is a very fine line between 'borrowing' and 'plagiarism'. Even with scales that have been printed in journals, it is likely that copyright is owned by either the author or the journal, or both, and permission may be required to use the items.

The source of items

If we do not 'borrow' items from other scales, then where can we get them? New items can come from five different sources: the patients or subjects themselves, clinical observation, theory, research, and expert opinion, although naturally the lines between these categories are not firm.

A point often overlooked in scale development is the fact that patients and potential research subjects are an excellent source of items. Whereas clinicians may be the best observers of the outward manifestations of a trait or disorder, only those who have it can report on the more subjective elements. Over the years, a variety of techniques have been developed, which can elicit these viewpoints in a rigorous and systematic manner; these procedures are used primarily by 'qualitative' researchers and are only now finding their way into more 'quantitative' types of studies. Here, we can touch only briefly on two of the more relevant techniques; greater detail is provided in texts such as Taylor and Bogden (1998) and Willms and Johnson (1993).

Focus groups

Willms and Johnson (1993) describe a focus group as (p. 61):

> a discussion in which a small group of informants (six to twelve people), guided by a facilitator, talk freely and spontaneously about themes considered important to the investigation. The participants are selected from a target group whose opinions and ideas are of interest to the researcher. Sessions are usually tape recorded and an observer (recorder) also takes notes on the discussion.

In the area of scale development, the participants would be patients who have the disorder or people who are representative of those whose opinions would be elicited by the instrument. At first, their task would not be to generate the specific items, but rather to suggest general themes that the research team members themselves can use to phrase the items. Usually, no more than two or three groups would be needed. Once the items have been written, focus groups can again be used to discuss whether these items are relevant, clear, unambiguous, written in terms that are understood by potential respondents, and if all the main themes have been covered. These groups are much more focused than those during the theme generation stage since there is a strong externally generated agenda, discussing the items themselves.

There are a number of advantages of focus groups over one-on-one interviews. The first, obviously, is efficiency; in the same length of time, the viewpoints of more people can be sampled. Second, the participants can react not only to the questions posed by the group leader, but also to what is said by the other members of the group, which often leads to more in-depth discussion. Third, in the majority of cases, the moderator is an 'outsider', in that they have not had the same experience of the disorder or condition of the members, so the latter may feel more comfortable discussing their experiences with peers. At the same time, the other group members can correct any misleading information from one individual.

Bear in mind, though, that focus groups cannot be used in all situations. There are some conditions that make it difficult for a person to interact with others, such as sociophobia or avoidant personality, and these obviously preclude group interactions. Further, it may be easier for people to talk about stigmatizing or embarrassing behaviours (e.g. sexual misconduct or inadequacies) in private rather than in public. More generally, care must always be taken in focus group settings to ensure that all participants have a chance to share their ideas and opinions, not just the ones most at ease at speaking in a group setting.

It may sound as if running focus groups is as simple as assembling a group of people in a room and asking them to talk. This is not the case. Many decisions need to be made, such as the composition of the group (homogeneous or heterogeneous with regard to, say, gender, age, diagnosis), the number of people in the group, how data will be recorded (taped and transcribed, taped only, memory of a recorder), and how they will be analysed. Helpful suggestions and examples are provided by Vogt et al. (2004) and Puchta and Potter (2004).

Key informant interviews

As the name implies, these are in-depth interviews with a small number of people who are chosen because of their unique knowledge. The use of key informants grew out of ethnographic and anthropological research, although early work in psychiatric epidemiology used them to estimate the prevalence of disorders in a community (Streiner and Cairney 2010). They are most often used when the people of interest cannot speak for themselves because of age, the nature of their condition (e.g. dementia), or a lack of familiarity with the language (e.g. recent immigrants). The informants can be patients who have, or have had, the disorder, for example, and who can articulate what they felt; clinicians who have extensive experience with the patients and can explain it from their perspective; or parents. The interviews can range from informal or unstructured ones, which are almost indistinguishable from spontaneous conversations, to highly structured ones, where the interviewer has a preplanned set of carefully worded questions. Generally, the less that is known about the area under study, the less structured is the interview. As with focus groups, it is best if the interviews are recorded for later analysis. There is no set number of people who should be interviewed. The criterion often used in this type of research is 'sampling to redundancy' or 'saturation'—that is, interviewing people until no new themes emerge.

Of course, these are not the only qualitative methods which could be used for generating ideas from target populations; the researchers are limited only by the bounds of their imagination (and time and funding). Cairney et al. (2018), when developing a measure of experiences during youth sport participation, used crowdsourcing techniques such as word boards and interactive booths with video/audio capture, while attending sport and coaching conferences as part of the item generation process. Ethnography, immersing oneself in an environment as a participant observer (e.g. Daynes and Williams 2018), is also a technique that can provide rich contextual information useful for scale constructors—even if the investigators do not collect the data themselves, ethnographic studies are part of the literature base that can be consulted at this phase of the process.

Clinical observation

Clinical observation is perhaps one of the most fruitful sources of items. Indeed, it can be argued that observation, whether of patients or students, precedes theory, research, or expert opinion. Scales are simply a way of gathering these clinical observations in a systematic fashion so that all the observers are ensured of looking for the same thing or all subjects are responding to the same items. As an example, Kruis et al. (1984) devised a scale to try to differentiate between irritable bowel syndrome (IBS) and organic bowel disease. The first part of their questionnaire consists of a number of items asked by the clinician of the patient—presence of abdominal pain and flatulence, alteration in bowel habits, duration of symptoms, type and intensity of pain, abnormality of the stools, and so forth. The choice of these items was predicated on the clinical experience of the authors, and their impressions of how IBS patients' symptomatology and presentation differ from those of other patients. Similarly, the *Menstrual Distress Questionnaire* (Moos 1984) consists of 47 symptoms, such as muscle stiffness, skin blemishes, fatigue, and feeling sad or blue, which have been reported clinically to be associated with premenstrual syndrome (PMS).

This is not to say that these groups of researchers are necessarily correct, in that the items they selected *are* different between patients with organic or functional bowel disease, or between the women who do and do not have PMS. In fact, perhaps the major drawback of relying solely on clinical observation to guide the selection of items is the real possibility that the clinicians may be wrong. The original rationale for electroconvulsive shock therapy (ECT), for instance, was based on a quite erroneous 'observation' that the incidence of epilepsy is far lower in the population with schizophrenia than that with the general population, so it was thought that inducing a seizure through ECT could cure the disorder. (It doesn't, although it is quite effective in some forms of depression.) Any scale that tried to capitalize on this association would be doomed to failure. A related problem is that a clinician, because of a limited sample of patients, or a narrow perspective imposed by a particular model of the disorder, may not be aware of other factors which may prove to be better descriptors or discriminators. Finally, even when clinicians may be quite accurate in their description of the signs and symptoms, they may not be fully aware of the impact of the disorder on the patients' lives. If this is a component of the scale, it would be better to talk to the patients themselves.

Theory

Clinical observation rarely exists in isolation. Individual laboratory results or physical findings convey far more information if they are components of a more global theory of an illness or behaviour. The term *theory*, in this context, is used very broadly, encompassing not only formal, refutable models of how things relate to one another but also vaguely formed hunches of how or why people behave, if only within a relatively narrow domain. A postulate that patients who believe in the efficacy of therapy will be more compliant with their physician's orders, for example, may not rival the theory of relativity in its scope or predictive power, but can be a fruitful source of items in this limited area. A theory or model can thus serve a heuristic purpose, suggesting items or subscales.

At first glance, it may appear as if theory is what we rely on until data are available; once studies have been done, it would be unnecessary to resort to theory and the scale developer can use facts to generate items or guide construction of the scale. Indeed, this was the prevailing attitude among test designers until relatively recently. However, there has been an increasing appreciation of the role that theory can play in scale and questionnaire development (Boorsboom et al. 2004). This is seen most clearly when we are trying to assess attitudes, beliefs, or traits. For example, if we wanted to devise a scale that could predict those post-myocardial infarction patients who would comply with an exercise regimen, our task would be made easier (and perhaps more accurate) if we had some model or theory of compliance (or behaviour change more broadly).

The Health Action Process Approach or HAPA model (Schwarzer et al. 2011), for instance, builds on Bandura's (1977) foundational work on self-efficacy, identifying three forms of perceived confidence that influence behaviour change, from intention to action—belief in one's ability to engage in a behaviour like exercise (task self-efficacy), the ability to maintain that behaviour over a long period (maintenance self-efficacy), and belief in one's ability to resume the behaviour if one goes off track (recovery self-efficacy). Each type of self-efficacy has specific implications for item wording. For example, a standard item measuring task self-efficacy involves asking respondents to rate how confident they are in being able to exercise, typically using a 10-point scale. Changing adjectives to include confidence in maintaining and reengaging or resuming the behaviour if stopped cover the other forms of efficacy in the model.

The obverse side is that a model which is wrong can lead us astray, prompting us to devise questions which ultimately have no predictive or explanatory power. While the inadequacy of the theory may emerge later in testing the validity of the scale, much time and effort can be wasted in the interim. For example, Patient Management Problems (PMPs) were based on the supposition that physician competence is directly related to the thoroughness and comprehensiveness of the history and physical examination. The problems, therefore, covered every conceivable question that could be asked of a patient and most laboratory tests that could be ordered. The scoring system similarly reflected this theory; points were gained by being obsessively compulsive, and lost if the right diagnosis were arrived at by the 'wrong' route, one which used short cuts. While psychometrically sound, the PMPs did not correlate with any other measure of clinical competence, primarily for the reason that the model was wrong—expert physicians do not function in the way envisioned by the test developers (Feightner 1985; Newble et al. 1982).

Research

Just as naked observations need the clothing of a theory, so a theory must ultimately be tested empirically. *Research findings* can be a fruitful source of items and subscales. For the purposes of scale construction, research can be of two types: a literature review of studies that have been done in the area or new research carried out specifically for the purpose of developing the scale. In both cases, the scale or questionnaire would be composed of items which have been shown empirically to be the characteristics of a group of people or which differentiate them from other people.

As an example of a scale based on previous research, the second part of the Kruis et al. (1984) scale for IBS is essentially a checklist of laboratory values and clinical history, e.g. erythrocyte sedimentation rate, leucocytes, and weight loss. These were chosen on the basis of previous research, which indicated that IBS and organic patients differed on these variables. This part of the scale, then, is a summary of empirical findings based on the research done by others.

In a different domain, Ullman and Giovannoni (1964) developed a scale to measure the 'process-reactive' continuum in schizophrenia. A number of items on the questionnaire relate to marriage and parenthood because there is considerable evidence that people with process schizophrenia, especially males, marry at a far lower rate than people with reactive schizophrenia. Another item relates to alcohol consumption, since among people with schizophrenia at least, those who use alcohol tend to have shorter hospital stays than those who do not drink.

When entering into a new area, though, there may not be any research that can serve as the basis for items. Under these circumstances, it may be necessary for the scale developer to conduct some preliminary research, which can then be the source of items. For example, Brumback and Howell (1972) needed an index to evaluate the clinical effectiveness of physicians working in federal hospitals and clinics. Existing scales were inadequate or inappropriate for their purposes and did not provide the kind of information they needed in a format that was acceptable to the raters. The checklist portion of the scale they ultimately developed was derived by gathering 2,500 descriptions of critical incidents from 500 people, classifying these into functional areas, and then using various item analytic techniques (to be discussed in Chapter 6) to arrive at the final set of 37 items. While this study is unusual in its size, it illustrates two points. First, it is sometimes necessary to perform research prior to the construction of the scale itself in order to determine the key aspects of the domain under investigation. Second, the initial item pool is often much larger than the final set of items. Again, the size of the reduction is quite unusual in this study (only 1.5 per cent of the original items were ultimately retained), but the fact that reduction occurs is common.

Expert opinion

The use of *expert opinion* in a given field was illustrated in a similar study by Cowles and Kubany (1959) to evaluate the performance of medical students. Experienced faculty members were interviewed to determine what they felt were the most important characteristics students should have in preparing for general practice, ultimately resulting in eight items. This appears quite similar to the first step taken by Brumback and Howell which was labelled 'research'; indeed, the line between the two is a very fine one, as is the difference between expert opinion and key informants; the distinctions are somewhat arbitrary. The important point is that, in all cases, information had to be gathered prior to the construction of the scale.

There are no hard and fast rules governing the use of expert judgements: how many experts to use, how they are found and chosen, or even more important, how differences among them are reconciled. The methods by which the opinions are gathered can run the gamut from having a colleague scribble some comments on a rough draft of the questionnaire to holding a conference of recognized leaders in the field, with explicit rules governing voting. Most approaches usually fall between these two extremes: somewhere in the neighbourhood of three to ten people known to the scale developer as experts are consulted, usually on an individual basis. Since the objective is to generate as many potential items as possible for the scale, those suggested by even one person should be considered, at least in the first draft of the instrument.

The advantage of this approach is that if the experts are chosen carefully, they probably represent the most recent thinking in an area. Without much effort, the scale developer has access to the accumulated knowledge and experience of others who have worked in the field. The disadvantages may arise if the panel is skewed in some way and does not reflect a range of opinions. Then, the final selection of items may represent one particular viewpoint, and there may be glaring gaps in the final product. Of course, too much heterogeneity (diversity or range of opinion) in the panel may lead to disagreement among experts, which in turn creates the problem of adjudicating disputed items.

For those working in the area of personality measurement, an unusual source of items exists—the International Personality Item Pool (IPIP). This is a collaborative endeavour of researchers around the world, who contribute or translate items that can then be used to develop scales (Goldberg et al. 2006). What is unique about this project is that the items are freely available from the website (<http://ipip.ori.org>). To date, over 300 scales have been derived from the scales (they are also available), including a number of well-validated instruments that have been widely used in research.

A similar initiative, called the Patient-Reported Outcomes Measurement Information System (PROMIS), exists for patient-reported outcomes (PROs). It is a collaborative effort sponsored by the National Institutes of Health in the United States to develop, validate, and standardize item banks to measure PROs initially in six areas relevant across common medical conditions: pain, fatigue, emotional distress, physical functioning, social role participation, and general health perception (Cella et al. 2007). This has since been expanded to social health (e.g. companionship, social isolation) as well as specific disorders, such as dyspnea, itch, gastrointestinal symptoms, sleep, and sexual functioning. There have also been PROs developed for children, and the items have been translated into many languages. The items are analysed using item response theory (see Chapter 12) so that they can be equated to one another. This item bank is publicly available (<http://www.nihpromis.org/>).

Delphi method

A technique that blends expert opinion and focus groups is the *Delphi method*, first developed by Norman Dalkey and Olaf Helmer (1963) of the Rand Corporation, and named for the Oracle of Delphi, who was an ancient Greek priestess at a temple of Apollo consulted for her prophecies. With it, there are several rounds of the scale that are sent to experts in the field. The responses are returned to the organizer, who then collates them and sends the summary out again. Often, the first round may ask respondents to simply propose potential items. Subsequent rounds would send them the items and the comments, and ask them to make further comment on the items, propose changes to wording, and vote to retain or eliminate certain ones. This can be done any number of times until there is general agreement, although four rounds are usually sufficient. This method was used to draft the Guidelines for Reporting Reliability and Agreement Studies (GRRAS; Kottner et al. 2010).

The advantages of the Delphi method are that it can be done digitally via the internet, obviating the need for in-person meetings; also, the responses and suggestions can be made anonymously, allowing for more honest (if sometimes more snarky) comments. Among the disadvantages are that one tardy respondent can slow the entire process, and the lack of face-to-face interaction may result in less discussion than would occur with in-person meetings.

It should be borne in mind that these are not mutually exclusive methods of generating items. A scale may consist of items derived from some or all of these sources. Indeed, it would be unusual to find any questionnaire derived from only one of them.

Content validity

Once the items have been generated from these various sources, the scale developer is ideally left with far more items than will ultimately end up on the scale. In Chapter 5, we will discuss various statistical techniques to select the best items from this pool. For the moment, though, we address the converse of this, ensuring that the scale has enough items and adequately covers the domain under investigation.

Traditionally, this has been referred to as *content validation*, but this is a very poor choice of terminology. As we will discuss in Chapter 10, the 'modern' (i.e. since the 1950s) definition of validity is that it refers to the conclusions we can draw from test results; that is, it is a property of the *test responses*, and not of the tests themselves (Messick 1975). As he stated, 'Content coverage is an important consideration in test construction and interpretation, to be sure, but in itself it does not provide validity' (p. 960). More accurate descriptors of what we are trying to achieve would be 'content relevance' and 'content coverage' (Messick 1980). We will continue to use the term 'content validity,' because it is widely known and less cumbersome than saying 'content relevance and coverage', but bear in mind that it is not truly a form of validity. (See Beckstead 2009 for an excellent discussion of the evolution of this concept.)

Concepts of content validity arose from achievement testing, where students are assessed to determine if they have learned the material in a specific content area; final examinations are the prime example. With this in mind, each item on the test should relate to one of the course objectives (content relevance). Items that are not related to the content of the course introduce error in the measurement, in that they discriminate among the students on some dimension other than the one purportedly tapped by the test—a dimension that can be totally irrelevant to the test. Conversely, each part of the syllabus should be represented by one or more questions (content coverage). If not, then students may differ in some important respects, but this would not be reflected in the final score. Table 3.1 shows how these two components of content validity can be checked in a course of, for example, cardiology. Each row reflects a different item on the test, and each column a different content area. Every item is examined in turn, and a mark placed in the appropriate column(s). Although a single number does not emerge at the end, as with other types of validity estimates, the visual display yields much information.

Table 3.1 Checking content validity for a course in cardiology

Question	Content area			
	Anatomy	**Physiology**	**Function**	**Pathology**
1		X		
2	X			
3			X	
4	X			
5				X
.				
.				
.				
20		X		

First, each item should fall into at least one content area represented by the columns. If it does not, then either that item is not relevant to the course objectives, or the list of objectives is not comprehensive. Second, each objective should be represented by at least one question; otherwise, it is not being evaluated by the test. Last, the number of questions in each area should reflect its actual importance in the syllabus (this is referred to as the *representativeness* of the content area). The reason for checking this is that it is quite easy to write items in some areas and far more difficult in others. In cardiology, for example, it is much easier to write multiple-choice items to find out if the students know the normal values of obscure enzymes than to devise questions tapping their ability to deal with the rehabilitation of cardiac patients. Thus, there may be a disproportionately large number of the former items on the test and too few of the latter in relation to what the students should know. The final score, then, would not be an accurate reflection of what the instructor hoped the students would learn.

Depending on how finely one defines the course objectives, it may not be possible to assess each one as this would make the test too long. Under these conditions, it would be necessary to *randomly sample* the domain of course objectives—that is, select them in such a way that each has an equal opportunity of being chosen. This indeed is closer to what is often done in measuring traits or behaviours, since tapping the full range of objectives may make the instrument unwieldy.

Although this matrix method was first developed for achievement tests, it can be applied equally well to scales measuring attitudes, behaviours, symptoms, and the like. In these cases, the columns are comprised of aspects of the trait or disorder that the investigator wants the scale to cover, rather than course objectives. Assume, for example, that the test constructor wanted to develop a new measure to determine whether living in a home containing elevated levels of formaldehyde leads to physical problems. The columns in this case would be those areas they felt would be affected by formaldehyde vapour (and perhaps a few that should *not* be affected, if they wanted to check on a general tendency to endorse symptoms). Therefore, based on previous research, theory, expert opinion, and other sources, these may include upper respiratory symptoms, gastrointestinal complaints, skin rash, sleep disturbances, memory problems, eye irritation, and so forth. This would then serve as a check that all domains were covered by at least one question, and that there were no irrelevant items. As can be seen, content validation applies to the scale as a whole, not to the separate items individually. Bear in mind, though, that content validation is a 'state' of the instrument, not a 'trait' (Messick 1993). That is, how relevant and representative the content is depends on the use to which the scale is put. One that has good content validity as a screening test for depression may have poor content coverage as a measure of response to treatment. Further, the content validity may decrease over time, as we learn more about the construct under study or as the nature of the underlying theory evolves (Haynes et al. 1995). For example, it was once believed that cardiovascular problems were associated with the 'Type-A personality', which was defined by a constellation of attitudes (e.g. time pressure, anger), behaviours (e.g. finishing the sentences of others), and physical characteristics. More recent research, though, has shown that only the destructive expression of anger is the key ingredient

(Seligman 1993). Consequently, any scale that tries to tap psychological correlates of heart disease, based on the old model of Type-A personality, would suffer from content irrelevance in light of more recent research.

Let us use a concrete example to illustrate how these various steps are put into practice. As part of a study to examine the effects of stress (McFarlane et al. 1980), a scale was needed to measure the amount of social support that the respondents felt they had. Although there were a number of such instruments already in existence, none met the specific needs of this project, or matched closely enough our theoretical model of social support. Thus, the first step, although not clearly articulated as such at the time, was to elucidate our *theory* of social support: what areas we wanted to tap, and which we felt were irrelevant or unnecessary for our purposes. This was augmented by *research* done in the field by other groups, indicating aspects of social support, which served as buffers, protecting the person against stress. The next step was to locate *previous instruments* and cull from them those questions or approaches that met our needs. Finally, we showed a preliminary draft of our scale to a number of highly experienced family therapists, whose *expert opinion* was formed on the basis of their years of *clinical observation*. This last step actually served two related purposes: they performed a *content validation* study, seeing if any important areas were missed by us, and also suggested additional items to fill these gaps. The final draft (McFarlane et al. 1981) was then subjected to a variety of reliability and validity checks, as outlined in subsequent chapters.

A more sophisticated approach to content validation is to use the *content validity ratio* (CVR) developed by Lawshe (1975) and modified by Waltz and Bausell (1981) and Lynn (1986). Each member of an expert panel, which may include content experts, theoreticians, and patients, is given an explicit description of the domains and a list of the items within them. The raters evaluate each item on a 4-point scale: 4 = Highly Relevant; 3 = Quite Relevant or Highly Relevant But Needs Rewording; 2 = Somewhat Relevant; and 1 = Not Relevant. The CVR for each item is defined as:

$$CVR = \frac{n_e - \frac{N}{2}}{N/2},$$

where n_e is the number of raters who deem the item to be essential (i.e. a rating of 3 or 4) and N is the total number of raters. The CVR can range between –1 and +1, and a value of 0 means that half of the panel feel that the item is essential. To ensure that the results are not due to chance, Lawshe recommended a value of 0.99 for five or six raters (the minimum number), 0.85 for eight raters, and 0.62 for ten raters; items with lower values would be discarded. At the same time that the raters evaluate relevance, they are also asked to comment on whether any aspects of the domain have been omitted. If there are, new items can be written, which further establishes content coverage.

The major problem with the CVR is that it does not correct for agreement by chance (this issue is discussed in detail in Chapter 8). Consequently, seemingly high values of the CVR may actually reflect poor agreement. A better measure would be the intraclass correlation, also discussed in Chapter 8. Furthermore, as Beckstead (2009) has determined, a minimum number of raters would be closer to 30 if they showed unanimous agreement, and over 50 if one disagreement can be tolerated.

Another method to select items is called the *item-sort task* (Anderson and Gerbing 1991). Anywhere between 5 and 30 raters are given a deck, with each item on a separate card. They are also given a list of constructs, one of which is the target plus two to five other, related ones. For example, in developing a scale tapping moral injury, there would also be constructs such as depression, post-traumatic distress, and one labelled 'other'. The raters' job is to simply place each card in the correct bin. Items with a sufficient proportion of placements would be candidate items. The raters can comment if they find the item to be confusing, double-barreled, or ambiguous. Further, if an item is factorially complex, in that it reflects two or more constructs, this will be revealed by the item having fewer placements in the target bin and some placed in other bins. It is also possible to apply statistical criteria. The formula for determining significance can get tedious to calculate, but Howard and Melloy (2016) provide a table for various numbers of raters. They state that if the statistical criterion is used, the results very closely parallel those from a factor analysis, which may not be possible to run because of sample size considerations.

Very comprehensive guides for determining content validity can be found in Haynes et al. (1995) and Howard (2018).

How many items should be written? At this first stage in scale development, our interest is in creating the item pool. Our aim is to be as inclusive as possible, even to the point of being overinclusive; poor items can be detected and weeded out later, but as we said in the opening paragraph of this chapter, nothing can be done after the fact to compensate for items we neglected to include. In a classic article on test construction, Loevinger (1957) wrote that (p. 659, italics in the original):

> *The items of the pool should be chosen so as to sample all possible contents which might comprise the putative trait according to all known alternative theories of the trait.*

Generic versus specific scales and the 'fidelity versus bandwidth' issue

Let us say you want to find or develop a test to measure the quality of life (QOL) of a group of patients with rheumatoid arthritis (RA). Should you look for (or develop) a QOL instrument that is tailored to the characteristics of these patients with RA, or should it be a scale which taps QOL for patients with a variety of disorders, of which RA is only one? Indeed, should we go even further and tailor the scale to the unique requirements of the individual patients? There are some scales (e.g. Guyatt et al. 1993) which are constructed by asking the patient to list five activities which they feel have been most affected by the disorder. Thus, the items on one patient's scale may be quite different from those on anyone else's instrument.

The argument in favour of disease-specific and patient-specific questionnaires is twofold. The first consideration is that if an instrument is designed to cover a wide range of disorders, many of the questions may be inappropriate or irrelevant for any one specific problem. A generic scale, for example, may include items tapping incontinence, shortness of breath, and problems in attention and concentration. These are areas which may present difficulties for patients with Crohn's disease, asthma, or depression, but rarely for arthritics. Consequently, these non-useful items contribute nothing but noise when the questionnaire is used for one specific disorder. This argument is simply carried to its logical extreme with patient-specific instruments; here, all of the items are, by definition, relevant for the patient, and there should be no items that are not applicable or should not change with effective therapy.

The second reason for using disease- or patient-specific scales follows directly from the first problem. In order to keep the length of a generic questionnaire manageable, there cannot be very many items in each of the areas tapped. Thus, there will be fewer relevant questions to detect real changes within patients, or differences among them.

On the opposite side of the argument, the cost of the greater degree of specificity is a reduction in generalizability (Aaronson 1988, 1989). That is, generic scales allow comparisons across different disorders, severities of disease, interventions, and perhaps even demographic and cultural groups (Patrick and Deyo 1989), as well as being able to measure the burden of illness of populations suffering from chronic medical and psychiatric conditions as compared with normal ones (McHorney et al. 1994). This is much harder, or even impossible, to do when each study uses a different scale. Especially, in light of the increase in the use of meta-analysis to synthesize the results of different studies (e.g. Glass et al. 1981), this can be a major consideration. Furthermore, since any one generic scale tends to be used more frequently than a given specific instrument, there are usually more data available regarding its reliability and validity.

Dowie (2002a, 2002b) raises a different argument in favour of generic scales. He states that researchers are most often interested in the 'main' effect of an intervention (i.e. did it improve the patient's condition?), relegating adverse or side effects to secondary outcomes. However, patients simply experience 'effects', which include the direct positive changes produced by the treatment; possibly other, indirect, gains (e.g. a greater feeling of independence following hip replacement); as well as any negative ones. Thus, from a clinical and decision-making perspective, disease-specific scales may overlook the aspects of the intervention that are important to the patient.

These problems are even more acute with patient-specific scales. Since no two people have exactly the same scale, it is difficult to establish psychometric properties such as reliability and validity or to make any comparisons across people, much less across different disorders. Another problem is a bit more subtle. All patients choose their most troublesome symptoms: this means that they will all start off with very similar scores, even if they differ among themselves quite considerably in other areas. That is, even if Patient A has problems in six areas, and Patient B in eleven, they will be identical on the scale if each can choose only the five most bothersome. Furthermore, since they both will start off at the test's ceiling, they have nowhere to go but down, making any intervention look effective.

Another way of conceptualizing the difference between specific and generic scales is related to what Cronbach (1990) labelled the 'bandwidth versus fidelity' dilemma. The term comes from the communication theory (Shannon and Weaver 1949) and refers to the problems faced in designing radios. If we build a receiver that covers all of the commercial radio stations plus the shortwave bands and also allows us to monitor police and fire calls, then we have achieved a wide bandwidth. The trade-off, though, is that no one station is heard very well. The opposite extreme is to design a receiver that will pick up only one station. The fidelity of the reception will be superb, since all of the components are designed for that one specific part of the spectrum, but the radio will be useless for any other station we may want to hear. Thus, we achieve bandwidth at the cost of fidelity and vice versa.

The issue is the proper balance between a narrow scale with low bandwidth and (presumably) good fidelity versus a generic scale with greater bandwidth but (again presumably) poorer fidelity. The literature comparing these two types of scales is somewhat limited. However, the general conclusion is that the advantages of disease-specific scales may be more apparent than real; well-designed, reliable, and valid generic questionnaires appear to yield results that are comparable to disease-specific ones across a number of illnesses and instruments (e.g. Bombardier et al. 1986; Liang et al. 1985; Parkerson et al. 1993) and the belief that disease-specific instruments are more sensitive than generic ones is not uniformly supported by the literature (Kaplan 1993).

The safest option, then, would likely be to use a generic instrument such as the 36-Item Short Form Health Survey (SF-36) (Ware et al. 1993) or the Sickness Impact Profile (Gilson et al. 1975) in all studies of QOL and to supplement it with a disease-specific one if it does not impose too much of a burden on the subjects.

Translation

Although it is not directly related to the problem of devising items, translation into another language is a problem that may have to be addressed. In most large studies, especially those located in major metropolitan centres, it is quite probable that English will not be the first language of a significant proportion of respondents. This raises one of two possible alternative strategies, both of which have associated problems. In the first, such respondents can be eliminated from the study. However, this raises the possibility that the sample will then not be a representative one, and the results may have limited generalizability. The second alternative is to translate the scales and questionnaires into the languages that are most commonly used within the catchment area encompassed by the study.

The goal of translation is to achieve equivalence between the original version and the translated version of the scale. In fact, some people do not talk of *translating* a scale, but rather *adapting* it. The first problem is what is meant by 'equivalence'. Herdman et al. (1997) list 19 different types of equivalencies that have been proposed by various authors, but most agree that there are five or six key ones (although they often differ regarding which five or six), and that they form a hierarchy (Herdman et al. 1998; Sechrest et al. 1972).

First it is necessary to establish *conceptual equivalence*; that is, do people in the two cultures see the concept in the same way? At one extreme, both the source and the target cultures completely agree on what the elements are that constitute the construct, indicating that the translators can proceed to the next step. At the other extreme, the concept may not exist in the target culture. Hunt (1986), for example, reported that poor Egyptian women had difficulty responding to an item about enjoying themselves because it did not have 'much existential relevance in a context where the concept of enjoyment is not present. Living in, or on, the edge of poverty, most of the day is taken up with work, finding food, doing chores, and just subsisting' (p. 156). Most often, what is found falls between these extremes; the concept exists in the target culture, but there may be differences with regard to the constituent elements or the weight given to each element. As an example, one of our students (Aracena et al. 2002) wanted to translate a child abuse scale into Spanish. As a first step, she conducted some focus groups to determine if the meaning of abuse was similar in Chile as in the United States, where the scale was developed. She found that behaviours that would be considered abusive (both physically and sexually) in North America were seen as part of the continuum of normal child-rearing practices in Chile. This meant that some of the items from the original scale should not be included in the translated version because they would not fall within the Chilean concept of abuse. It should be borne in mind that this goes both ways; scales originally developed in different societies may not translate well into ours. For example, Lau et al. (2020) constructed a scale to measure resilience among residents of China. Some of the items performed poorly in the English translation, because resilience in China includes the ability to recover and persevere despite hunger, dehydration, and tiredness, whereas the Western conceptualization of the construct is limited to the psychological domain.

There are many other, often subtle, concepts that either do not exist in other cultures or take on different forms that are difficult or impossible to translate meaningfully. Living in monotheistic North and South America and Europe, we often forget that other religions, such as Shintoism, and Hinduism, are polytheistic and reflect very different relationships between the secular and the spiritual than are found in the Abrahamic religions. Conversely, there are concepts in other cultures that have no direct counterpart in ours, such as *amae*: a Japanese feeling that goes beyond emotional dependency that is almost, but not quite, captured by terms such as 'guilt' or 'social embarrassment'; and the Danish/Norwegian word *hygge*, meaning (roughly) a mood of coziness, wellness, contentment, and conviviality.

Conceptual equivalence can be determined in a number of ways (Stewart and Nápoles-Springer 2000): through a review of the ethnographic and anthropological literature about the target group, interviews and focus groups, and consultations with a broad range of experts.

If conceptual equivalence exists, even partially, it is possible to move to looking for *item equivalence*. This determines whether the specific items are relevant and acceptable in the target population. It does not make sense, for instance, to ask about a person's ability to climb a flight of stairs if the questionnaire will be used in a setting consisting solely of single-storey dwellings. Also, it may be taboo in some cultures to enquire about certain topics, such as sexual problems, negative feelings directed towards family members, or income. These questions may have to be reworded or replaced before the translation can begin. Item equivalence is established in much the same way as conceptual equivalence.

Semantic equivalence refers to the meaning attached to each item. For example, we generally associate the colour blue with sadness, and black with depression. In China, though, white is the colour of mourning, a shade we use to connote purity.

Consequently, a literal translation of the phrase 'I feel blue' or 'The future looks black to me' would not convey the same semantic meaning in many other cultures. Similarly, Anglo-Saxons often associate mild physical discomfort with stomach problems, whereas the French would be more prone to attribute it to their liver, and Germans to their circulation. Sometimes, a literal translation renders a question moot. Hambleton (1994) gives an example of a multiple choice item: 'Where is a bird with webbed feet most likely to live? (a) mountains, (b) woods, (c) sea, (d) desert.' The problem in translating this item into Swedish is that the term for 'webbed feet' is 'swimming feet', so the stem gives away the answer (except perhaps to those who think it is possible to swim in the desert). This problem exists even within the same language as spoken in different countries. Oscar Wilde wrote that 'We have really everything in common with America nowadays except, of course, language' and George Bernard Shaw similarly said, 'England and America are two countries separated by a common language'. This is well illustrated with a scale developed in England, one item of which reads, 'I have been feeling in need of a good tonic'. While someone in the United Kingdom would know that a tonic is a medicinal substance, a person in North America may wonder why a health questionnaire is asking about a type of soda usually added to gin. This problem exists even within the same language as spoken in different countries. The word 'comadre' has the dictionary definition of a child's godmother; in Mexican and Texan Spanish, though, it means a close personal advisor and friend; but in Nicaragua, it can also refer to 'the other woman'. Obviously, a scale measuring who is available for social support will yield different responses (and reactions) when used in these different countries. Similarly, idioms derived from sports (e.g. 'getting to first base', 'out in left field', or 'a sticky wicket') do not translate well. Semantic equivalence can be established in a number of ways. First, people can be given the translated version and asked to rephrase the question in their own words, or say what they think the item means (a process of cognitive testing described in Chapter 6, under the heading 'Testing the items'). Second, the process of translation and back-translation, outlined later in this chapter, will often uncover discrepancies in interpretation between the two versions.

Operational equivalence goes beyond the items themselves and looks at whether the same format of the scale, the instructions, and the mode of administration can be used in the target population. For example, it is impolite in many North American First Nations groups to ask a direct question, and in some Asian and African cultures for younger people to question their elders. Needless to say, self-administered scales would be totally inappropriate in places with low literacy levels. Even the format of the items may present difficulties. We found that older people in Canada had difficulty grasping the concept of putting an X on a 10-cm line (a visual analogue scale, discussed in Chapter 4) corresponding to their degree of discomfort. They were able to use this type of scale reliably only when we turned it on its side and made it resemble a thermometer that could be filled in with a red marker (Mohide et al. 1990). Others have found that people from different cultures, ranging from Japan and China to El Salvador, had difficulty with ordered response options (e.g. 'Strongly agree' to 'Disagree') and avoided negative options (Lee et al. 2002) or preferred dichotomous responses (Flaskerud

1988). When gathering data involving dates, remember that formats are not consistent between countries or even within the same country. The number 09/02/08 could variously refer to September 2, 2008, February 9, 2008, February 8, 2009, or August 2, 2009. It is best to explicitly ask for the day, month, and year.

Finally, *measurement equivalence* investigates whether the psychometric properties of the test—its various forms of reliability and validity—are the same in both versions. Of course, this can be done only after the test has been translated.

Once it has been determined that the scale can be translated (i.e. if conceptual equivalence exists, and items that may present problems for item and semantic equivalence can be changed), it is time to begin the translation process itself. Guillemin et al. (1993) recommend at least two independent translations and state that it is even better if each translation is done by a team. The people should translate into their native tongue and should be aware of the intent of each item and the scale as a whole. This allows them to go beyond a strictly semantic translation and to use more idiomatic language that would be better understood by the respondents. These people not only should be fluent in both languages, but also have a deep understanding of both cultures. This would allow them to spot problems with items such as 'I like to go to dances' if the culture does not permit dancing, as is the case with some fundamentalist religions.

The next step is called 'back-translation'. Each item is now translated back into the source language, again by independent teams who have not seen the originals and are not aware of the purpose of the scale. This time, the members should be familiar with idiomatic use of the source language. Finally, a committee should look at the original and the back-translated items, and resolve any discrepancies. Needless to say, all of the people involved in the translation, back-translation, and reconciliation phases should be fluent in both languages. In the translation phase, their first language should be the target language; in the back-translation phase, it should be the source language; and the composition of the committee should be mixed.

One problem with the translation and back-translation process has to do with the translators themselves. They are usually better educated and have a higher reading level than those who will ultimately be completing the scale (Hambleton 1994); and their familiarity with two languages (and perhaps two cultures) may make it easier for them to grasp the intended meaning of the question (Mallinckrodt and Wang 2004). Consequently, it is necessary to have a group of unilingual people, similar in terms of sociodemographic characteristics to the target population, check the items using the procedures outlined in Chapter 5.

As mentioned under *measurement equivalence*, it is now necessary to establish the psychometric properties of the translated scale. This can be as simple as determining its reliability and doing some validity studies. A more thorough testing would also see if the norms and cut points used in the original scale are appropriate for the translated one. At the most sophisticated level, statistical testing using confirmatory factor analysis (CFA) and the differential item functioning (DIF) component of item response theory (IRT) can be used to determine if the individual items perform in the same way in both versions. IRT is explained in more detail in Chapter 12, and a very brief description of CFA is given in Appendix B; people who are interested in a basic introduction can read Norman and Streiner (2014) or Byrne (2016) for a more detailed explanation.

If the researcher has access to a large ($N > 30$) bilingual sample from the target culture and the item statistics from a larger group ($N > 300$) in the original language, a quantitative approach for verifying the semantic equivalence of a translated measure has been proposed by Mallinckrodt and Wang (2004):

1. Construct two versions of the scale: each would have half of the items from the original version and half of the items from the translated form. Ideally, each version would itself have two forms: one where the items in the original language are presented first and one where the translated items are presented first, thus resulting in four forms.

2. The bilingual subjects get one form, assigned randomly, along with scales that can be used for construct validation.

3. Optionally, this would be repeated 2 weeks later (without the scales for validation) to allow for test–retest reliability.

This allows the researcher to determine: (1) the split-half reliability, comparing the translated to the original version (this and other terms will be defined more fully in other chapters of this book); (2) the internal consistency of each version; (3) the test–retest reliability; and (4) some preliminary construct validity. Further, the performance of each item in the translated version can be compared to those in the original language, using the data from the large, normative sample.

The question that therefore arises is whether translating a scale is worth the effort. It requires the translation itself, back-translation, and then re-establishing the reliability and validity within the new context—in essence, exactly the same steps that are required for developing a new scale. The only difference is that the devising of new items has been replaced by the translating of old ones. The advantage of translating a scale is that, if psychometric equivalence is established between the two versions, it then becomes possible to compare different countries or cultures regarding the construct being measured. For example, the EQ-5D, a scale that assesses quality of life, is available in approximately 30 languages (<https://euroqol.org/>).

Many scales have been translated, but problems still remain. For example, in two studies we have been involved in (O'Brien et al. 1994; Streiner et al. 1994), we used 'validated' versions of tests translated into French. The results, though, showed a lower incidence of migraine headaches in one study, and a higher self-reported quality of life in the other. The unresolved issue is whether these differences are due to cultural and other factors or reflect subtle variations in the wording of the instruments used to measure them. Although questions may not have arisen had the prevalence rates been similar, there would still have been the issue of whether there actually are differences, but our translated instrument may have missed them.

The conclusion is that translating an instrument *can* be done, but it is as time-consuming as developing a new tool. Further, both similarities and differences in results must be interpreted with extreme caution.

Further reading

Aday, L.A. and Cornelius, L.J. (2006). *Designing and conducting health surveys: A comprehensive guide* (3rd edn). Wiley, New York.

Brislin, R.W. (1970). Back-translation for cross-cultural research. *Journal of Cross-Cultural Psychology*, **1**, 185–216.

Del Greco, L., Walop, W., and Eastridge, L. (1987). Questionnaire development: 3. Translation. *Canadian Medical Association Journal*, **136**, 817–18.

DeVellis, R.F. and Thorpe, C.T. (2022). *Scale development: Theory and applications* (5th edn). Sage, Thousand Oaks, CA.

Oppenheim, A.N. (2000). *Questionnaire design and attitude measurement* (New edn). Heinemann, London.

Payne, S.L. (1951). *The art of asking questions*. Princeton University Press, Princeton, NJ.

Roid, G.H. and Haladyna, T.M. (1982). *A technology for test-item writing*. Academic Press, New York.

Sudman, S. and Bradburn, N.M. (2004). *Asking questions* (Rev. edn). Jossey-Bass, San Francisco, CA.

References

Aaronson, N.K. (1988). Quantitative issues in health-related quality of life assessment. *Health Policy*, **10**, 217–30.

Aaronson, N.K. (1989). Quality of life assessment in clinical trials: Methodological issues. *Controlled Clinical Trials*, **10**, 195S–208S.

Anderson, J.C. and Gerbing, D.W. (1991). Predicting the performance of measures in a confirmatory factor analysis with a pretest assessment of their substantive validities. *Journal of Applied Psychology*, **76**, 732–40.

Angleitner, A., John, O.P., and Löhr, F.-J. (1986). It's *what* you ask and how you ask it: An item metric analysis of personality questionnaires. In *Personality assessment via questionnaires* (eds. A. Angleitner and J.S. Wiggins), pp. 61–107. Springer, New York.

Aracena, M., Balladares, E., Román, F., and Weiss, C. (2002). Conceptualización de las pautas de crianza de buentrato y maltrato infantil, en familias del estrato socioeconómico bajo: Una mirada cualitativa. *Revista de Psicología de la Universidad de Chile*, **11**, 39–53.

Bandura, A. (1977). Self-efficacy: Toward a unifying theory of behavioral change. *Psychological Review*, **84**, 191–215.

Beckstead, J.W. (2009). Content validity is naught. *International Journal of Nursing Studies*, **46**, 1274–83.

Bombardier, C., Ware, J., Russell, I.J., Larson, M., Chalmers, A., and Read, J.L. (1986). Auranofin therapy and quality of life in patients with rheumatoid arthritis: Results of a multicenter trial. *American Journal of Medicine*, **81**, 565–78.

Boorsboom, D., Mellenbergh, G.J., and van Heerden, J. (2004) The concept of validity. *Psychological Review*, **111**, 1061–71.

Brumback, G.B. and Howell, M.A. (1972). Rating the clinical effectiveness of employed physicians. *Journal of Applied Psychology*, **56**, 241–4.

Byrne, B.M. (2016). *Structural equation modeling with AMOS: Basic concepts, applications, and programming* (3rd edn). Routledge, New York.

Cairney, J., Clark, H.J., Kwan, M.Y.W., Bruner, M., and Tamminen, K. (2018). Measuring sport experiences in children and youth to better understand the impact of sport on health and positive youth development: Designing a brief measure for population health surveys. *BMC Public Health*, **18**, 446.

Cella, D., Yount, S., Rothrock, N., Gershon, R., Cook, K., Reeve, B., *et al.* (2007). The Patient-Reported Outcomes Measurement Information System (PROMIS): Progress of an NIH roadmap cooperative group during its first two years. *Medical Care*, **45**(Suppl. 1), S3–11.

Cowles, J.T. and Kubany, A.J. (1959). Improving the measurement of clinical performance of medical students. *Journal of Clinical Psychology*, **15**, 139–42.

Cronbach, L.J. (1990). *Essentials of psychological testing* (5th edn). Harper and Row, New York.

Dalkey, N. and Helmer, O. (1963). An experimental application of the Delphi method to the use of experts. *Management Science*, **9**, 458–67.

Daynes, S. and Williams, T.M. (2018). *On ethnography*. Polity Press, Cambridge.

Dowie, J. (2002a). Decision validity should determine whether a generic or condition-specific HRQOL measure is used in health care decisions. *Health Economics*, **11**, 1–8.

Dowie, J. (2002b). 'Decision validity . . .': a rejoinder. *Health Economics*, **11**, 21–2.

Feightner, J.W. (1985). Patient management problems. In *Assessing clinical competence* (eds. V.R. Neufeld and G.R. Norman), pp. 183–200. Springer, New York.

Flaskerud, J.H. (1988). Is the Likert scale format culturally biased? *Nursing Research*, **37**, 185–6.

Gilson, B.S., Gilson, J.S., Bergner, M., Bobbit, R.A., Kressel, S., Pollard, W.E., *et al.* (1975). The Sickness Impact Profile: Development of an outcome measure of health care. *American Journal of Public Health*, **65**, 1304–10.

Glass, G.V., McGraw, B., and Smith, M.L. (1981). *Meta-analysis in social research*. Sage, Beverly Hills, CA.

Goldberg, L.R. (1971). A historical survey of personality scales and inventories. In *Advances in psychological assessment* (Vol. **2**) (ed. P. McReynolds), pp. 293–336. Science and Behavior, Palo Alto, CA.

Goldberg, L.R., Johnson, J.A., Eber, H.W., Hogan, R., Ashton, M.C., Cloninger, C.R., *et al.* (2006). The international personality item pool and the future of public-domain personality measures. *Journal of Research in Personality*, **40**, 84–96.

Guillemin, F., Bombardier, C., and Beaton, D. (1993). Cross-cultural adaptation of health-related quality of life measures: Literature review and proposed guidelines. *Journal of Clinical Epidemiology*, **46**, 1417–32.

Guyatt, G.H., Eagle, D.J., Sackett, B., Willan, A., Griffith, L., McIlroy, W., *et al.* (1993). Measuring quality of life in the frail elderly. *Journal of Clinical Epidemiology*, **46**, 1433–44.

Hambleton, R.K. (1994). Guidelines for adapting educational and psychological tests: A progress report. *European Journal of Psychological Assessment*, **10**, 229–44.

Hathaway, S.R. and McKinley, J.C. (1951). *Manual for the Minnesota Multiphasic Personality Inventory* (Rev. edn). Psychological Corporation, New York.

Haynes, S.N., Richard, D.C.S., and Kubany, E.S. (1995). Content validity in psychological assessment: A functional approach to concepts and methods. *Psychological Assessment*, **7**, 238–47.

Herdman, M., Fox-Rushby, J., and Badia, X. (1997). 'Equivalence' and the translation and adaptation of health-related quality of life questionnaires. *Quality of Life Research*, **6**, 237–47.

Herdman, M., Fox-Rushby, J., and Badia, X. (1998). A model of equivalence in the cultural adaptation of HRQoL instruments: The universalist approach. *Quality of Life Research*, **7**, 323–35.

Howard, M.C. (2018). Scale pretesting. *Practical Assessment, Research & Evaluation*, **23**, No. 5.

Howard, M.C. and Melloy, R.C. (2016). Evaluating item-sort task methods: The presentation of a new statistical significance formula and methodological best practices. *Journal of Business Psychology*, **31**, 173–86.

Hunt, S.M. (1986). Cross-cultural issues in the use of socio-medical indicators. *Health Policy*, **6**, 149–58.

Kaplan, R.M. (1993). *The Hippocratic predicament: Affordability, access and accountability in health care*. Academic Press, San Diego, CA.

Kottner, J., Audigé, L., Brorson, S., Donner, A., Gajewski, B.J., Hrøbjartsson, A., *et al*. (2010). Guidelines for Reporting Reliability and Agreement Studies (GRRAS) were proposed. *Journal of Clinical Epidemiology*, **64**, 96–106.

Kruis, W., Thieme, C., Weinzierl, M., Schuessler, P., Holl, J., and Paulus, W. (1984). A diagnostic score for the irritable bowel syndrome: Its value in the exclusion of organic disease. *Gastroenterology*, **87**, 1–7.

Lau, C., Chiesi, F., Saklofske, D.H., Yan, G., and Li, C. (2020). How essential is the essential resilience scale? Differential item functioning of Chinese and English versions and criterion validity. *Personality and Individual Differences*, **155**, Article 109666.

Lawshe, C.H. (1975). A quantitative approach to content validity. *Personnel Psychology*, **28**, 563–75.

Lee, J.W., Jones, P.S., Mineyama, Y., and Zhang, X.E. (2002). Cultural differences in responses to a Likert scale. *Research in Nursing & Health*, **25**, 295–306.

Liang, M.H., Larson, M.G., Cullen, K.E., and Schwartz, J.A. (1985). Comparative measurement efficiency and sensitivity of five health status instruments for arthritis research. *Arthritis and Rheumatism*, **28**, 542–7.

Loevinger, J. (1957). Objective tests as instruments of psychological theory. *Psychological Reports*, **3**, 635–94.

Lynn, M.R. (1986). Determination and quantification of content validity. *Nursing Research*, **35**, 382–5.

Mallinckrodt, B. and Wang, C.-C. (2004). Quantitative methods for verifying semantic equivalence of translated research instruments: A Chinese version of the experiences in close relationships scale. *Journal of Counseling Psychology*, **51**, 368–79.

McFarlane, A.H., Norman, G.R., Streiner, D.L., Roy, R.G., and Scott, D.J. (1980). A longitudinal study of the influence of the psychosocial environment on health status: A preliminary report. *Journal of Health and Social Behavior*, **21**, 124–33.

McFarlane, A.H., Neale, K.A., Norman, G.R., Roy, R.G., and Streiner, D.L. (1981). Methodological issues in developing a scale to measure social support. *Schizophrenia Bulletin*, **7**, 90–100.

McHorney, C.A., Ware, J.E., Lu, J.F.R., and Sherbourne, C.D. (1994). The MOS 36-item short form health survey (SF-36): III. Tests of data quality, scaling assumptions, and reliability across diverse patient groups. *Medical Care*, **32**, 40–66.

Messick, S. (1975). The standard problem: Meaning and values in measurement and evaluation. *American Psychologist*, **30**, 955–66.

Messick, S. (1980). Test validity and the ethics of assessment. *American Psychologist*, **35**, 1012–27.

Messick, S. (1993). Validity. In *Educational measurement* (2nd edn) (ed. R.L. Linn), pp. 13–104. Oryx Press, Phoenix, AZ.

Mohide, E.A., Pringle, D.M., Streiner, D.L., Gilbert, J.R., Muir, G., and Tew, M. (1990). A randomized trial of family caregiver support in the home management of dementia. *Journal of the American Geriatric Society*, **38**, 446–54.

Moos, R.H. (1984). *Menstrual distress questionnaire*. Stanford University Medical Center, Palo Alto, CA.

Newble, D.I., Hoare, J., and Baxter, A. (1982). Patient management problems: Issues of validity. *Medical Education*, **16**, 137–42.

Norman, G.R. and Streiner, D.L. (2014). *Biostatistics: The bare essentials* (4th edn). PMPH USA, Shelton, CT.

O'Brien, B., Goeree, R., and Streiner, D.L. (1994). Prevalence of migraine headache in Canada: A population-based survey. *International Journal of Epidemiology*, **23**, 1020–6.

Parkerson, G.R., Connis, R.T., Broadhead, W.E., Patrick, D.L. Taylor, T.R., and Tse, C.J. (1993). Disease-specific versus generic measurement of health-related quality of life in insulin-dependent diabetic patients. *Medical Care*, **31**, 629–39.

Patrick, D.L. and Deyo, R.A. (1989). Generic and disease-specific measures in assessing health status and quality of life. *Medical Care*, **27**(3 Suppl.), S217–32.

Puchta, C. and Potter, J. (2004). *Focus group practice*. Sage, Thousand Oaks, CA.

Schwarzer, R., Lippke, S., and Luszczynska, A. (2011). Mechanisms of health behavior change in persons with chronic illness or disability: The Health Action Process Approach (HAPA). *Rehabilitation Psychology*, **56**, 161–70.

Sechrest, L., Fay, T.L., and Hafeez Zaidi, S.M. (1972). Problems of translation in cross-cultural research. *Journal of Cross-Cultural Psychology*, **3**, 41–56.

Seligman, A.W. (1993). Cardiovascular consequences of expressing, experiencing, and repressing anger. *Journal of Behavioral Medicine*, **16**, 539–69.

Shannon, C. and Weaver, W. (1949). *The mathematical theory of communication*. University of Illinois Press, Urbana, IL.

Slade, T., Grove, R., and Burgess, P. (2011). Kessler Psychological Distress Scale: Normative data from the 2007 Australian National Survey of Mental Health and Wellbeing. *Australian and New Zealand Journal of Psychiatry*, **45**, 308–16.

Stewart, A.L. and Nápoles-Springer, A. (2000). Health-related quality-of-life assessments in diverse population groups in the United States. *Medical Care*, **38**(Suppl. II), II–102–24.

Streiner, D.L. and Cairney, J. (2010). The social science contribution to psychiatric epidemiology. In *Mental disorder in Canada: An epidemiological perspective*. (eds. J. Cairney and D.L. Streiner), pp. 11–28. University of Toronto Press, Toronto, ON.

Streiner, D.L., O'Brien, B., and Dean, D. (1994). *Quality of life in major depression: A comparison of instruments*. Paper presented at the 19th Annual Meeting of the Collegium Internationale Neuro-Psychopharmacologicum, Washington, DC.

Taylor, J.A. (1953). A personality scale of manifest anxiety. *Journal of Abnormal and Social Psychology*, **48**, 285–90.

Taylor, S.J. and Bogden, R. (1998). *Introduction to qualitative research methods: A guidebook and resources* (3rd edn). Wiley, New York.

Ullman, L.P. and Giovannoni, J.M. (1964). The development of a self-report measure of the process-reactive continuum. *Journal of Nervous and Mental Disease*, **138**, 38–42.

Vogt, D.W., King, D.W., and King, L.A. (2004). Focus groups in psychological assessment: Enhancing content validity by consulting members of the target population. *Psychological Assessment*, **16**, 231–43.

Waltz, C.W. and Bausell, R.B. (1981). *Nursing research: Design, statistics and computer analysis.* F.A. Davis, Philadelphia, PA.

Ware, J.E. Jr., Snow, K.K., Kosinski, M., and Gandek, B. (1993). *SF-36 health survey manual and interpretation guide.* The Health Institute, New England Medical Center, Boston, MA.

Wechsler, D. (1958). *The measurement and appraisal of adult intelligence* (4th edn). Williams and Wilkins, Baltimore, MD.

Willms, D.G. and Johnson, N.A. (1993). *Essentials in qualitative research: A notebook for the field.* Unpublished manuscript. McMaster University, Hamilton, ON.

Chapter 4

Scaling responses

Introduction to scaling responses

Having devised a set of questions using the methods outlined in Chapter 3, we must choose a method by which responses will be obtained. The choice of method is dictated, at least in part, by the nature of the question asked. For example, a question like 'Have you ever gone to church?' leads fairly directly to a response method consisting of two boxes, one labelled 'Yes' and the other 'No'. By contrast, the question 'How religious are you?' does not dictate a simple two-category response, and a question like 'Do you believe that religious instruction leads to racial prejudice?' may require the use of more subtle and sophisticated techniques to obtain valid responses.

There has been a bewildering amount of research in this area, in disciplines ranging from psychology to economics. Often the results are conflicting, and the correct conclusions are frequently counter-intuitive. In this chapter, we describe a wide variety of scaling methods, indicate their appropriate use, and make recommendations regarding a choice of methods.

Some basic concepts

In considering approaches to the development of response scales, it is helpful to first consider the kinds of possible responses which may arise. A basic division is between those responses that are categorical, such as race, religion, or marital status, and those that are continuous variables, like haemoglobin, blood pressure, or the amount of pain recorded on a 100-mm line. The second related feature of response scales is commonly referred to as the *level of measurement*. If the response consists of named categories, such as particular symptoms, a job classification, or religious denomination, the variable is called a *nominal* variable, because the response alternatives are names, rather than numbers. Numbers can be assigned to the names, but they are arbitrary and can be considered to be alternative names. Ordered categories, such as staging in breast cancer and educational level (less than high school, high school diploma, some college or university, university degree, postgraduate degree), are called ordinal variables because, unlike nominal variables, they can be placed in order. By contrast, variables in which the interval between values is constant and known are called *interval* variables. Temperature, measured in degrees Celsius or Fahrenheit, is an interval variable. Strictly speaking, rating scales, where the response is on a 5-point or 7-point scale, are not considered interval level measurement, since we can never be sure that the distance between 'strongly disagree' and 'disagree' is the same as between 'agree' and 'strongly agree'. However, as we will discuss under General issues in the construction of continuous scales, rating scales are usually analyzed as if they were interval (that is, using parametric statistics). Also, if this is a concern, methods have been devised to achieve interval level measurement with subjective scales, as will be discussed in the chapter on Item response theory. Finally, variables where there is a meaningful zero point, so that the ratio of two responses has some meaning, are called *ratio* variables. Temperature measured in Kelvin is a ratio variable, whereas the temperatures in Fahrenheit or Celsius are not. That is, 100° Kelvin is twice as hot as 50° Kelvin, because the zero point for the Kelvin scale (Absolute zero) is when all molecular motion ceases. But 100° Fahrenheit is not twice as hot as 50° Fahrenheit. To show this, let's convert those temperatures into Celsius: 100°F = 37.8°C and 50°F = 10°C. Now the 2:1 ratio doesn't hold, even though the temperatures are the same. The issue is that the zero point in Fahrenheit and Celsius is arbitrary and different.

What is the significance of these distinctions? The important difference lies between nominal and ordinal data on one hand, and interval and ratio variables on the other. In the latter case, measures such as means, standard deviations, and differences among the means can be interpreted, and the broad class of techniques called 'parametric statistics' can, therefore, be used for analysis. By contrast, since it makes no sense to speak of the average religion or average sex of a sample of people, nominal and ordinal data must be considered as frequencies in individual categories, and 'non-parametric' statistics must be used for analysis. The distinction between these two types of analysis is described in any introductory statistics book, such as those listed in 'Further reading' at the end of this chapter.

Categorical judgements

One form of question frequently used in health sciences requires only a categorical judgement by the respondent, either as a 'yes/no' response, or as a simple check. The responses would then result in a *nominal* scale of measurement. Some examples are shown in Fig. 4.1. Care must be taken to ensure that questions are written clearly and unambiguously, as discussed in Chapter 5. However, there is little difficulty in deciding on the appropriate response method.

Have you ever had a chest X-ray?   yes — no —

Which of the following symptoms are you currently experiencing?

    Headaches —
    Dizziness   —
    Cough   —
    Colds   —
    Other   (please write in) ————————————

Are you able to climb the stairs?   yes — no —

I think that people are watching me.   true — false —

Fig. 4.1 Examples of questions requiring categorical judgements.

Perhaps the most common error when using categorical questions is that they are frequently employed in circumstances where the response is not, in fact, categorical. Attitudes and behaviours often lie on a continuum. When we ask a question like 'Do you have trouble climbing stairs?', we ignore the fact that there are varying degrees of trouble. Even the best athlete might have difficulty negotiating the stairs of a sky-scraper at one run without some degree of discomfort. What we wish to find out pre-sumably is *how much* trouble the respondent has in negotiating an ordinary flight of stairs.

Ignoring the continuous nature of many responses leads to three difficulties. The first one is fairly obvious: since different people may have different ideas about what constitutes a positive response to a question, there will likely be error introduced into the responses, as well as uncertainty and confusion on the part of respondents.

The second problem is perhaps more subtle. Even if all respondents have a similar conception of the category boundaries, there will still be error introduced into the measurement because of the limited choice of response levels. For example, the state-ment in Fig. 4.2 might be responded to in one of two ways, as indicated in (a) and (b): the first method effectively reduces all positive opinions, ranging from strong to mild, to a single number, and similarly for all negative feelings. The effect is a potential loss of information and a corresponding reduction in reliability.

The third problem, which is a consequence of the second, is that dichotomizing a continuous variable leads to a loss of *efficiency* of the instrument and a reduction in its correlation with other measures. A more efficient instrument requires fewer obser-vations than a less efficient one to show an effect. Suissa (1991) calculated that a di-chotomous outcome is, at best, 67 per cent as efficient as a continuous one; depending on how the measure was dichotomized, this can drop to under 10 per cent. Under the best of circumstances, that is, when the cut point is at the median, then, if you needed 67 subjects to show an effect when the outcome is measured along a continuum, you would need 100 subjects to demonstrate the same effect when the outcome is dichot-omized. When circumstances are not as ideal, the inflation in the required sample size can be 10 or more. Similarly, Hunter and Schmidt (1990) showed that if the dichotomy resulted in a 50–50 split, with half of the subjects in one group and half in the other, the correlation of that instrument with another is reduced by 20 per cent. Any other split results in a greater attenuation; if the result is that 10 per cent of the subjects are in one group and 90 per cent in the other, then the reduction is 41 per cent.

Doctors carry a heavy responsibility					
(a) agree __	disagree __				
(b) strongly agree	agree	mildly agree	mildly disagree	disagree	strongly disagree
__	__	__	__	__	__

Fig. 4.2 Example of a continuous judgement.

We have demonstrated this result with real data on several occasions. In a recent study of the certification examinations in internal medicine in Canada, the reliability of the original scores, inter-rater and test–retest, was 0.76 and 0.47, respectively. These scores were then converted to a pass–fail decision and the reliability recalculated. The comparable statistics for these decisions were 0.69 and 0.36, a loss of about 0.09 in reliability.

There are two common, but invalid, objections to the use of multiple response levels. The first is that the researcher is only interested in whether respondents agree or disagree, so it is not worth the extra effort. This argument confuses measurement with decision-making: the decision can always be made after the fact by establishing a cut-off point on the response continuum, but information lost from the original responses cannot be recaptured.

The second argument is that the additional categories are only adding noise or error to the data; people cannot make finer judgements than 'agree–disagree'. Although there may be particular circumstances where this is true, in general, the evidence indicates that people are capable of much finer discriminations; this will be reviewed in a later section of the chapter (see General issues in the construction of scales) where we discuss the appropriate number of response steps.

Continuous judgements

Accepting that many of the variables of interest to healthcare researchers are continuous rather than categorical, methods must be devised to quantify these judgements.

The approaches that we will review fall into three broad categories:

1. *Direct estimation* techniques, in which subjects are required to indicate their response by a mark on a line (along a continuum of responses) or by selecting a response category (putting a check in a box or selecting a category from a dropdown menu).

2. *Comparative* methods, in which subjects choose among a series of alternatives that have been previously calibrated by a separate criterion group.

3. *Econometric* methods, in which the subjects describe their preference by anchoring it to extreme states (perfect health–death).

Direct estimation methods

Direct estimation methods are designed to elicit from the subject a direct quantitative estimate of the magnitude of an attribute. The approach is usually straightforward, as in the example used earlier, where we asked for a response on a 6-point scale ranging from 'strongly agree' to 'strongly disagree'. This is one of many variations, although all share many common features. We begin by describing the main contenders; then we will explore their advantages and disadvantages.

Visual analogue scales

The visual analogue scale (VAS) is the essence of simplicity—a line of fixed length, usually 100 mm, with anchors like 'No pain' and 'Pain as bad as it could be' at the extreme ends and no words describing intermediate positions. An example is shown in Fig. 4.3. Respondents are required to place a mark, usually an 'X' or a vertical line, on the line corresponding to their perceived state. The VAS technique was introduced over 100 years ago (Hayes and Patterson 1921), at which time it was called the 'graphic rating method', but became popular in clinical psychology only in the 1960s. The method has been used extensively in medicine to assess a variety of constructs: pain (Huskisson 1974), mood (Aitken 1969), and functional capacity (Scott and Huskisson 1978), among many others.

The VAS has also been used for the measurement of change (Scott and Huskisson 1979). In this approach, researchers are interested in the perceptions of the degree to which patients feel that they have improved as a result of treatment. The strategy used is to show patients, at the end of a course of treatment, where they had marked the line prior to commencing treatment, and then asking them to indicate, by the second line, their present state. There are a number of conceptual and methodological issues in the measurement of change, by VAS or other means, which will be addressed in Chapter 11.

Proponents are enthusiastic in their writings regarding the advantages of the method over its usual rival, a scale in which intermediate positions are labelled (e.g. 'mild', 'moderate', 'severe'); however, the authors frequently then demonstrate a substantial correlation between the two methods (Downie et al. 1978), suggesting that the advantages are more perceived than real. One also suspects that the method provides an illusion of precision, since a number given to two decimal places (e.g. a length measured in millimetres) has an apparent accuracy of 1 per cent. Of course, although one can measure a response to this degree of precision, there is no guarantee that the response accurately represents the underlying attribute to the same degree of resolution. In fact, Jensen et al. (1994) found that when pain patients were given a 101-point numerical scale, almost all of the people grouped the numbers in multiples of 5 or 10—in essence treating it as if it were an 11- or 21-point scale. Moreover, little information was lost using these 'coarser' gradations.

The simplicity of the VAS has contributed to its popularity, although there is some evidence that patients may not find it as simple and appealing as researchers; in one study described earlier in this section (Huskisson 1974), 7 per cent of patients were unable to complete a VAS, as against 3 per cent for an adjectival rating scale. Similarly, Bosi Ferraz et al. (1990) found that in Brazil, illiterate subjects had more difficulty with a VAS than with numerical or adjectival scales; their test–retest reliabilities, although statistically significant, were below an acceptable level. Some researchers in gerontology have concluded that there may be an age effect

---

How severe has your arthritic pain been today?

pain as   no
bad as it _____ pain
could be

Fig. 4.3 Example of a visual analogue scale (VAS).

in the perceived difficulty in using the VAS, leading to a modification of the technique. Instead of a horizontal line, they have used a vertical 'thermometer', which is apparently easier for older people to complete. At the other end of the age continuum, children preferred a Likert scale (described shortly) over a VAS with numbers underneath, and rated the unnumbered VAS as their least preferred option (van Laerhoven et al. 2004).

Even among people who are comfortable with the method, the VAS has a number of serious drawbacks. Scale constructors tend to give little thought to the wording of the end-points, yet patients' ratings of pain are highly dependent on the exact wording of the descriptors (Seymour et al. 1985). While the lower limit is often easy to describe (none of the attributes being measured), the upper end is more problematic. What is the maximum amount of dizziness?: is it a function of time (e.g. 'dizzy all of the time'), or of intensity (we have no idea how to word that), or both? For that matter, how does a person know what is 'The most intense pain imaginable' if they have never experienced it? Does a mark half-way along the VAS indicate pain half the time, half the intensity, half the frequency, or something else? This also means that everyone may have a different end-point that is dependent on their imagination.

Perhaps the most serious problem with the VAS is not inherent in the scale at all. In many applications of the VAS in health sciences, the attribute of interest, such as pain, is assessed with a single scale, as in the example shown earlier. However, the reliability of a scale is directly related to the number of items in the scale, so that the one-item VAS test is likely to demonstrate low reliability in comparison to longer scales. The solution, of course, is to lengthen the scale by including multiple VASs to assess related aspects of the attribute of interest.

An interesting hybrid approach is to combine adjectival and VAS formats in the same measure—what has been called a modified VAS approach (Cairney et al. 2018). In the PLAYfun tool for example, a measure of motoric competence designed for children and youths, raters score a set of motor competences using a scale which is subdivided into four boxes, each reflecting a stage of development for that particular motor skill—initial, emerging, competent, proficient (Cairney et al. 2018; Caldwell et al. 2021). The child performs a standardized motor task and the observer (rater) first decides what box (stage of development) best describes the child's performance. From there, the observer can mark an 'X' at any point within the box, as would be done with a standard VAS. The total length of the boxes end to end is 100 mm, so, as with a standard VAS, the child's score on that particular task can range from 0 to 100. The modification was designed to orient observers to the appropriate stage of development of the skill, while still providing for a range of scoring within each domain. Proponents argue the scoring provides advantages over other measures of motor skill that often use binary ratings of proficiency—the child can either do the skill or not (Cairney et al. 2018). It is also interesting to note that there are 18 items (skills to be rated) in the measure, so unlike traditional pain measures, this tool also addresses the limitations of using single item measures.

In conclusion, although the VAS approach has the merit of simplicity, there is sufficient evidence that other methods may yield more precise measurement and possibly increased levels of satisfaction among respondents. It remains to be seen whether

How much of a role should the courts have in deciding whether to end life-support measures?

No role at all	A minor role	A major role	They should be the sole deciders
☐	☐	☐	☐

How much of a role should the courts have in deciding whether to end life-support measures?

| No role
at all | A very
minor role | A minor
role | A major
role | A very
major role | They should be
the sole deciders |

Fig. 4.4 Examples of adjectival scales.

combining VAS scaling with more traditional adjectival scaling offers a solution to the inherent limitations of the VAS approach.

Adjectival scales

Adjectival scales, as the name implies, use descriptors along a continuum, rather than simply labelling the end-points, as with the VAS. Two examples of this scale are shown in Fig. 4.4. The top scale uses discrete boxes, forcing the respondent to select among the four alternatives (the actual number of boxes is arbitrary), while the bottom scale looks more like a continuous line, allowing the person to place the mark even on a dividing line. The latter option gives an illusion of greater flexibility but in reality, it is the person who scores the scale who usually imposes some rule to assign the answer into one of the existing categories (e.g. always use the category on the left, or the one closer to the middle). Adjectival scales are used very often in rating scales, such as those used for student evaluations (e.g. unsatisfactory/satisfactory/excellent/superior) or self-reported health (excellent/very good/good/fair/poor).

A variant of this, used primarily for estimating the probability of an event, is called the *Juster scale* (Hoek and Gendall 1993). As seen in Fig. 4.5, it combines adjectival descriptors of probabilities with numerical ones and appears to have good psychometric properties.

It is evident that the rating scale, with continuous responses, bears close resemblance to the VAS, with the exception that additional descriptions are introduced at intermediate positions. Although proponents of the VAS eschew the use of descriptors, an opposite position is taken by psychometricians regarding rating scales. Guilford (1954) states, 'Nothing should be left undone to give the rater a clear, unequivocal conception of the continuum along which he is to evaluate objects' (p. 292).

Likert scales

Likert scales (Likert 1932) are similar to adjectival scales, with one exception. Adjectival scales are unipolar, in that the descriptors range from none or little of

10	Certain, practically certain	(99 in 100 chance)
9	Almost sure	(9 in 10 chance)
8	Very probably	(8 in 10 chance)
7	Probable	(7 in 10 chance)
6	Good possibility	(6 in 10 chance)
5	Fairly good possibility	(5 in 10 chance)
4	Fair possibility	(4 in 10 chance)
3	Some possibility	(3 in 10 chance)
2	Slight possibility	(2 in 10 chance)
1	Very slight possibility	(1 in 10 chance)
0	No chance, almost no chance	(1 in 100 chance)

Fig. 4.5 Example of a Juster scale.

Reproduced with permission from Hoek, J.A. and Gendall, P.J., A new method of predicting voting behavior, *Journal of the Market Research Society* (www.mrs.org.uk/ijmr), Volume 35, Number 4, pp. 361–73, Copyright © 1993 Market Research Society.

the attribute at one end to a lot or the maximal amount at the other. In contrast, Likert scales are bipolar, as in Fig. 4.6. The descriptors most often tap agreement (Strongly agree–Strongly disagree), but it is possible to construct a Likert scale measuring almost any attribute, such as acceptance (Most agreeable–Least agreeable), similarity (Most like me–Least like me), or probability (Most likely–Least likely).

There are two important points in designing Likert scales. The first is that the adjectives should be appropriate for the stem. Test constructors often want to keep the labels under the boxes the same from one item to another in order to reduce the burden on the respondents. However, this may lead to situations where descriptors for agreement appear on items that are better described with adjectives for similarity (e.g. 'I am very easy going'). It is far better to have the stem and adjectives make sense than to have consistency. The second point is what to label the middle position. It should reflect a

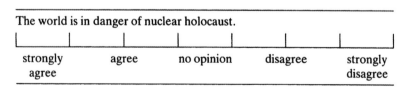

Fig. 4.6 Example of a Likert scale.

middle amount of the attribute and not an inability to answer the question. For instance, 'Cannot say' may reflect the following:

1. A middle amount.
2. Wanting to answer 'It all depends'.
3. That the item does not apply.
4. That the person does not understand the item.
5. That the person is unable to make up their mind.
6. The person does not want to answer that question.

Better terms would be 'Neither agree nor disagree' or 'Neutral'. However, there is some research that indicates that most people who opt for 'Neither agree nor disagree' would really rather say 'It all depends', and that endorsement of this option is more closely associated with the item than to characteristics of the person (Kulas and Stachowski 2009, 2013). When given the option of 'Uncertain', many respondents said that they were in fact certain but the other available options did not apply (Conn and Rieke 1994). This would indicate that the stem is worded too broadly, and greater contextualization is required. Cognitive interviewing, which is discussed in Chapter 6, would likely reveal this during pre-testing.

Another implication of the middle category not always reflecting a middle amount of the attribute is that assigning consecutive numbers to the response options (e.g. 'Strongly agree' = 1, 'Agree' = 2, 'Neutral' = 3, 'Disagree' = 4, and 'Strongly disagree' = 5) may not always be appropriate, and could result in a distorted estimate of the construct (Murray et al. 2016). They recommend using item response theory (discussed in Chapter 12) to determine if it actually belongs in the centre and, if not, combining it with one of the adjacent categories.

There is one final point to note: Rensis Likert's name 'is among the most mispronounced in [the] field' (Latham 2006, p. 15). Most English-speaking people say it as 'Like-urt', but it is more properly pronounced as 'Lick-urt'.

A variant of the Likert scale, used primarily with children, is called a *Harter scale* (Harter 1982). A typical item is shown in Fig. 4.7. The child first decides whether they are more like the kid on the right or on the left, and then whether the description is True or Really true for them; there is no neutral position. Harter claims that this format reduces bias in responding because contrasting two types of children reduces the possibility that one of the alternatives is seen as less normal or desirable than the other. We have successfully used this format with children as young as 8 years of age.

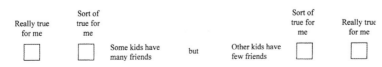

Fig. 4.7 Example of a Harter scale.
Adapted from Harter, S., The Perceived Competence Scale for Children, *Child Development*, Volume 53, Number 1, pp. 87–97, Copyright © 1982, with permission from Blackwell Publishing, Inc.

By the same token, their parents, who filled out the scale as they thought their kids would, did not feel that the format was too 'infantile' for them (Ronen et al. 2003).

There are a number of issues that have to be considered in constructing Likert scales, such as the number of boxes or scale divisions, whether there should be a neutral category and, if so, where it should be placed, and whether all of the divisions need be labelled. These will be discussed later in the chapter in the section 'General issues in the construction of continuous scales'.

Face scales

A major problem with Likert and adjectival scales is that they require some degree of reading ability, making them inappropriate for young children, and difficult for those with any type of cognitive disorder, such as retardation or Alzheimer's disease. To try to get around this problem, there have been attempts to use faces to measure primarily pain or unhappiness. Some scales, such as the *Oucher*, use photographs that are supposed to show increasing degrees of distress (Beyer 1984; Beyer et al. 1992). However, most of the scales use line drawings that lack indicators of gender or ethnicity, making them applicable to a wider range of subjects. An example of one such scale is the Wong–Baker FACES Pain Scale (Wong and Baker 1988). It consists of six circles—others use five (e.g. Pothman 1990) or seven (Bieri et al. 1990)—ranging from a smiling face with the label 'No Hurt', to one depicting a crying face with the label 'Hurts Worst'. Because the wording with this type of scale is either very simple or non-existent, many of them have been used with children from a number of different countries. In order to avoid the problem that the FACES is copyrighted and it may be necessary to pay to use it in some circumstances, He et al. (2022) developed a similar 6-point scale using emojis that are in the public domain. Preliminary data show that it is highly correlated with a VAS and adjectival scale.

Although seemingly simple and straightforward, these scales illustrate some of the problems with non-verbal instruments. For example, the 'No Hurt' and 'Hurts Little Bit' faces are smiling, so that children may feel they have to pick the 'Hurts Little More' face if they are experiencing any pain. At the other end of the scale, children may feel they have to be crying before they can select the 'Hurts Worst' face. Further, boys and those from certain cultures may be biased against selecting a face that shows tears (Champion et al. 1998). For the most part, though, these scales have at least preliminary evidence that they have good psychometric properties (Stinson et al. 2006).

One pole or two

The major difference between VAS and adjectival scales on the one hand and Likert scales on the other is the number of 'poles' of the factor being assessed. VAS and adjectival scales are unipolar, in that they assess the magnitude of a feeling or belief from zero or little to very much or a maximum. Likert scales are bipolar; one end reflects strong endorsement of an idea, and the other end strong endorsement of its opposite. Which format to use usually is obvious from what is being evaluated: the amount of pain or the ability to perform some action would require a unipolar format, whereas endorsement of a belief or attitude is often bipolar—strongly agree or in favour to strongly disagree or reject. However, some attributes are not as clear-cut, and there are significant implications in the choice that is made.

The problem is perhaps most acute in the assessment of affect. What is the opposite of 'happiness'?; is it 'unhappiness' (or at the extreme, 'depression') or is it 'no happiness'? The answer depends on your theory of mood states. There are some who argue vehemently that positive and negative affects (e.g. upset/calm, displeased/pleased) are opposite ends of a continuum (e.g. Russell and Carroll 1999a, 1999b), while others, with just as much vehemence, insist that they are separate states (e.g. Watson and Tellegen 1999; Zautra et al. 1997) and that you can be, for example, both happy and unhappy or pleased and displeased to varying degrees at the same time. Needless to say, where you stand in this debate influences whether you would use one bipolar or two unipolar scales to measure this state (or these states).

Less obvious, though, is that the debate may be fuelled by the fact that people may misinterpret unipolar scales as bipolar. For example, if the stem of an item were 'Indicate how happy you feel right now', and the response options ranged from 'Not At All' to 'Extremely', what would the lowest score indicate: a lack of happiness or a degree of unhappiness? The problem is that respondents do not attend to just the item; they are influenced by, among other things, the format of the scale itself (Knäuper and Turner 2003). As a result, the response depends on the interpretation each individual gives to the way the scale is constructed. When shown similar scales, different respondents labelled the points differently, but most placed 'neutral' somewhere in the centre of the scale, not at the left end (Russell and Carroll 1999a). The only way to disentangle a person's response is to ask two two-part questions: (1a) Do you feel happy? (1b) If so, how much?; and then (2a) Do you feel unhappy? (2b) If so, how much?

There are (at least) two morals to this story. First, your choice of the response format is dependent on your implicit theory of the attribute you are trying to measure. Second, without adequate pre-testing of the items (discussed at the end of Chapter 6), you may not be aware that scales that you intend to be unipolar may be interpreted as bipolar.

General issues in the construction of continuous scales

Regardless of the specific approach adopted, there are a number of questions that must be addressed in designing a rating scale to maximize precision and minimize bias.

1. *How many steps should there be?* The choice of the number of steps or boxes on a scale is not primarily an aesthetic issue. We indicated earlier in the discussion of categorical ratings that the use of two categories to express an underlying continuum will result in a loss of information. The argument can be extended to the present circumstances; if the number of levels is less than the rater's ability to discriminate, the result will be a loss of information. Although the ability to discriminate would appear to be highly contingent on the particular situation, there is evidence that this is not the case. A number of studies have shown that for reliability coefficients in the range normally encountered, from 0.4 to 0.9, the reliability drops as fewer categories are used. Nishisato and Torii (1970) studied this empirically by generating distributions of two variables with known correlations, ranging from 0.1 to 0.9 in steps of 0.2. They then rounded off the numbers as if they were creating a scale of a particular number of steps. For example, if the original numbers fell in

the range from 1.000 to 10.000, a 2-point scale was created by calling any number less than 5.000 a 0 and any number greater than or equal to 5.000 a 1. A 10-point scale was created by rounding off up to the decimal point, resulting in discrete values ranging from 1 to 10. The final step in this simulation was to recalculate the correlation using the rounded numbers. Since the rounding process resulted in the loss of precision, this should have the effect of reducing the correlation between the sets of numbers. The original correlation corresponds to the test–retest reliability of the original data, and the recalculated correlation using the rounded-off numbers is equivalent to the reliability which would result from a scale with 2, 5, or 10 boxes, with everything else held constant.

As can be seen from Fig. 4.8, the loss in reliability for seven and ten categories is quite small. However, the use of five categories reduces the reliability by about 12 per cent, and the use of only two categories results in an average reduction of the reliability coefficient of 35 per cent. These results were confirmed by other studies and suggested that the minimum number of categories used by raters should be in the region of five to seven. Of course, a common problem of ratings is that raters seldom use the extreme positions on the scale, and this should be taken into account when designing the scale, as discussed in Chapter 6.

Two other considerations are the preference of the respondents, and how easy they find it to complete scales with different numbers of options. Jones (1968) and Carp (1989) found that even though they were the easiest to use, people 'consistently disliked' dichotomous items. They found them less 'accurate', 'reliable', and 'interesting', and more 'ambiguous' and 'restrictive' than items with more options. The exception to this may be that some cultural groups and those with less education and familiarity with scales have difficulty with ordered categories (Flaskerud 1988), much as was found with VASs, as we discussed in the section on 'Visual

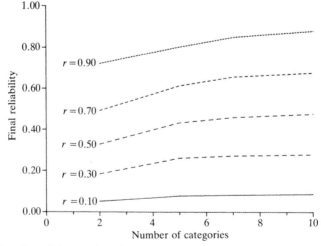

Fig. 4.8 The effect of the number of scale categories on reliability.

analogue scales'. At the other end, Preston and Colman (2000) said that respondents found scales with 10 or 11 options less easy to use, and they required more time to fill out than that required for the scales with fewer steps. Moreover, test–retest reliability tended to decrease for scales with more than 10 response categories. Thus, respondent preferences are congruent with statistical results; five to nine steps are ideal in most circumstances. Even if it is found that some options are not used, it is better to combine them in the analysis phase than to reduce the options to a dichotomy.

2. *How should categories be combined?* As we just mentioned, there are times when, despite our best efforts in writing good items, some response categories are endorsed very rarely or not at all. This can present problems in the data analysis stage, because there may not be a sufficient number of respondents to allow us to derive accurate information about some response options. In these situations, it may be best to eliminate or combine adjacent categories. This will not adversely affect the psychometric properties of the scale, because the options aren't being used in any case. This issue is the best way to do this. The simplest situation occurs when there is an end-aversion bias (discussed in Chapter 6), in which people avoid using the most extreme options, such as Very Strongly Agree or Very Strongly Disagree. Here the solution is to simply combine the extreme response with the next one (e.g. Very Strongly Agree with Strongly Agree). If the under-utilized category appears in the middle of the other categories, there are a few possible strategies. One is to combine it with an option to which it is semantically related (Disagree with Strongly Disagree). A second approach would be to combine it with an adjacent category so that the number of respondents to each option is more or less the same. Finally, the distribution of responses may be so skewed that all you can do is dichotomize or trichotomize the answers. A plot of the distribution may help you choose the cut point(s), or there may be a logical place to make the division, such as between Agree and Disagree.

3. *Is there a maximum number of categories?* From a purely statistical perspective, the answer is 'No', since the actual reliability approaches the theoretical maximum asymptotically. However, there is good evidence that, in a wide variety of tasks, people are unable to discriminate much beyond seven levels. In a now classic article entitled 'The magic number seven plus or minus two: Some limits on our capacity for processing information', Miller (1956) showed that the limit of short-term memory is of the order of seven 'chunks' (hence seven-digit telephone numbers in the United States and Canada). Interestingly, the first two-thirds of the article are devoted to discussion of discrimination judgements. In an impressive number of situations, such as judging the pitch or loudness of a sound, the saltiness of a solution, the position of a point on a line, or the size of a square, the upper limit of the number of categories that could be discriminated was remarkably near seven (plus or minus two).

There is certainly no reason to presume that people will do any better in judgements of sadness, pain, or interpersonal skill. Thus it is reasonable to presume that the upper practical limit of useful levels on a scale, taking into account human foibles, can be set at seven. Indeed, Hawthorne et al. (2006) found that nine categories resulted in cognitive overload because of 'channel capacity limitation', and reducing the number of response options to five did not adversely affect the scale. Similarly, in an attempt to reduce ceiling effects, Keeley et al. (2013) used rating scales with five through nine steps. There was a slight superiority of seven rather than five steps, and a negligible increase with nine. Certainly these findings clearly suggest that the 'one in a hundred' precision of the VAS is illusory; people are probably mentally dividing it into about seven segments.

There are two caveats to this recommendation. First, recognizing the common 'end-aversion bias' described in Chapter 6, where people tend to avoid the two extremes of a scale, there may be some advantage to designing nine levels on the scale. Conversely, when a large number of individual items are designed to be summed to create a scale score, it is likely that reducing the number of levels to five or three will not result in significant loss of information.

4. *Should there be an even or odd number of categories?* Where the response scale is unipolar, that is to say, scale values range from zero to a maximum, then the question is of little consequence and can be decided on stylistic grounds. However, for bipolar scales (like Strongly agree–Strongly disagree) the provision of an odd number of categories allows raters the choice of expressing no opinion. Conversely, an even number of boxes forces the raters to commit themselves to one side or the other. Bear in mind, though, what we said in the discussion of Likert scales. Neutral is often used as a dumping ground for a host of possible alternatives; and Uncertain may indicate that the stem is overly broad and the respondent really means 'It all depends'. There is no absolute rule; depending on the needs of the particular research it may or may not be desirable to allow a neutral position.

5. *Should all the points on the scale be labelled, or only the ends?* Most of the research indicates that there is relatively little difference between scales with adjectives under each box and end-anchored scales (e.g. Dixon et al. 1984; Newstead and Arnold 1989). In fact, subjects seem to be more influenced by the adjectives on the ends of the scales than those in the intermediate positions (e.g. Frisbie and Brandenburg 1979; Wildt and Mazis 1978). Respondents, though, are more satisfied when many or all of the points on the scale are labelled (Dickinson and Zellinger 1980). There is some tendency for end-anchored scales to pull responses to the ends, producing greater variability. Similarly, if only every other box is defined (usually because the scale constructor cannot think of enough adjectives), the labelled boxes tend to be endorsed more often than the unlabelled ones. The conclusion seems to be that it is better to label all of the points if you are able to think of descriptors.

6. *Should the neutral point always be in the middle?* As with many of the recommendations, the answer is a very definite 'It all depends'. In situations where positive and negative responses to the item are equally likely, it makes sense to have the neutral option (e.g. neither agree nor disagree) in the middle; and respondents tend to place themselves near the centre of rating scales, where they assume the 'typical' or 'normal' person falls (Schwarz et al. 1985). However, ratings of students or residents, of satisfaction with care, and of many other targets show a very strong skew

towards the positive end. For example, Erviti et al. (1979) found a mean score of 3.3 on a 4-point scale rating medical students; and Linn (1979) reported a mean of 4.11 with a 5-point scale. This is understandable to a large degree. We do not have to make judgements about how unsatisfactory the bad students actually are; just that they do not pass muster. Ideally they are (we hope) weeded out early, leaving us to make distinctions among the remaining ones, who are at least satisfactory. The result is, in essence, that the bottom half of the scale is not used at all, truncating a 7-point scale into a 2- or 3-point one. The phenomenon is not unique to rating scales; after all, while final examinations typically have a pass mark of 50 per cent or 60 per cent, most or all students end up in the top half.

Earlier, we recommended an unbalanced scale in such circumstances, with one box for the negative end and five or six for the positive side, to allow the raters to make finer distinctions (Streiner 1985). There is some evidence that, combined with more points on the scale, this leads to greater discrimination, a lower mean score, and higher correlations with a gold standard (Klockars and Yamagishi 1988), although the effect is relatively modest (Klockars and Hancock 1993). We discuss this further, and give some examples of unbalanced scales, in Chapter 6.

7. *Do the adjectives always convey the same meaning?* Many adjectival scales use words or phrases like 'Almost always', 'Often', 'Seldom', or 'Rarely' in order to elicit judgements about the frequency of occurrence of an event or the intensity of a feeling. The question that arises from this is as follows: to what extent do people agree on the meanings associated with these adjectives? Most research regarding agreement has focused on people's estimations of probabilities which they assign to words like 'Highly probable' or 'Unlikely', and the data are not encouraging. In some studies (Bryant and Norman 1980; Lichtenstein and Newman 1967), the estimated probability of a 'Highly probable' event ranged from 0.60 to 0.99. Other phrases yielded even more variability: 'Usually' ranged from 0.15 to 0.99, 'Rather unlikely' from 0.01 to 0.75, and 'Cannot be excluded' from 0.07 to 0.98. A part of the problem is the vagueness of the terms themselves. Another difficulty is that the meanings assigned to adjectives differ with the context. For example, the term 'Often' connotes a higher absolute frequency for common events as opposed to rare ones; and 'Not too often' carries different meanings depending on whether the activity described is an exciting or a boring one (Schaeffer 1991). As Parducci (1968) showed, the meaning of 'Often' is different depending on whether one is describing the frequency of contraceptive failure or missing classes. Further, the interpretation of quantifiers such as 'Quite a bit' or 'Hardly ever' is strongly influenced by the respondents' own frequency of engaging in such behaviours. When asked how much television they watch, those who have the TV on most of the day have a different interpretation of 'Often' from those who watch only 1 hour a day (Wright et al. 1994), much like the definition of an alcoholic as 'Someone who drinks more than I do'. The conclusion is that it is difficult to make comparisons among people when vague quantifiers of frequency are used. Under such circumstances, it would be better to use actual numbers, except when the objective is to measure the person's *perception* of frequency. Bear in mind, though, that the format of the frequency scale itself may influence the responses because it serves as a frame of reference

(Schwarz 1999). People tend to think that values in the middle of the range reflect 'average' or 'typical' frequencies. When the answers consisted of low-frequency options in the middle, only 16.2 per cent of respondents reported watching TV more than 2½ hours a day; when higher-frequency options were in the middle, 37.5 per cent of the respondents reported doing so (Schwarz et al. 1985).

8. *Do numbers placed under the boxes influence the responses?* Some adjectival scales also put numbers under the words, to help the respondent find an appropriate place along the line. Does it matter whether the numbers range from 1 to 7 or from −3 to +3? What little evidence exists suggests that the answer is 'Yes'. Schwarz et al. (1991) gave subjects a scale consisting of a series of 11-point Likert scales. In all cases, one extreme was labelled 'Not at all successful' and the other end 'Extremely successful'. However, for some subjects, the numbers under the adjectives went from −5 to +5, while for others they went from 0 to 10. Although the questionnaire was completed anonymously, minimizing the chances that the respondents would attempt to present themselves well to the examiner (see social desirability bias in Chapter 6), the numbers made a large difference. When only positive integers were used, 34 per cent of the subjects used the lower (relatively unsuccessful) half of the scale (0 to 5) and had a mean value of 5.96. However, when the −5 to +5 numbering scheme was used, only 13 per cent used the lower half, and the mean value was pushed up to 7.38. The same results were found by Mazaheri and Theuns (2009) in ratings of satisfaction. Thus, it appeared as if the subjects were using the numbers to help them interpret the meaning of the adjectives, and that the negative scale values conveyed a different meaning from the positive ones.

9. *Should the order of successive question responses change?* Some scales reverse the order of responses at random, so that successive questions may have response categories which go from low to high or high to low, in order to avoid 'yea-saying' bias (discussed in Chapter 6). In essence, the reverse scoring also serves as a 'speed bump' (or 'road hump' in the United Kingdom), slowing the respondents down so that they concentrate more on the item. Note that this does *not* involve using negatively worded items (e.g. 'I am not anxious'), because these introduce yet other problems, discussed in Chapter 5. The dilemma is that a careless subject may not notice the change, resulting in almost totally uninterpretable responses. Of course, with reversed order, the researcher will know that the responses are uninterpretable due to carelessness, whereas if order is not reversed the subject looks consistent whether or not they paid attention to individual questions. It is probably best to have all of the items keyed in the same direction, and to randomly insert a number of items to check if the person is paying attention, such as 'For this item, place a mark in the box labelled Agree'. This is discussed in more detail in Chapter 6.

10. *Do questions influence the response to other questions?* The answer is definitely 'Yes'. Not only do earlier questions affect people's responses to later ones (e.g. Schuman and Presser 1981), but also, when the person is able to go back and forth in the questionnaire, later ones can influence previous ones (Schwarz and Hippler 1995).

There are at least three reasons for this. First, people try to appear consistent. If they believe that the answer to one question may contradict their response to a previous one, they may alter the earlier response to remove the inconsistency, and similarly, may respond to a new question in light of how they answered previously. Second, as Schwarz (1999) points out, respondents try to intuit what the intention of the questionnaire is, in order to respond appropriately. If later items change their interpretation, they may again go back and modify their responses in light of this different understanding. Finally, according to cognitive theory, people do not retrieve all of their relevant knowledge about a topic at one time, but only what is *temporarily accessible* (Higgins 1996). Subsequent questions may alter what is remembered and thus influence their responses.

11. *Can it be assumed that the data are interval?* As we indicated earlier in this chapter under 'Some basic concepts', one issue regarding the use of rating scales is that they are, strictly speaking, on an ordinal level of measurement. Although responses are routinely assigned numerical values, so that 'Strongly agree' becomes a 7 and 'Strongly disagree' becomes a 1, we really have no guarantee that the true distance between successive categories is the same—i.e. that the distance between 'Strongly agree' and 'Agree' is really the same as the distance between 'Strongly disagree' and 'Disagree'. The matter is of more than theoretical interest, since the statistical methods that are used to analyse the data, such as analysis of variance, rest on this assumption of equality of distance. Considerable debate has surrounded the dangers inherent in the assumption of interval properties. The arguments range from the extreme position that the numbers themselves are interval (e.g. 1, 2, …, 7) and can be manipulated as interval level data regardless of their relationship to the underlying property being assessed (Gaito 1982), to the opposite view that the numbers must be demonstrated to have a linear relationship with the underlying property before interval level measurement can be assumed (Townsend and Ashby 1984). Again, though, recall what we said about the middle category in Likert scales; this may violate the assumption that the responses are in strictly ascending or descending order. In fact, although the argument that the data must be shown to be linear in order to justify the assumption of interval level measurement is frequently used as an argument for treating the data as ordinal, it is not that hard to show that the data from both Likert scales (Carifio 1976, 1978; Vickers 1999) and VASs (Myles et al. 1999) *do* have linear properties. So from a pragmatic viewpoint, it appears that under most circumstances, unless the distribution of scores is severely skewed, one can analyse data from rating scales as if they were interval without introducing severe bias. However, for a contrary view, see Liddell and Kruschke (2018).

   In Chapter 12, we will discuss statistical methods that allow us to determine the degree to which rating scales approach interval level status.

12. *Can I use parametric statistics like analysis of variance to analyse data from rating scales?* The question obviously is related to Question 11. It deserves mention, as the opposition to treating rating scale data with parametric statistics is frequently framed as 'the data are not normally distributed, so you can't use them'. Indeed,

while related to the previous question, it is not exactly identical, since data can be perfectly interval, but not normally distributed: income levels or days in hospital are obvious examples. However, there are several related counter-arguments to this statement:

  a. *The central limit theorem*: when we all took our Intro Stats course, at some point the professor talked about the 'Central Limit Theorem', which says that, for sample sizes sufficiently large (and in this case, that is 5 or 10 per group) the distribution of means is normally distributed regardless of the original distribution. So parametric statistical tests of differences between groups, which rely on the distribution of means, are perfectly acceptable.

  b. *Items and scales*: by exactly the same argument, when we devise a questionnaire consisting of a number of Likert-scale items and add them up into a score, the scores will be normally distributed, regardless of the distribution of individual item responses (Carifio and Perla 2007). So statistics like regression and correlation, which depend on the variability, not the means, are still acceptable.

  c. *Robustness of the test*: related to the discussion of the central limit theorem, it is likely not surprising that a number of simulation studies have shown that, in fact, statistics like the Pearson correlation (Havlicek and Peterson 1976) and the F test (Glass et al. 1972) are very robust with respect to ordinal measurement and non-normality.

13. *Can I add up the items to create a total score?* With the majority of scales, the scores for each item are summed to create a total score. The issue is whether this is legitimate or not. As we will discuss in more detail in Chapter 5, there is a hierarchy of scales, ranging from *parallel indicators* through *tau (τ)-equivalent* and *congeneric*. Very briefly, with parallel indicator and τ-equivalent scales, all of the items have roughly the same correlation with the construct, but they do not with congeneric scales. That means that, with congeneric scales (which we have to assume all scales are, unless proven otherwise), some items contribute more to the total score than others. Strictly speaking, then, it would be wrong to simply add up the items. However, Wainer (1976) showed that, in multiple regression, once there are more than about 10 variables, weighting does not materially affect the predictive power of the equation. By analogy, we could argue that once a scale has more than about 10 or so items, the fact that the items correlate differently with the construct becomes less and less important. With shorter scales, though, this could be problematic.

14. *What is the youngest age group with which these methods can be used?* Age is probably less of a factor than cognitive ability, which is highly variable at a younger age, and dependent on factors such as gender, socioeconomic status, and other variables we know nothing about (but most certainly not listening to Mozart *in utero*). Having said that, a few general statements are possible. Our experience has been that children under 8, which corresponds to Grade 2 in North America, have difficulty with Harter-type scales, which are entirely verbal (Ronen et al. 2003). Most studies of the effect of age have used various instruments for rating pain. One

small study found that children under 7 had difficulty with numerical rating scales (Beyer and Aradine 1988). The data are inconclusive regarding VASs. McGrath et al. (1985) reported good results in children as young as 5, but Bernston and Svensson (2001), in a small study, found them to be less reliable than a 4-point adjectival scale in children 10–17 years of age. The consensus, though, seems to be that at 7 years, the child is old enough to handle the cognitive demands of a VAS (Beyer and Aradine 1988). Scales that show faces have been used successfully at much younger ages. Champion et al. (1998) report good validity for these scales with children as young as 5 years, and Bieri et al. (1990) state that children as young as 3 adequately comprehend them.

Critique of direct estimation methods

Direct estimation methods, in various forms, are pervasive in research involving subjective judgements. They are relatively easy to design, require little pre-testing in contrast to the comparative methods described next, and are easily understood by subjects. Nevertheless, the ease of design and administration is both an asset and a liability: because the intent of questions framed on a rating scale is often obvious to both researcher and respondent, it can result in a bias in the response. The issue of bias is covered in more detail in Chapter 6, but we mention some problems briefly here. One bias of rating scales is the *halo effect*; since items are frequently ordered in a single column on a page it is possible to rapidly rate all items on the basis of a global impression, paying little attention to the individual categories. People also rarely commit themselves to the extreme categories on the scale, effectively reducing the precision of measurement. Finally, it is common in ratings of other people, staff or students, to have a strong positive skew, so that the average individual is rated well above average, again sacrificing precision. (Note that this definition of skew, used in describing the response to items, is opposite that used in statistics. We agree it is confusing.)

In choosing among specific methods, the scaling methods we have described differ for historical rather than substantive reasons, and it is easy to find examples that have features of more than one approach. The important point is to follow the general guidelines—specific descriptors, seven or more steps, and so forth—rather than becoming preoccupied with choosing among alternatives.

Comparative methods

Although rating scales have a number of advantages—simplicity, ease, and speed of completion—there are occasions where their simplicity would be a deterrent to acquiring useful data. For example, in a study of predictors of child abuse (Shearman et al. 1983), one scale questioned parents on the ways they handled irritating child behaviours. A number of infant behaviours were presented, and parents had to specify how they dealt with each problem. Casting this scale into a rating format (which was not done) might result in items like those in Fig. 4.9.

The ordered nature of the response scale would make it unlikely that parents would place any marks to the left of the neutral position. Instead, we would like the respondent to simply indicate their likely action, or select it from a list. If we could then

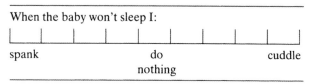

Fig. 4.9 Possible scaling of a question about child abuse.

assign a value to each behaviour, we could generate a score for the respondent based on the sum of the assigned values.

The approach that was used was one of a class of *comparative* methods, called the *paired-comparison* technique, whereby respondents were simply asked to indicate which behaviour—'punish', 'cuddle', 'hit', 'ignore', 'put in room'—they were likely to exhibit in a particular circumstance. These individual responses were assigned a numerical value in advance on the basis of a survey of a group of experts (in this case day-care workers), who had been asked to compare each parental response to a situation to all other possible responses, and select the most appropriate response for each of these pairwise comparisons.

The comparative methods also address a general problem with all rating scales, the ordinal nature of the scale. Comparative methods circumvent the difficulty by directly scaling the value of each description before obtaining responses, to ensure that the response values are on an interval scale.

There are three comparative methods that have been used in the literature: *Thurstone's method* of equal-appearing intervals, the *paired-comparison* technique, and *Guttman scaling*. Thurstone's method has just about disappeared from view, but we have kept it in the book as a point of comparison for the other methods. Each of these methods is discussed in the following sections.

Thurstone's method of equal-appearing intervals

The method begins with the selection of 100–200 statements relevant to the topic about which attitudes are to be assessed. Following the usual approaches to item generation, these statements are edited to be short and to the point. Each statement is then typed on a separate card, and a number of judges are asked to sort them into a single pile from the lowest or least desirable to highest. Extreme anchor statements, at the opposite ends of the scale, may be provided. Following the completion of this task by a large number of judges, the median rank of each statement is computed, which then becomes the scale value for each statement.

As an example, if we were assessing attitude to doctors, we might assemble a large number of statements like 'I will always do anything my doctor prescribes', 'I think doctors are overpaid', and 'Most doctors are aware of their patients' feelings'. Suppose we gave these statements to nine judges (actually, many more would be necessary for stable estimates) and the statement 'I think nurses provide as good care as doctors' was ranked respectively by the nine judges 17, 18, 23, 25, 26, 27, 28, 31, and 35 of 100 statements. The median rank of this statement is the rank of the fifth person, in this case 26, so this would be the value assigned to the statement.

The next step in the procedure is to select a limited number of statements, about 25 in number, in such a manner that the intervals between successive items are about equal and they span the entire range of values. These items then comprise the actual scale.

Finally, in applying the scale to an individual, respondents are asked to indicate which statements apply to them. The respondents' score is then calculated as the average score of items selected. As is obvious from this description, Thurstone scales are extremely labour-intensive to construct. Added to the fact that they are not noticeably better than Likert scales in terms of their interval properties and that most statistical techniques are fairly robust to violations of intervalness in any case, this technique exists only in museums of scale development (if such museums exist), although the odd example does occasionally pop up (e.g. Krabbe 2008).

Paired-comparison technique

The paired-comparison method is directed at similar goals and uses a similar approach to the Thurstone method. In both methods, the initial step is to calibrate a limited set of items so that they can be placed on an interval scale. Subjects' responses to these items are then used in developing a score by simply summing or averaging the calibration weights of those items endorsed by a subject.

Where the two methods differ is in their approach to calibration. Thurstone scaling begins with a large number of items and asks people to judge each item against all others by explicitly ranking the items. By contrast, the paired-comparison method, as the name implies, asks judges to explicitly compare each item one at a time to each of the remaining items and simply judge which of the two has more of the property under study. Considering the example which began this chapter, our child-care workers would be asked to indicate the more desirable parental behaviour in pairwise fashion as follows:

punish–spank

punish–cuddle

punish–ignore

spank–cuddle

spank–ignore

cuddle–ignore.

In actual practice, a larger sample of parental behaviours would be used, order from right to left would be randomized, and the order of presentation of the cards would be randomized. This is one reason why the technique is little used. The number of pairs each person must evaluate is $n(n - 1)/2$, where n is the number of behaviours. So, if there are 10 of them, there would be 45 pairs; for 20 behaviours, 190 pairs. Furthermore, the researcher would have to prepare twice as many cards in order to balance the order of the behaviours.

If such a list of choices were given to a series of ten judges, the data would be then displayed as in Table 4.1, indicating the proportion of times each alternative was chosen over each other option.

Table 4.1 Probability of selecting behaviour in column over behaviour in row

Behaviour	1 Punish	2 Spank	3 Ignore	4 Cuddle
1. Punish	0.50	0.60	0.70	0.90
2. Spank	0.40	0.50	0.70	0.80
3. Ignore	0.30	0.30	0.50	0.70
4. Cuddle	0.10	0.20	0.30	0.50

Reading down the first column, the table shows, for example that 'punish' was chosen over 'spank' by 40 per cent of the subjects. Note that the diagonal entries are assumed equal to 0.50, that is, 'punish' is selected over 'punish' 50 per cent of the time; also, the top right values are the 'mirror image' of those in the bottom left (i.e. 1 minus the value of the bottom left).

The next step is to use the property of the normal curve to convert this table to z-values. This bit of sleight-of-hand is best illustrated by reference to Fig. 4.10, which shows the 40 per cent point on a normal curve—that is, the point on the curve where 40 per cent of the distribution falls to the left. If the mean of the curve is set to zero and the standard deviation to 1, this occurs at a value of −0.26. As a result, the probability value of 0.40 is replaced by a z-value of −0.26. In practice, these values are determined by consulting a table of the normal curve in any statistical text. The resulting values are shown in Table 4.2.

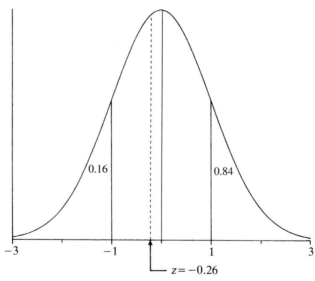

Fig. 4.10 The normal curve.

Table 4.2 z-values of the probabilities

Behaviour	1	2	3	4
1. Punish	0.00	0.26	0.53	1.28
2. Spank	-0.26	0.00	0.53	0.85
3. Ignore	-0.53	-0.53	0.00	0.53
4. Cuddle	-1.28	-0.85	-0.53	0.00
Total z	-2.07	-1.12	+0.53	+2.66
Average z	-0.52	-0.28	+0.13	+0.66

The z-scores for each column are then summed and averaged, yielding the z-score equivalent to the average probability of each item being selected over all other items. The resulting z-score for 'punish' now becomes −0.52, and for 'cuddle' it is +0.66. The range of negative and positive numbers is a bit awkward, so a constant (usually 3) is often added to all the values to avoid negative weights. These weights can be assumed to have interval properties.

All this manipulation is directed to the assignment of weights to each option. To use these weights for scoring a subject is straightforward; the score is simply the weight assigned to the option selected by the subject. If the questionnaire is designed in such a way that a subject may endorse multiple response options, for example by responding to various infant behaviours like crying, not going to sleep, or refusing to eat, the weights for all responses can be added or averaged since they are interval level measurements.

The Guttman method

In Guttman scales, the goal is to produce response alternatives to a stem so that the endorsement of one presupposes: (1) endorsement of all less difficult responses and (2) non-endorsement of all of the more difficult ones. For example, in assessing a child's mobility, the stem 'My child is able to' might have the options: (a) crawl, (b) stand, (c) walk, and (d) run. If the mother chooses 'walk', it implies that the child can also crawl and stand, but not yet run.

The Guttman method begins, as does the Thurstone method, with a large sample of items. However, this is reduced by judgement of the investigator to a relatively small sample of 10–20 items, which are thought to span the range of the attitude or behaviour assessed. As we shall see, in Guttman scaling, it is crucial that the items address only a single underlying attribute, since an individual score arises from the accumulated performance on all items.

These items are then administered directly to a sample of subjects, who are asked to endorse those items applicable to them. Unlike the alternative methods discussed in this section, there is no separate calibration step. The items are then tentatively ranked according to increasing amount of the attribute assessed, and responses are displayed in a subject-by-item matrix, with 1's indicating those items endorsed by a subject and 0's indicating the remaining items.

Table 4.3 Guttman scaling

I am able to:	Subject				
	A	B	C	D	E
Walk across the room	1	1	1	1	1
Climb the stairs	1	1	1	1	0
Walk one block outdoors	1	1	0	0	0
Walk more than one mile	1	0	0	0	0

As an example, suppose we were assessing function of the lower limbs in a sample of people with osteoarthritis. A display of the responses of five subjects to four items might resemble Table 4.3.

In this example, subject A gets a score of 4, subject B a score of 3, C and D attain scores of 2, and subject E a score of 1. This is an idealized example, since no 'reversals' occur, in which a subject endorsed a more difficult item (e.g. walk more than a mile) but not an easier one (e.g. climb the stairs). In reality, such reversals do occur, detracting from the strict ordering of the items implied by the method. There are a number of indices which reflect how much an actual scale deviates from perfect cumulativeness, of which the two most important are the *coefficient of reproducibility* and the *coefficient of scalability*.

The first, reproducibility, indicates the degree to which a person's scale score is a predictor of their response pattern. To calculate it, we must know the total number of subjects (N), the number for whom there was some error in the ordering (n_e), and the number of items (I). The coefficient is then as follows:

$$\text{Reproducibility} = 1 - \frac{n_e}{I \times N}$$

If we gave our 4-item scale to 150 people and found that the order was correct for 109 cases and incorrect for 41, then the coefficient in this case would be given as:

$$1 - \frac{41}{150 \times 4} = 0.932.$$

Reproducibility can vary between 0 and 1 and should be higher than 0.9 for the scale to be valid.

The coefficient of scalability reflects whether the scale is truly unidimensional and cumulative. Its calculation is complex and best left to computer programs. It, too, varies between 0 and 1 and should be at least 0.6.

Guttman scaling is best suited to behaviours that are developmentally determined (e.g. crawling, standing, walking, running), where mastery of one behaviour virtually guarantees mastery of lower-order behaviours. Thus it is useful in assessing development in children, decline due to progressively deteriorating disease, functional ability, and the like. It is *not* appropriate in assessing the kind of loss in function due to focal lesions that arises in stroke patients, where the impairment of some function may be unrelated to the impairment of other functions. Unlike the other methods discussed in this section, Guttman scales are unlikely to have interval scale properties.

Guttman scaling is also the basis of *item response theory* (discussed in Chapter 12), which has emerged as a very powerful scaling method and begins with a similar assumption of ordering of item difficulty and candidate ability. However, in contrast to Guttman scaling, item response scaling explicitly assigns values to both items and subjects on an interval scale and also successfully deals with the random processes which might result in departures from strict ordering demanded by the Guttman scale.

Critique of comparative methods

It is clear that any of the three comparative methods we have described requires considerably more time for development than any of the direct scaling methods. Nevertheless, this investment may be worthwhile under two circumstances:

1. If it is desirable to disguise the ordinal property of the responses, as in the earlier child abuse example, then the additional resources may be well spent.

2. The Thurstone and paired-comparison methods guarantee interval level measurement, which may be important in some applications, particularly when there are relatively few items in the scale.

With regard to choice among the methods, as we have indicated, the Guttman method has several disadvantages in comparison to other methods. It is difficult to select items with Guttman properties, and the scale has only ordinal properties. The choice between Thurstone and paired-comparison is more difficult. However, the Thurstone method is more practical when there are a large number of items desired in the scale, since the number of comparisons needed in the paired-comparison technique is roughly proportional to the square of the number of items.

Econometric methods

The final class of scaling methods we will consider has its roots in a different discipline, economics, and has become increasingly popular in the medical literature in applications ranging from clinical trials to decision analysis. The problem for which these methods were devised involves assigning a numerical value to various health states. This arises in economics and health in the course of conducting cost/benefit studies, where it becomes necessary to scale benefits along a numerical scale so that cost/benefit ratios can be determined.

Note that economists are generally not interested in a specific individual's choice, but rather tend to obtain ratings of health states by averaging judgements from a large number of individuals in order to create a utility score for the state. Thus the focus of measurement is the described health state, not the characteristic of the individual respondent. This creates interesting problems for the assessment of reliability, which are explicitly dealt with in Chapter 9.

For example, consider a clinical trial comparing medical management of angina to coronary bypass surgery. Surgery offers a potential benefit in quality of life, but the trade-off is the finite possibility that the patient may not survive the operation or immediate postoperative period. How, then, does one make a rational choice between the two alternatives?

The first approach to the problem was developed in the 1950s and is called the *Von Neumann–Morgenstern standard gamble* (SG) (Von Neumann and Morgenstern 1953). The subject is asked to consider the following scenario:

> You have been suffering from 'angina' for several years. As a result of your illness, you experience severe chest pain after even minor physical exertion such as climbing stairs, or walking one block in cold weather. You have been forced to quit your job and spend most days at home watching TV. Imagine that you are offered a possibility of an operation that will result in complete recovery from your illness. However, the operation carries some risk. Specifically, there is a probability 'p' that you will die during the course of the operation. How large must 'p' be before you will decline the operation and choose to remain in your present state?

Clearly, the closer the present state is to perfect health, the smaller the risk of death one would be willing to entertain. Having obtained an estimate of 'p' from subjects, the value of the present state can be directly converted to a 0–1 scale by simply subtracting 'p' from 1, so that a tolerable risk of 1 per cent results in a value (called a 'utility') of 0.99 for the present state, and a risk of 50 per cent results in a utility of 0.50. Thus, a utility is a number representing the strength of a person's preference for various health outcomes under conditions of uncertainty; and the preference reflects the degree of the person's satisfaction, distress, or desirability with these outcomes (Revicki and Kaplan 1993). Using utilities, it is possible to derive another index, called *quality-adjusted life years*, or QALYs (Zeckhauser and Shepard 1976). One year in a health state that has a utility of 1.0 equals 1 QALY; if another health state has a utility of 0.5, one year living with it yields a QALY of ½. So, if a 40-year-old person in a given health state (e.g. irritable bowel syndrome; IBS) is expected to live another 20 years, and IBS has a utility of 0.4, then that person will have 8 QALYs (i.e. 20 × 0.4). By deriving QALYs for a wide variety of health states, health economists have drawn up *league tables*, expressing the incremental cost-effectiveness of different interventions in terms of cost per QALY gained. For example, Maynard (1991) estimated that neurosurgical interventions for head injury cost £240 per QALY (in 1990 British pounds), kidney transplants cost £4,710 per QALY, and hospital haemodialysis cost £21,970 per QALY. This takes into account (1) the person's expected life expectancy, (2) the cost of the intervention, and (3) the utility of the health state. Attempts have been made to ration healthcare on the basis of these tables, but these have often failed because it is perceived as 'rationing' (Lamb 2004).

One difficulty with the SG is that few people, aside from statisticians and professional gamblers, are accustomed to dealing in probabilities. In order to deal with this problem, a number of devices are used to simplify the task. Subjects may be offered specific probabilities—e.g. 10 per cent chance of perioperative death and 90 per cent chance of complete recovery—until they reach a point of indifference between the two alternatives. Visual aids, such as 'probability wheels', have also been used.

This difficulty in handling probabilities led to the development of an alternative method, called the *time trade-off technique* (TTO; Torrance et al. 1972), which avoids the use of probabilities. One begins by estimating the likely remaining years of life for a healthy subject, using actuarial tables; that is, if the patient is 30 years old we could estimate that they have about 40 years remaining. The previous question would then be rephrased as follows:

> Imagine living the remainder of your natural lifespan (40 years) in your present state. Contrast this with the alternative that you can return to perfect health for fewer years. How many years would you sacrifice if you could have perfect health?

In practice, the respondent is presented with the alternatives of 40 years in his present state versus 0 years of complete health. The upper limit is decreased and the lower limit increased until a point of indifference is reached. The more years a subject is willing to sacrifice in exchange for a return to perfect health, presumably the worse they perceive their present health. The response (call it Y) can be converted to a scaled utility by the following simple formula:

$$U = (40 - Y)/40$$

A thorough example of the application of this method in a clinical trial of support for relatives of demented older people is given in Mohide et al. (1988).

Both the SG and the TTO use a 'holistic' approach, in that the rater is given as full a description of the condition as is feasible, including the symptoms, difficulties with daily activities, psychological and social sequelae, and so forth. Another approach, used in instruments such as the Health Utility Index (HUI; Torrance 1986) and the Quality of Wellbeing Scale (QWB; Kaplan and Bush 1982), is to 'decompose' the health state into its various components, such as its effects on vision, ambulation, dexterity, pain, emotions, and so forth. Using weights generated from large population surveys, these are weighted and summed into a global utility score.

Critique of econometric methods

We have presented the various methods as a means to measure the utilities attached to individual health states. Although they are limited to the measurement of health states, they have been used both with real patients and with normal, healthy individuals imagining themselves to be ill.

The TTO and SG methods are quite difficult to administer and require a trained interviewer, so it remains to see whether they possess advantages over simpler techniques. One straightforward alternative would be a direct estimation of health state, using an adjectival or visual analogue scale. The HUI and QWB are an amalgam of econometric and psychometric approaches and attempt to address some of the difficulties with the first two methods. Torrance (1976) has shown that the TTO and SG methods yield similar results, which differed from the direct estimation method, suggesting that these methods may indeed be a more accurate (or at least a different) reflection of the underlying state.

However, the methods are based on the notion that people make rational choices under conditions of uncertainty. There is an accumulation of evidence, reviewed in Chapter 6, which suggests that responses on rating scales can be influenced by a variety of extraneous factors. Tversky and Kahneman (1974; Kahneman 2011) have shown that humans are far from the rational decision-makers assumed by economic theorists and developers of econometric measures. The methods reviewed in this section are no more immune to seemingly irrational behaviour, as reviewed by Llewellyn-Thomas and Sutherland (1986). As one example, framing a question in terms of 40 per cent survival instead of 60 per cent mortality will result in a shift of values. The problem addressed by the econometric methods assumed that context-free values could be elicited. It seems abundantly clear that such 'value-free' values are illusory, and a deeper understanding of the psychological variables which influence decisions and choices is necessary. Moreover, it appears that real patients assign higher (more positive) utilities to states of ill health than those assigned by non-patients who imagine themselves in that state, casting doubt on these analogue studies and the league tables that are based on the judgements of non-patients, as most are.

Ever since Von Neumann and Morgenstern's (1953) theoretical work, one of the main selling points of econometric methods is that they yield results that are at an interval or ratio level of measurement. This was an unproven (and for many years, unprovable) assertion. However, with the introduction of item response theory (discussed in Chapter 12), techniques have been developed to evaluate whether scales actually do have interval or ratio level properties. The limited research is not encouraging. Cook et al. (2001) found that 'None of the utility scales functioned as interval-level scales in our sample' (p. 1275).

Last, the lower anchor is usually assumed to be death. There has been little work to examine conditions which some people (e.g. Richard Dreyfuss in the movie *Whose Life Is It Anyway?*) see as worse than death.

On psychometric grounds, the SG may not bear close scrutiny, either. While early studies appeared to show that the test–retest reliability of the SG was superior to a rating scale (RS) (Torrance 1987), it turns out that this may have been a consequence of an incorrect approach to computing reliability, as we will discuss in Chapter 9. More recent studies have shown that the test–retest reliability of the SG is worse than the RS (0.45 versus 0.67; Moore et al. 1999). Juniper et al. (2001) showed substantially lower concurrent validity than the RS against a disease-specific quality of life measure (−0.08 to +0.12 versus +0.21 to +0.46), as did Rutten-van Molken et al. (1995; 0.13 to 0.19 versus 0.47 to 0.59). Of course, it could be claimed that the SG remains the gold standard, since it alone is consistent with rational choice theory. Perhaps, but one suspects that while the researchers may appreciate these theoretical distinctions, they are lost on participants. Indeed, one problem with the SG and TTO is that respondents find them difficult to complete. In one study, it took 3 years of schooling to complete the RS against 6 years for the SG.

From our perspective, perhaps the final nail in the coffin of econometric methods was a study by Krabbe et al. (1997). They compared the SG, TTO, and a third technique (willingness to pay) with rating scales. Their conclusions were that: (1) rating scales were the most feasible and reliable and (2) with a simple power transformation it is possible to go from scores derived from rating scales to those from the other techniques. Given this, in addition to the other limitations we described, we see no need for the more complex and cognitively demanding econometric methods.

To rate or to rank

The goal of many of the techniques discussed so far, such as adjectival and Likert scales, VASs, and the various econometric methods, is to assign a numerical value to an item; that is, the respondents rate themselves as to the degree to which they have an attribute or endorse a statement. Even the comparative techniques (Thurstone's method, Guttman scaling, and paired-comparison), which begin by ranking items, have as their ultimate aim the construction of a scale that has specific numbers (i.e. ratings) assigned to each item or step. However, in some areas, particularly the assessment of values, another approach is possible: that of *ranking* a series of alternatives. For example, one of the measures in our study of the effect of social support on morbidity (McFarlane et al. 1980) tapped how highly people valued good health in relation to nine other qualities. We gave the respondents ten index cards, on each of which was printed one quality, such as Wealth, Happiness, and Health, and their task was to arrange the cards from the most highly valued to the least. The outcome measure was the rank assigned to Health.

One major advantage of ranking, as opposed to rating, is that it forces people to differentiate among the responses. If the respondents are poorly motivated, or are low in 'cognitive sophistication', they can minimize their effort in responding (a phenomenon called *satisficing*, which we discuss in more detail in Chapter 6) by rating all qualities equally high or low (Krosnick and Alwin 1988). This problem exists because of other factors, too, such as *yea-saying* or *nay-saying* biases, *social desirability*, or the *halo effect*, also discussed in Chapter 6. Forcing the respondents to rank the attributes in order of desirability or value lessens the possibility of non-differentiation because the person must make choices among the alternatives. It does not totally eliminate the problem of poor motivation, as the subject can simply order them randomly, but this can be detected by having the person do the task twice.

However, there is a price to pay for this. First, it is cognitively more difficult to rank order a list of items than to rate each one. In face-to-face interviews, subjects can be given cards, with one attribute on each, and they can rearrange them until they are satisfied. Some computer-administered questionnaires allow the respondent to rank order lists by automatically adjusting the values. This cannot be done, though, if the questionnaire is mailed, especially if it is administered over the telephone. A more important problem is statistical in nature. If all of the values are used (as opposed to the situation in the example, where only the value of Health was recorded), then the scale becomes *ipsative*. An ipsative scale has the property that the sum of the individual items is always the same, and therefore it is also the same for every person. For example, if the respondent has to rank five attributes, then the sum of the ranks will be 15 (i.e. $1 + 2 + 3 + 4 + 5$; more generally, with k items, the sum will be $k(k + 1)/2$, and the mean will be $(k + 1)/2$). This means that there must be a negative correlation among the items (Jackson and Alwin 1980), and the sum of the correlations between individual items and some other variable will always be zero (Clemans 1966). Related to this is another problem, that the rankings are not independent. If we know the ranks assigned to four of the five attributes, then we would be able to perfectly predict the last one. This lack of independence violates assumptions of most statistical tests.

Ipsative scores make sense if the objective is to compare the *relative* strength of various attributes within one individual, but are useless (1) in making comparisons between individuals, and (2) examining the *absolute* magnitude of different traits. For example, a musically inclined physicist may have a low score on a scale of Aesthetics, simply because their score on the Theoretical scale is higher (Hicks 1970).

Alwin and Krosnick (1985) conclude that the correlation between ratings and rankings is extremely high, but the relationships among the individual items are quite different. Because of the statistical problems mentioned earlier as well as others (e.g. traditional forms of techniques such as factor analysis, the intra-class correlation, and generalizability theory—all discussed in later chapters—cannot be used with ranked data), ratings are usually preferred. However, recent developments in item response theory (discussed in Chapter 12) have breathed new life into this method, by overcoming many of its shortcomings (Brown and Maydeu-Olivares 2013).

Multidimensional scaling

In the previous sections of this chapter, we discussed various techniques for creating scales, which differentiate attributes along one dimension, such as a Guttman scale, which taps mobility. However, there are situations in which we are interested in examining the similarities of different 'objects', which may vary along a number of separate dimensions. These objects can be diagnoses, occupations, social interactions, stressful life events, pain experiences, countries, faces, or almost anything else we can imagine (Weinberg 1991). The dimensions themselves are revealed by the analysis; that is, they are 'hidden' or 'latent', in that they are not directly observable from the data but inferred from the patterns that emerge in the way the objects group together. (For a more complete description of latent variables, see the chapter on factor analysis in Norman and Streiner (2014).) The family of techniques for performing this type of analysis is called *multidimensional scaling* (MDS). Very briefly, MDS begins with some index of how 'close' each object is to every other object and then tries to determine how many dimensions underlie these evaluations of closeness.

To illustrate the technique, imagine that we want to determine what dimensions may underlie the similarities or differences among nine symptoms experienced by patients with various types of depression. The first step is to construct a *similarity matrix* (also called a *proximity matrix*). This can be done in a number of different ways. First, patients or clinicians can be given all possible pairs of symptoms, as with the paired-comparison technique. But now, rather than choosing one or the other, they would indicate how similar the two symptoms are on, say, a 10-point scale, with 1 meaning not at all similar to 10 meaning most similar. Another way of constructing the matrix is to determine the frequency with which the symptoms co-occur in a sample of patients. A third method may be to ask patients to rate the perceived severity of each of the nine symptoms on some form of scale and then correlate each symptom with all of the others. The mathematics of MDS do not care how the similarity matrix is formed—rating or judgements, frequency of co-occurrence, correlations, or any one of a number of other techniques. The difference shows up only in terms of how we interpret the results.

For the purpose of this example, let us assume that we used the frequency of co-occurrence and obtained the results shown in Table 4.4. A score of 1 means that the symptoms always occur together, and 0 indicates that they never occur together. As would be expected, the maximum coefficient occurs along the main diagonal; sadness is more related to itself than to any other symptom. Conversely, coefficients of 0 reflect mutually exclusive symptoms, such as insomnia and hypersomnia.

In actuality, this *similarity* or *proximity* matrix is transformed to its opposite: a *distance* or *dissimilarity* matrix, where the entries would indicate how far apart or dissimilar the objects are. MDS uses this matrix to determine the number of dimensions that underlie the similarities among the symptoms. There are a number of different computer programs which do this. They vary according to various assumptions which are made: whether the objects are differentiated holistically or in terms of separate attributes; and whether the proximities among the objects are measured on an ordinal or an interval scale. A description of the programs is given in an article by Weinberg (1991) and a monograph by Kruskal and Wish (1978). Irrespective of which program

Table 4.4 Similarity matrix of nine symptoms of depression

	A	B	C	D	E	F	G	H	I
A	1.00								
B	0.865	1.00							
C	0.495	0.691	1.00						
D	0.600	0.823	0.612	1.00					
E	0.125	0.135	0.402	0.127	1.00				
F	0.201	0.129	0.103	0.111	0.000	1.00			
G	0.125	0.581	0.513	0.578	0.713	0.399	1.00		
H	0.312	0.492	0.192	0.487	0.303	0.785	0.000	1.00	
I	0.105	0.223	0.332	0.201	0.592	0.762	0.414	0.185	1.00

A = Feeling of sadness
B = Pessimism
C = Decreased libido
D = Suicidal ideation
E = Weight gain
F = Weight loss
G = Hypersomnia
H = Early morning wakening
I = Psychomotor retardation

is used, the results are usually displayed in a graph, with each axis representing one dimension. The researcher then tries to determine what the dimensions represent, in terms of the underlying properties of the objects. For example, assume that the dissimilarity matrix yielded just two interpretable dimensions. We can then plot the location of each symptom along these two dimensions, as in Fig. 4.11.

The closer the symptoms are on the graph, the more similar they are to one another. It would appear as if the first dimension is differentiating symptoms which are primarily psychological from those which are more physiological in nature, while the second dimension reflects a continuum of psychomotor retardation versus agitation. As with all such techniques, there are diagnostic tests to determine how well the data fit the model. In MDS, this goodness of fit is called *stress*, and the usual rule of thumb is that it should be ≤0.1 and not above 0.15.

Most researchers stop at this point and are content to have determined the number and characteristics of the underlying dimensions. The scale developer, however, can use MDS as a first step, to reveal the 'psychological dimensions' people use in evaluating different stimuli, which are then used to construct scales that measure the various dimensions separately.

MDS and exploratory factor analysis (EFA) are very similar in terms of what they hope to accomplish: reduce a large number of variables into a smaller number of latent, explanatory factors. In fact, EFA is a special case of one form of MDS, called smallest space analysis (Guttman 1982). The question, then, is when to use each. If the responses are dichotomous (e.g. True/False, Yes/No), then the choice is obvious: traditional forms of EFA should never be used with dichotomous items, and MDS is definitely an option (e.g. Brazill and Grofman 2002). An advantage of MDS is that it can handle non-linear relationships among variables, nominal or ordinal data, and does not require multivariate

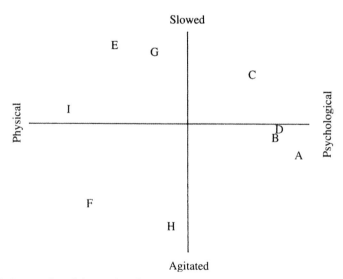

Fig. 4.11 Scatter plot of the results of MDS.

normality as most other techniques do (Jaworska and Chupetlovska-Anastasova 2009). When the data are continuous and appropriate for EFA, then it appears that MDS results in fewer factors than EFA. Some argue that this makes the solution easier to interpret, but carries the risk that some important factors may be overlooked.

Further reading

Dunn-Rankin, P., Knezek, G.A., Wallace, S.R., and Zhang, S. (2004). *Scaling methods* (2nd edn). Erlbaum, Mahwah, NJ.

Furr, R.M. (2021). *Psychometrics: An introduction* (4th edn). Sage, Thousand Oaks, CA.

Gorsuch, R.L. (2014). *Factor analysis* (2nd edn). Lawrence Erlbaum, Hillsdale, NJ.

TenBrink, T.D. (1974). *Evaluation: A practical guide for teachers*. McGraw-Hill, New York.

References

Aitken, R.C.B. (1969). A growing edge of measurement of feelings. *Proceedings of the Royal Society of Medicine*, **62**, 989–92.

Alwin, D.F. and Krosnick, J.A. (1985). The measurement of values in surveys: A comparison of ratings and rankings. *Public Opinion Quarterly*, **49**, 535–52.

Bernston, L. and Svensson, E. (2001). Pain assessment in children with juvenile chronic arthritis: A matter of scaling and rater. *Acta Paediatrica*, **90**, 1131–6.

Beyer, J. (1984). *The Oucher: A user's manual and technical report*. Hospital Play Equipment Company, Evanston, IL.

Beyer, J. and Aradine, C. (1988). Convergent and discriminant validity of a self-report measure of pain intensity for children. *Child Health Care*, **16**, 274–81.

Beyer, J., Denyes, M., and Villarruel, A. (1992). The creation, validation, and continuing development of the Oucher: A measure of pain intensity in children. *Journal of Pediatric Nursing*, **7**, 335–46.

Bieri, D., Reeve, R., Champion, G., Addicoat, L., and Ziegler, J. (1990). The faces pain scale for the self-assessment of the severity of pain experienced by children: Development, initial validation, and preliminary investigation for ratio scale properties. *Pain*, **41**, 139–50.

Bosi Ferraz, M., Quaresma, M.R., Aquino, L.R.L., Atra, E., Tugwell, P., and Goldsmith, C.H. (1990). Reliability of pain scales in the assessment of literate and illiterate patients with rheumatoid arthritis. *Journal of Rheumatology*, **17**, 1022–4.

Brazill, T.J. and Grofman, B. (2002). Factor analysis versus multi-dimensional scaling: Binary choice roll-call voting and the US Supreme Court. *Social Networks*, **24**, 201–29.

Brown, A. and Maydeu-Olivares, A. (2013). How IRT can solve problems of ipsative data in forced-choice questionnaires. *Psychological Methods*, **18**, 36–52.

Bryant, G.D. and Norman, G.R. (1980). Expressions of probability: Words and numbers. *New England Journal of Medicine*, **302**, 411.

Cairney, J., Veldhuizen, S., Graham, J.D., Rodriquez, C., Bedard, C., Bremer, E., *et al.* (2018). A construct validation study of PLAYfun. *Medicine and Science in Sport and Exercise*, **50**, 855–62.

Caldwell, H.A., Cristofaro, N.A., Cairney, J., Bray, S.R., and Timmons, B.W. (2021). Measurement properties of the Physical Literacy Assessment for Youth (PLAY) Tools. *Applied Physiology, Nutrition and Metabolism*, **46**, 571–8.

Carifio, J. (1976). Assigning students to career education programs by preference: Scaling preference data for program assignments. *Career Education Quarterly*, **1**, 7–26.

Carifio, J. (1978). Measuring vocational preferences: Ranking versus categorical rating procedures. *Career Education Quarterly*, **1**, 34–66.

Carifio, J. and Perla, R.J. (2007). Ten common misunderstandings, misconceptions, persistent myths and urban legends about Likert scales and Likert response formats and their antidotes. *Journal of Social Sciences*, **3**, 106–16.

Carp, F.M. (1989). Maximizing data quality in community studies of older people. In *Special research methods for gerontology* (eds. M.P. Lawton and A.R. Herzog), pp. 93–122. Baywood Publishing, Amityville, NY.

Champion, G.D., Goodenough, B., von Baeyer, C.L., and Thomas, W. (1998). Measurement of pain by self-report. In *Measurement of pain in infants and children: Progress in pain research and management*, Vol. **10**. (eds. G.A. Finley and P.J. McGrath), pp. 123–60. IASP Press, Seattle, WA.

Clemans, W.V. (1966). *An analytical and empirical examination of some properties of ipsative measures*. Psychometric Monographs Number 14. Psychometric Society, Richmond, VA.

Conn, S.R. and Rieke, M.L. (1994). *The 16 PF fifth edition technical manual*. Institute for Personality and Ability Testing, Champaign, IL.

Cook, K.F., Ashton, C.M., Byrne, M.M., Brody, B., Geraci, J., Giesler, R.B., *et al.* (2001). A psychometric analysis of the measurement level of the rating scale, time trade-off, and standard gamble. *Social Science & Medicine*, **53**, 1275–85.

Dickinson, T.L. and Zellinger, P.M. (1980). A comparison of the behaviorally anchored rating mixed standard scale formats. *Journal of Applied Psychology*, **65**, 147–54.

Dixon, P.N., Bobo, M., and Stevick, R.A. (1984). Response differences and preferences for all-category-defined and end-defined Likert formats. *Educational and Psychological Measurement*, **44**, 61–6.

Downie, W.W., Leatham, P.A., Rhind, V.M., Wright, V., Branco, J.A., and Anderson, J.A. (1978). Studies with pain rating scales. *Annals of Rheumatic Diseases*, **37**, 378–81.

Erviti, V., Fabrey, L.J., and Bunce, J.V. (1979). The development of rating scales to assess the clinical performance of medical students. In *Proceedings, 18th Annual Conference on Research in Medical Education*, pp. 185–9, Washington, DC.

Flaskerud, J.H. (1988). Is the Likert scale format culturally biased? *Nursing Research*, **37**, 185–6.

Frisbie, D.A. and Brandenburg, D.C. (1979). Equivalence of questionnaire items with varying response formats. *Journal of Educational Measurement*, **16**, 43–8.

Gaito, J. (1982). Measurement scales and statistics: Resurgence of an old misconception. *Psychological Bulletin*, **87**, 564–7.

Glass, G.V., Peckham, P.D., and Sanders, J.R. (1972). Consequences of failure to meet assumptions underlying the analyses of variance and covariance. *Review of Educational Research*, **42**, 237–88.

Guilford, J.P. (1954). *Psychometric methods*. McGraw-Hill, New York.

Guttman, L. (1982). Facet theory, smallest space analysis, and factor analysis. *Perceptual and Motor Skills*, **54**, 491–3.

Harter, S. (1982). The Perceived Competence Scale for Children. *Child Development*, **53**, 87–97.

Havlicek, L.L. and Peterson, N.L. (1976). Robustness of the Pearson correlation against violations of assumptions. *Perceptual and Motor Skills*, **43**, 1319–34.

Hawthorne, G., Mouthaan, J., Forbes, D., and Novaco, R.W. (2006). Response categories and anger measurement: Do fewer categories result in poorer measurement? Development of the DAR5. *Social Psychiatry and Psychiatric Epidemiology*, **41**, 164–72.

Hayes, M.H.S. and Patterson, D.G. (1921). Experimental development of the graphic rating method. *Psychological Bulletin*, **18**, 98–9.

He, S., Renne, A., Argandykov, D., Convissar, D., and Lee, J. (2022). Comparison of an emoji-based visual analog scale with a numeric rating scale for pain assessment. *JAMA*, **328**, 208–9.

Hicks, L.E. (1970). Some properties of ipsative, normative, and forced-choice normative measures. *Psychological Bulletin*, **74**, 167–84.

Higgins, E.T. (1996). Knowledge activation: Accessibility, applicability, and salience. In *Social psychology: Handbook of basic principles* (eds. E.T. Higgins and A. Kruglanski), pp. 133–68. Guilford Press, New York.

Hoek, J.A. and Gendall, P.J. (1993). A new method of predicting voting behavior. *Journal of the Market Research Society*, **35**, 361–73.

Hunter, J.E. and Schmidt, F.L. (1990). Dichotomization of continuous variables: The implications for meta-analysis. *Journal of Applied Psychology*, **75**, 334–49.

Huskisson, E.C. (1974). Measurement of pain. *Lancet*, **ii**, 1127–31.

Jackson, D.J. and Alwin, D.F. (1980). The factor analysis of ipsative measures. *Sociological Methods and Research*, **9**, 218–38.

Jaworska, N. and Chupetlovska-Anastasova, A. (2009). A review of multidimensional scaling (MDS) and its utility in various psychological domains. *Tutorials in Quantitative Methods for Psychology*, **5**, 1–10.

Jensen, M.P., Turner, J.A., and Romano, J.M. (1994). What is the maximum number of levels needed in pain intensity measurement? *Pain*, **58**, 387–92.

Jones, R.R. (1968). Differences in response consistency and subjects' preferences for three personality response formats. In *Proceedings of the 76th annual convention of the American Psychological Association*, pp. 247–8, Washington, DC.

Juniper, E.F., Norman, G.R., Cox, F.M., and Roberts, J.N. (2001). Comparison of the standard gamble, rating scale, AQLQ and SF-36 for measuring quality of life in asthma. *European Respiratory Journal*, **18**, 38–44.

Kahneman, D. (2011). *Thinking, fast and slow*. Farrar Straus Giroux, New York.

Kaplan, R.M. and Bush, J. (1982). Health-related quality of life measurement for evaluation research and policy analysis. *Health Psychology*, **1**, 61–80.

Keeley, J.W., English, T., Irons, J., and Henslee, A.M. (2013). Investigating halo and ceiling effects in student evaluations of instruction. *Educational and Psychological Measurement*, **73**, 440–57.

Klockars, A.J. and Hancock, G.R. (1993). Manipulations of evaluative rating scales to increase validity. *Psychological Reports*, **73**, 1059–66.

Klockars, A.J. and Yamagishi, M. (1988). The influence of labels and positions in rating scales. *Journal of Educational Measurement*, **25**, 85–96.

Knäuper, B. and Turner, P.A. (2003). Measuring health: Improving the validity of health assessments. *Quality of Life Research*, **12**(Suppl. 1), 81–9.

Krabbe, P.F.M. (2008). Thurstone scaling as a measurement method to quantify subjective health outcomes. *Medical Care*, **46**, 357–65.

Krabbe, P.F.M., Essink-Bot, M.-L., and Bonsel, G.J. (1997). The comparability and reliability of five health-state valuation methods. *Social Science and Medicine*, **45**, 1641–52.

Krosnick, J.A. and Alwin, D.F. (1988). A test of the form-resistant correlation hypothesis: Ratings, rankings, and the measurement of values. *Public Opinion Quarterly*, **52**, 526–38.

Kruskal, J.B. and Wish, M. (1978). *Multidimensional scaling*. Sage, Beverly Hills, CA.

Kulas, J.T. and Stachowski, A.A. (2009). Middle category endorsement in odd-numbered Likert response scales: Associated item characteristics, cognitive demands, and preferred meanings. *Journal of Research in Personality*, **43**, 489–93.

Kulas, J.T. and Stachowski, A.A. (2013). Respondent rationale for *neither agreeing nor disagreeing*: Person and item contributors to middle category endorsement intent on Likert personality indicators. *Journal of Research in Personality*, **47**, 254–62.

Lamb, E.J. (2004). Rationing of medical care: Rules of rescue, cost-effectiveness, and the Oregon plan. *American Journal of Obstetrics and Gynecology*, **190**, 1636–41.

Latham, G.P. (2006). *Work motivation: History, theory, research, and practice*. Sage, Thousand Oaks, CA.

Lichtenstein, S. and Newman, J.R. (1967). Empirical scaling of common verbal phrases associated with numerical probabilities. *Psychonomic Science*, **9**, 563–4.

Liddle, T.M. and Kruschke, J.K. (2018). Analyzing ordinal data with metric models: What could possibly go wrong? *Journal of Experimental Social Psychology*, **79**, 328–48.

Likert, R.A. (1932). A technique for the development of attitudes. *Archives of Psychology*, **22**, 1–55.

Linn, L. (1979). Interns' attitudes and values as antecedents of clinical performance. *Journal of Medical Education*, **54**, 238–40.

Llewellyn-Thomas, H. and Sutherland, H. (1986). Procedures for value assessment. In *Recent advances in nursing: Research methodology* (ed. M. Cahoon), pp. 169–85. Churchill-Livingstone, London.

Maynard, A. (1991). Developing the health care market. *The Economic Journal*, **101**, 1277–86.

Mazaheri, M. and Theuns, P. (2009). Effects of varying response formats on self-ratings of life-satisfaction. *Social Indicators Research*, **90**, 381–95.

McFarlane, A.H., Norman, G.R., Streiner, D.L., Roy, R. G., and Scott, D.J. (1980). A longitudinal study of the influence of the psychosocial environment on health status: A preliminary report. *Journal of Health and Social Behavior*, **21**, 124–33.

McGrath, P., de Veber, L., and Hearn, M. (1985). Multidimensional pain assessment in children. In *Advances in pain research and therapy*, Vol. 9 (ed. H.L. Fields), pp. 387–93. Raven Press, NY.

Miller, G.A. (1956). The magic number seven plus or minus two: Some limits on our capacity for processing information. *Psychological Bulletin*, **63**, 81–97.

Mohide, E.A., Torrance, G.W., Streiner, D.L., Pringle, D.M., and Gilbert, J.R. (1988). Measuring the well-being of family caregivers using the time trade-off technique. *Journal of Clinical Epidemiology*, **41**, 475–82.

Moore, A.D., Clarke, A.E., Danoff, D.S., Joseph, L., Belisle, P., Neville, C., *et al.* (1999). Can health utility measures be used in lupus research? A comparative validation and reliability study of 4 indices. *Journal of Rheumatology*, **26**, 1285–90.

Murray, A.L., Booth, T., and Molenaar, D. (2016). When middle really means "top" or "bottom": An analysis of the 16PFS using Bock's nominal response model. *Journal of Personality Assessment*, **98**, 319–31.

Myles, P.S., Troedel, S., Boquest, M., and Reeves, M. (1999). The pain visual analog scale: Is it linear or nonlinear? *Anesthesia and Analgesia*, **89**, 1517–20.

Newstead, S.E. and Arnold, J. (1989). The effect of response format on ratings of teachers. *Educational and Psychological Measurement*, **49**, 33–43.

Nishisato, N. and Torii, Y. (1970). Effects of categorizing continuous normal distributions on the product-moment correlation. *Japanese Psychological Research*, **13**, 45–9.

Norman, G.R. and Streiner, D.L. (2014). *Biostatistics: The bare essentials* (4th edn). PMPH USA, Shelton, CT.

Parducci, A. (1968). Often is often. *American Psychologist*, **25**, 828.

Pothman, R. (1990). Comparison of the visual analog scale (VAS) and a smiley analog scale (SAS) for the evaluation of pain in children. *Advances in Pain Research and Therapy*, **15**, 95–9.

Preston, C.C. and Colman, A.M. (2000). Optimal number of response categories in rating scales: Reliability, validity, discriminating power, and respondent preferences. *Acta Psychologica*, **104**, 1–15.

Revicki, D.A. and Kaplan, R. M. (1993). Relationship between psychometric and utility-based approaches to the measurement of health-related quality of life. *Quality of Life Research*, **2**, 477–87.

Ronen, G.M., Streiner, D.L., Rosenbaum, P., and the Canadian Pediatric Epilepsy Network (2003). Health-related quality of life in childhood epilepsy: The development of self-report and proxy-response measures. *Epilepsia*, **44**, 598–612.

Russell, J.A. and Carroll, J.M. (1999a). On the bipolarity of positive and negative affect. *Psychological Bulletin*, **125**, 3–30.

Russell, J.A. and Carroll, J.M. (1999b). The phoenix of bipolarity: Reply to Watson and Tellegen (1999). *Psychological Bulletin*, **125**, 611–17.

Rutten-van Molken, M.P.M.H., Custers, F., van Doorslaer, E.K.A., Jansen, C.C.M., Heurman, L., Maesen, F.P., *et al.* (1995). Comparison of performance of four instruments in evaluating the effects of salmeterol on asthma quality of life. *European Respiratory Journal*, **8**, 888–98.

Schaeffer, N.C. (1991). Hardly ever or constantly? Group comparisons using vague quantifiers. *Public Opinion Quarterly*, **55**, 395–423.

Schuman, H. and Presser, S. (1981). *Questions and answers*. Academic Press, New York.

Schwarz, N. (1999). Self-reports: How the questions shape the answers. *American Psychologist*, **54**, 93–105.

Schwarz, N. and Hippler, H.J. (1995). Response alternatives: The impact of their choice and ordering. In *Measurement error in surveys* (eds. P. Biemer, R. Groves, N. Mathiowetz, and S. Sudman), pp. 41–56. Wiley, New York.

Schwarz, N., Hippler, H.J., Deutsch, B., and Strack, F. (1985). Response scales: Effects of category range on report behavior and subsequent judgments. *Public Opinion Quarterly*, **49**, 388–95.

Schwarz, N., Knauper, B., Hippler, H.-J., Noelle-Neumann, E., and Clark, L. (1991). Rating scales: Numeric values may change the meaning of scale labels. *Public Opinion Quarterly*, **55**, 570–82.

Scott, P.J. and Huskisson, E.C. (1978). Measurement of functional capacity with visual analog scales. *Rheumatology and Rehabilitation*, **16**, 257–9.

Scott, P.J. and Huskisson, E.C. (1979). Accuracy of subjective measurements made with and without previous scores: An important source of error in serial measurement of subjective states. *Annals of the Rheumatic Diseases*, **38**, 558–9.

Seymour, R.A., Simpson, J.M., Charlton, J.E., and Phillips, M.E. (1985). An evaluation of length and end-phrase of visual analog scales in dental pain. *Pain*, **21**, 177–85.

Shearman, J.K., Evans, C.E.E., Boyle, M.H., Cuddy, L.J., and Norman, G.R. (1983). Maternal and infant characteristics in abuse: A case control study. *Journal of Family Practice*, **16**, 289–93.

Stinson, J.N., Kavanagh, T., Yamada, J., Gill, N., and Stevens, B. (2006). Systematic review of the psychometric properties, clinical utility and feasibility of self-report pain measures for use in clinical trials in children and adolescents. *Pain*, **125**, 143–57.

Streiner, D.L. (1985). Global rating scales. In *Clinical competence* (eds. V.R. Neufeld and G.R. Norman), pp. 119–41. Springer, New York.

Suissa, S. (1991). Binary methods for continuous outcomes: A parametric alternative. *Journal of Clinical Epidemiology*, **44**, 241–8.

Torrance, G. (1976). Social preferences for health states: An empirical evaluation of three measurement techniques. *Socio-Economic Planning Sciences*, **10**, 129–36.

Torrance, G.W. (1986). Measurement of health state utilities for economic appraisal. *Journal of Health Economics*, **5**, 1–30.

Torrance, G.W. (1987). Utility approach to measuring health-related quality of life. *Journal of Chronic Diseases*, **40**, 593–600.

Torrance, G., Thomas, W.H., and Sackett, D.L. (1972). A utility maximization model for evaluation of health care programs. *Health Services Research*, **7**, 118–33.

Townsend, J.T. and Ashby, F.G. (1984). Measurement scales and statistics: The misconception misconceived. *Psychological Bulletin*, **96**, 394–401.

Tversky, A. and Kahneman, D. (1974). Judgment under uncertainty: Heuristics and biases. *Science*, **185**, 1124–31.

Van Laerhoven, H., van der Zaag-Loonen, H.J., and Derkx, B.H.F. (2004). A comparison of Likert scale and visual analogue scales as response options in children's questionnaires. *Acta Paediatrica*, **93**, 830–5.

Vickers, A. (1999). Comparison of an ordinal and a continuous outcome measure of muscle soreness. *International Journal of Technology Assessment in Health Care*, **15**, 709–16.

Von Neumann, J. and Morgenstern, O. (1953). *The theory of games and economic behavior*. Wiley, New York.

Wainer, H. (1976). Estimating coefficients in linear models: It don't make no nevermind. *Psychological Bulletin*, **83**, 213–17.

Watson, D. and Tellegen, A. (1999). Issues in the dimensional structure of affect—effects of descriptors, measurement error, and response formats: Comment on Russell and Carroll (1999). *Psychological Bulletin*, **125**, 601–10.

Weinberg, S.L. (1991). An introduction to multidimensional scaling. *Measurement and Evaluation in Counseling and Development*, **24**, 12–36.

Wildt, A.R. and Mazis, A.B. (1978). Determinants of scale response: Label versus position. *Journal of Marketing Research*, **15**, 261–7.

Wong, D. and Baker, C. (1988). Pain in children: Comparison of assessment scales. *Pediatric Nursing*, **14**, 9–17.

Wright, D.B., Gaskell, G.D., and O'Muircheartaigh, C.A. (1994). How much is 'Quite a bit'? Mapping between numerical values and vague quantifiers. *Applied Cognitive Psychology*, **8**, 479–496.

Zautra, A.J., Potter, P.T., and Reich, J.W. (1997). The independence of affects is context-dependent: An integrative model of the relationship between positive and negative affect. *Annual Review of Gerontology and Geriatrics*, **17**, 75–102.

Zeckhauser, R. and Shepard, D. (1976). Where now for saving lives? *Law and Contemporary Problems*, **40**, 5–45.

Chapter 5

Selecting the items

Introduction to selecting items

In Chapters 1 through 4, we discussed how to develop items that would be included in the new scale. Obviously, not all of the items will work as intended; some may be confusing to the respondent, some may not tell us what we thought they would, and so on. Here we examine various criteria used in determining which ones to retain and which to discard.

Interpretability

The first criterion for selecting items is to eliminate any items that are ambiguous or incomprehensible. Problems can arise from any one of a number of sources: the words are too difficult; they contain jargon terms that are used only by certain groups of people, such as health professionals; or they are 'double-barrelled'.

Reading level

Except for scales that are aimed at a selected group whose educational level is known, the usual rule of thumb is that the scale should not require reading skills beyond that of a 12-year-old. This may seem unduly low, but many people who are high-school graduates are unable to comprehend material much above this level. There is some evidence that many people have reading levels three or four levels below their highest completed grade (Cutilli 2007). Many ways have been proposed to assess the reading level required to understand written material. Some methods, like the 'cloze' technique (Taylor 1957), eliminate every nth word to see at what point meaning disappears; the easier the material, the more words can be removed and accurately 'filled in' by the reader. Other methods are based on the number of syllables in each word or the number of words in each sentence (e.g. Flesch 1948; Fry 1968). However, these procedures can be laborious and time-consuming, and others may require up to 300 words of text (e.g. McLaughlin 1969). These are usually inappropriate for scales or questionnaires where each item is an independent passage and meaning may depend on one key word.

Within recent years, a number of computer packages have appeared that purport to check the grammar and style of one's writing. Some of these programs further provide one or more indices of reading level, and these have also been incorporated into various word processing packages. Since the procedures used in the programs are based on the techniques we just mentioned, their results should probably be interpreted with great caution when used to evaluate scales.

Another method is to use a list of words that are comprehensible at each grade level (e.g. Dale and Eichholz 1960). While it may be impractical (and even unnecessary) to check every word in the scale, those which appear to be difficult can be checked. Even glancing through one of these books can give the scale-developer a rough idea of the complexity of Grade 6 words. Approaching the problem from the other direction, Payne (1954) compiled a very useful list of 1,000 common words, indicating whether each was unambiguous, problematic, or had multiple meanings. There are also directories of words or phrases to avoid and their more readable alternatives (e.g. use 'about' rather than 'approximately', or 'help' rather than 'facilitate', and remember that wise bit of advice: You should never utilize 'utilize' when you can use 'use'). These include websites such as plainlanguage.gov (<http://www.plainenglish.co.uk/files/alternative.pdf>) and one that translates 'medicalese' into English (<https://apps.lib.umich.edu/medical-dictionary/>).

Ambiguity

Ambiguity can occur in the phrasing of the item, the response alternatives, or both. It can arise if terms are vague (e.g. 'many', 'frequently'), have multiple meanings (e.g. 'cheap' can mean inexpensive or stingy), the stem is double-barrelled, and so forth. At the extreme are 'contranyms'—words that have two opposite meanings, such as 'cleave' (which can mean either to split or to adhere to), 'overlook' (to fail to notice or to supervise), or 'sanction' (to authorize or to penalize). Even a seemingly straightforward item such as 'I like my mother' can pose a problem if the respondent's mother is dead. Some people answer by assuming that the sentence can also be read in the past tense, while others may simply say 'no', reflecting the fact that they cannot like her now. On a questionnaire designed to assess patients' attitudes to their recent hospitalization, one item asked about information given to the patient by various people. A stem read 'I understand what was told to me by:', followed by a list of different healthcare professionals, with room to check either 'yes' or 'no'. Here, a 'no' response opposite 'social worker', for instance, could indicate any one of the following:

1. The patient did not understand what the social worker said.
2. They never saw a social worker.
3. They do not remember whether they saw the social worker or not.
4. They don't know what a social worker is.

While these latter three possibilities were not what the test developer intended, the ambiguity of the question and the response scheme forced the subject to respond with an ambiguous answer.

Ambiguity can also arise by the vagueness of the response alternatives. The answer to the question 'Have you seen your doctor recently' depends on the subject's interpretation of 'recently'. One person may feel that it refers to the previous week, another to the past month, and a third person may believe it covers the previous year. Even if we rephrase the question to use a seemingly more specific term, ambiguity can remain. 'Have you seen your doctor during the past year?' can mean any one of the following:

1. During the last 12 months, more or less.

2. Since this date 1 year ago.

3. Since 1 January of this year.

The message is to avoid vague terms such as 'often', 'lately', or 'recently'. If a specific time-frame (or any other variable) is called for, it should be spelled out explicitly. We will return to the problems of recall in the next chapter.

Double-barreled question

A 'double-barreled' item is one that asks two or more questions at the same time, each of which can be answered differently. Consider an item like 'My eyes are red and teary'. How should one answer if one's eyes are red but not teary, or teary but not red? Since some people will say 'yes' only if both parts are true, while others will respond this way if either symptom was present, the final result may not reflect the actual state of affairs. A more subtle instance of a double-barreled question would be 'I do not smoke because of the fear of lung cancer'. This item has one part that measures the occurrence or non-occurrence of a behaviour ('I do not smoke') and a second part that taps motivation ('because of the fear of lung cancer'). People who do not smoke for other reasons, such as religious beliefs, concern about impaired lung functioning, fear of heart disease, dislike of the smell, and so forth, are in a quandary. They may be reluctant to answer 'False' because that might imply that they do smoke; yet they cannot answer 'True' because the rationale stated in the item does not correspond to their motivation for not smoking. Unfortunately, many disease-specific quality of life scales have fallen into the trap of using these subtle double-barreled questions. For example, the *Calgary Sleep Apnea Quality of Life Index* (Flemons and Reimer 1998) asks patients how much their apnoea contributes to them 'being easily upset'. Assuming the person does in fact become easily upset, how do they apportion a certain amount to their apnoea as opposed to other factors going on in their life?

As we mentioned in Chapter 3, Dowie (2002a, 2002b) states that patients experience effects of disorders and improvements more globally, so it may be specious to expect them to be able to divide emotions among various causes. One of the most extreme examples of an item with many parts is one on the *Sleep Impairment Index* (Morin 1993), which reads 'How noticeable to others do you think your sleep problem is in terms of impairing the quality of your life?' As Fox et al. (2007) point out, not only is it very long (a point we will touch on soon), but also the respondent must consider the following four ideas: (1) is there a sleep problem? (2) if so, does it impair quality of life? (3) if it does, is this noticeable to others? and finally (4) if it is, how noticeable? An answer of 'No' could arise at any of the steps (and the test administer will not know where in the chain this occurred) or more likely because the respondent just gave up trying to keep all these ideas in mind.

Although it would increase the length of the questionnaire or interview, it would be much better to break a question like this into more manageable chunks (see Box 5.1).

> ## Box 5.1 Example of a question using branching to reduce cognitive load.
>
> Question A. Do you have a sleep problem?
>
>   No. Please go to Question B.
>
>   Yes. ↓
>
> Does it impair your quality of life?
>
>   No. Please go to Question B.
>
>   Yes. ↓
>
> Do you think others notice that it impairs your quality of life?
>
>   No. Please go to Question B.
>
>   Yes. ↓
>
> How much do you think they notice?
>
> Not At All _____Very Much
>
> Question B.

The bottom line is to beware of items that contain words such as 'and', 'or', or 'because'. As we will discuss later in this chapter, pre-testing with a group similar to the intended audiences could reveal that a problem may exist.

Jargon

Jargon terms can slip into a scale or questionnaire quite insidiously. Since we use technical vocabulary on a daily basis, and these terms are fully understood by our colleagues, it is easy to overlook the fact that these words are not part of the everyday vocabulary of others or may have very different connotations. Terms like 'lesion', 'care-giver', or 'range of motion' may not be ones that the average person understands. Even more troublesome are words which *are* understood, but in a manner different from what the scale developer intended. 'Hypertension', for example, means 'being very tense' to some people; and asking someone what colour their stool is may elicit the response that the problem is with their gut, not their furniture. Samora et al. (1961) compiled a list of 50 words which physicians said they used routinely with their patients and then asked 125 patients to define them. Words that were erroneously defined at least 50 per cent of the time included 'nutrition', 'digestion', 'orally', and 'tissue'—words that most clinicians would assume their patients knew. The range of definitions given for *appendectomy* included a cut rectum, sickness, the stomach, a pain or disease, taking off an arm or leg, something contagious, or something to do with the bowels, in addition to surgical removal of the appendix. Patients and physicians differ even in terms of what should be called a disease. Campbell et al. (1979) state that 'the medically qualified were consistently more generous in their acceptance of disease connotation than the laymen' (p. 760). Over 90 per cent of general practitioners, for instance, called duodenal ulcers a disease, while only 50 per cent of lay people did. Boyle (1970) found the greatest disagreement between physicians and patients to be in the area of the location of internal organs. Nearly 58 per cent of patients had the heart occupying the entire thorax, or being adjacent to the left shoulder (almost 2 per cent had it near the right shoulder). Similarly, the majority of patients placed the stomach over the belly button, somewhat south of its actual location. Not surprisingly, knowledge of medical terms and the aetiology, treatment, and symptoms of various disorders is strongly associated with educational level (Seligman et al. 1957).

The ubiquity of medical information available via the internet has increased the use and understanding (and misuse and misunderstanding) of many medical terms that would have been obscure just a decade or so ago (Armstrong and Powell 2009; Fage-Butler and Jensen 2015). Nevertheless, assessing the level of health literacy of respondents may not always be feasible, so avoiding jargon whenever possible is still sage advice. Again, pre-testing is desirable, with the interviewer asking the people not whether they had the complaint, but rather what they think the term means.

Value-laden words

A final factor affecting the interpretation of the question is the use of value-laden terms. Items such as 'Do you often go to your doctor with trivial problems?' or 'Do physicians make too much money?' may prejudice the respondents, leading them to answer as much to the tenor of the question as to its content. (Both items also contain ambiguous terms, such as 'often', 'trivial', and 'too much'.) Perhaps the second-most egregious real example of value-laden words was found in a survey of physicians by a company flogging its product. The last question reads 'Given that [the product] will provide substantial cost savings to your hospital, would you be willing to use [the product] for your cataract procedures?' The most egregious was from a poll conducted by a conservative organization on behalf of an even more conservative politician who was in favour of limiting lawsuits against large companies. The question read 'We should stop excessive legal claims, frivolous lawsuits and overzealous lawyers'. Can you guess how people responded? Naturally, such value-laden terms should be avoided.

Positive and negative wording

We design scales and questionnaires assuming highly motivated people, who read each item carefully, ponder the alternatives, and put down an answer reflecting their true beliefs or feelings. Unfortunately, not all respondents fit this ideal picture. As we discuss in more depth in Chapter 6, some people, because of a lack of motivation or poor cognitive skills, take an easy way out; they may say 'Yes' to everything, or just go down the right-hand column of response alternatives. In order to minimize any such response set, some people have recommended balancing the items so that some are worded positively and others negatively (e.g. Anastasi 1982; Likert

1932). However, research has shown that this is generally a bad idea. Negatively worded items—that is, those that use words such as 'not' or 'never' or have words with negative prefixes (e.g. in-, im-, or un-)—should be avoided whenever possible for a number of reasons. First, simply reversing the polarity of an item does not necessarily reverse the meaning. Answering 'Yes' to the question 'I feel well' connotes a positive state; whereas saying 'No' to 'I do not feel well' reflects the absence of a negative one, which is not always the same thing. Second, children and lower-functioning adults have difficulty grasping the concept that they have to disagree with an item in order to indicate a positive answer, such as reporting being in good health by having to say 'No' to 'I feel unwell much of the time' (Benson and Hocevar 1985; Melnick and Gable 1990). Indeed, because negatively worded items have been estimated to occupy about twice as much space in working memory as positively worded ones (Tamir 1993), even very bright students sometimes failed easy multiple choice items while correctly answering much harder ones (Chiavaroli 2017). Third, there is a tendency for respondents to endorse a negative item rather than reject a positive one (Campostrini and McQueen 1993; Reiser et al. 1986). Fourth, there is a 'method effect' due to the wording. When scales with both positively and negatively worded items are factor analysed, two factors usually emerge: one consisting of the positive items and the other of the negative items, irrespective of their content (e.g. Horan et al. 2003; Lindwall et al. 2012); needless to say, this is not a good property of a scale. Finally, negatively worded items have lower validity coefficients than positively worded ones (Holden et al. 1985; Schriesheim and Hill 1981); and scales that have stems with both positive and negative wording are less reliable than those where all the stems are worded in the same direction (Barnette 2000). Using item response theory (discussed in Chapter 12), Sliter and Zickar (2013) found that negatively worded items were more difficult and were less discriminating than positively worded ones. Thus, to create a balanced scale, all of the items should be positively worded, but one half should tap one direction of the trait and the other half should tap the opposite direction of it.

Length of items

Items on scales should be as short as possible, although not so short that comprehensibility is lost. Item validity coefficients tend to fall as the number of letters in the item increases. Holden et al. (1985) found that, on average, items with 70–80 letters had validity coefficients under 0.10, while items containing 10–20 characters had coefficients almost four times higher. Similarly, there was a negative correlation between the average number of words in an item and the proportion of people responding to it the same way across two administrations of the scale (Wiggins and Goldberg 1965).

A very different approach to testing questions has been developed by Graesser et al. (2006). They developed a Web-based tool called QUAID (Question Understanding Aid; available at <http://www.psyc.memphis.edu/quaid.html>) that detects and diagnoses up to five different types of problems with questionnaire or survey items. It does not cure the problems, but then again, it does not charge for its services either. Using various databases of word frequency and familiarity, it flags terms that may not be understood by most respondents. Needless to say, its advice must be tempered by considering the intended audience; while most people may not know what *dialysis* means, physicians and patients with end-stage renal disease would. Second, QUAID identifies vague or imprecise predicates, such as *many*, *often*, or *rarely*. Third, it looks for vague or ambiguous noun phrases, such as words that may have two or more meanings. The fourth problem it looks for is complex syntax, for example, many words before the verb or two or more adjectives in a noun phrase. Finally, it decides if the item may impose a high load on working memory, such as by including many *ifs* or *nots*, or by requiring the respondent to keep a large number of words in mind.

Face validity

One issue that must be decided before the items are written or selected is whether or not they should have *face validity*. That is, do the items appear on the surface to be measuring what they actually are? As is often the case, there are two schools of thought on this issue, and the 'correct' answer often depends on the purpose that the measure will be used for.

Those who argue for face validity state, quite convincingly, that it serves at least five useful functions. It:

1. increases motivation and cooperation among the respondents
2. may attract potential candidates
3. reduces dissatisfaction among users
4. makes it more likely that policy makers and others accept the results
5. improves public relations, especially with the media and the courts (Nevo 1985).

If the item appears irrelevant, then the respondent may very well object to it or omit it, irrespective of its possibly superb psychometric properties. For example, it is commonly believed that some psychiatric patients manifest increased religiosity, especially during the acute phase of their illness. Capitalizing on this fact, the MMPI contains a few items tapping into this domain. Despite the fact that these items are psychometrically quite good, it has opened the test to much (perhaps unnecessary) criticism for delving into seemingly irrelevant, private matters.

On the other hand, it may be necessary in some circumstances to disguise the true nature of the question, lest the respondents try to 'fake' their answers, an issue we will return to in greater detail in Chapter 6. For example, patients may want to appear worse than they actually are in order to ensure that they will receive help; or better than they really feel in order to please the doctor. This is easy to do if the items have face validity—that is, their meaning and relevance are self-evident—and much harder if they do not. Rather than asking patients if they have lost or gained weight recently, you may want to ask if their shirts still fit. This is a non-objectionable question that does not have face validity. Thus, the ultimate decision depends on the nature and purpose of the instrument.

If it is decided that the scale should have face validity (which is usually the case), then the issues become as follows:

1. Who should assess it, and
2. How.

Because face validity pertains to how respondents and other users of the test perceive it, it should be judged by them and not by experts in the field; further, it is sufficient to ask them to simply rate it on a 5-point scale, ranging from Extremely Suitable to Irrelevant (Nevo 1985).

Frequency of endorsement and discrimination

After the scale has been pre-tested for readability and absence of ambiguity, it is then given to a large group of subjects to test for other attributes, including the endorsement frequency. (The meaning of 'large' is variable, but usually 50 subjects would be an absolute minimum.) The frequency of endorsement is simply the proportion of people (p) who give each response alternative to an item. For dichotomous items, this reduces to simply the proportion saying 'yes' (or conversely, 'no'). A multiple-choice item has a number of 'frequencies of endorsement': the proportion choosing alternative A, one for alternative B, and so forth.

In achievement tests, the frequency of endorsement is a function of the *difficulty* of the item, with a specific response alternative reflecting the correct answer. For personality measures, the frequency of endorsement is the 'popularity' of that item—the proportion of people who choose the alternative which indicates more of the trait, attitude, or behaviour (Allen and Yen 1979).

Usually, items where one alternative has a very high (or low) endorsement rate are eliminated. If p is over 0.95 (or under 0.05), then most people are responding in the same direction or with the same alternative. Since we can predict what the answer will be with greater than 95 per cent accuracy, we learn very little by knowing how a person actually responded. Such questions do not improve a scale's psychometric properties and may actually detract from them while making the test longer. In practice, only items with endorsement rates between 0.20 and 0.80 are used.

Using this criterion, which is quite liberal, may result in items that are highly skewed, in that the responses bunch up at one end of the continuum or the other. However, this does not have a major deleterious effect on the psychometric properties of the scale (assuming, of course, that p is somewhere between 0.2 and 0.8). Especially when the mean inter-item correlation is high (at least 0.25 or so), we can live with highly skewed items (Bandalos and Enders 1996; Enders and Bandalos 1999; Feldt 1993). Thus, items should not be thrown out simply on the basis of the skewness of the distribution of responses.

There are some scales, though, which are deliberately made up of items with a high endorsement frequency. This is the case where there may be some question regarding the subject's ability or willingness to answer honestly. A person may not read the item accurately because of factors such as illiteracy, low intelligence, a lack of motivation, or difficulties in concentration; or may not answer honestly because of an attempt to 'fake' a response for some reason. Some tests, like the MMPI or the *Personality Research Form* (Jackson 1984), have special scales to detect these biases, comprised of a heterogeneous group of items which have only one thing in common: an endorsement frequency of 90–95 per cent. To obtain such high rates, the questions have to be either quite bizarre (e.g. 'I have touched money') or extremely banal (e.g. 'I eat most days'). A significant number of questions answered in the 'wrong' direction is a flag that the person was not reading the items carefully and responding as most people would do. This may temper the interpretation given to other scales that the person completes. We discuss the issues of biased and random responding, and how to detect these, in greater detail in Chapter 6.

Another index of the utility of an item, closely related to endorsement frequency, is its *discrimination*, which is an index of the extent to which people who score high on the rest of the scale endorse the item and those who score low do not endorse it. It is related to endorsement frequency in that, from a psychometric viewpoint, items which discriminate best among people have values of *p* near the cut point of the scale, and items that are endorsed by very many or very few people will not discriminate. It differs in that it looks at the item in relation to all of the other items on the scale, not just in isolation.

A simple item discrimination index is given by the following formula:

$$d_i = \frac{U_i - L_i}{n_i}$$

where U_i is the number of people above the median who score positive on item i, L_i is the number of people below the median who score positive on item i, and n_i is the number of people above (or below) the median.

Had the developers of the National Eye Institute Visual Functioning Questionnaire (Mangione et al. 1998), the most widely used quality of life scale in ophthalmology, checked for frequency of endorsement, they may likely have thought twice about some of their response options. Note that this is a self-administered scale (see Box 5.2).

Box 5.2 One question from the National Eye Institute Visual Functioning Questionnaire.

2. At the present time, would you say your eyesight using both eyes (with glasses or contact lenses, if you wear them) is **excellent, good, fair, poor, very poor**, or are you **completely blind?**

    (Circle one)

    Excellent 1
    Good 2
    Fair 3
    Poor 4
    Very Poor 5
    Completely Blind 6

National Eye Institute Visual Functioning Questionnaire—25 (VFQ-25), version 2000 (Interviewer Administered Format) is reproduced here (in part) with permission from the RAND Corporation. Copyright © the RAND Corporation. RAND's permission to reproduce the survey is not an endorsement of the products, services, or other uses in which the survey appears or is applied.

We wonder how many people were able to circle option 6? This emphasizes, yet again, the necessity to pre-test questionnaires with people who will actually complete the scale.

Homogeneity of the items

In most situations, whenever we are measuring a trait, behaviour, or symptom, we want the scale to be homogeneous. That is, all of the items should be tapping different aspects of the same attribute and not different parts of different traits. (Later in this chapter, in the section titled 'Multifactor inventories', we deal with the situation where we want the test to measure a variety of characteristics.) For example, if we were measuring the problem-solving ability of medical students, then each item should relate to problem-solving. A high degree of homogeneity is desirable in a scale because it 'speaks directly to the ability of the clinician or the researcher to interpret the composite score as a reflection of the test's items' (Henson 2001). This has two implications:

1. The items should be moderately correlated with each other.
2. Each should correlate with the total scale score.

Indeed, these two factors form the basis of the various tests of homogeneity or 'internal consistency' of the scale.

A hierarchy of scales

Before the mechanics of measuring internal consistency are discussed, we have to take a bit of a detour and discuss a hierarchy of scales. At first glance, it may appear as if all scales are more or less alike; they all have a number of items (although the response options may differ), most of them have a total score derived from summing the items, and so forth. But, from a psychometric perspective, there can be major differences among them which influences how—and even whether—we can measure homogeneity.

The major assumption underlying most scales is that they are measuring a single underlying *construct*, such as anxiety, pain, or depression. We will discuss what a construct is in more detail in Chapter 10, but for now, suffice it to say that it is something that we cannot see directly, but can only observe its effects on measurable variables. For example, we do not see 'intelligence', but rather we can measure its observable manifestations, such as the size of one's vocabulary, problem-solving ability, or knowledge of the world. We can diagram this as in Fig. 5.1, where the oval represents the underlying construct, the rectangles the measured items or variables, and the circles reflect the errors for a 3-item scale. The important point to note is that the arrows come *from* the construct *to* the items; that is, the responses to the items are due to the amount of the construct that each person has. The λs (the Greek letter lambda) are the correlations of each item with the construct (the *factor loading* in factor analysis; see Appendix B), and the εs are the errors.

In a *parallel indicators* scale, all of the items have similar factor loadings and the error terms are likewise similar. That is, $\lambda_1 = \lambda_2 = \lambda_3$, and $\varepsilon_1 = \varepsilon_2 = \varepsilon_3$. (Of course they won't be exactly the same, but they should be relatively the same in magnitude—a term

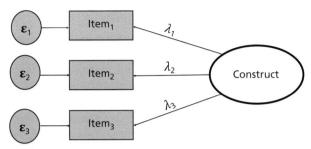

Fig. 5.1 Representation of how a construct influences measured variables.

we can't really quantify.) If the scales are τ (tau)-*equivalent*, then the factor loadings are similar, but the errors differ from one item to the next: $\lambda_1 = \lambda_2 = \lambda_3$, but $\varepsilon_1 \neq \varepsilon_2 \neq \varepsilon_3$. Finally, with *congeneric* scales, neither the factor loadings nor the errors are similar across items: $\lambda_1 \neq \lambda_2 \neq \lambda_3$, and $\varepsilon_1 \neq \varepsilon_2 \neq \varepsilon_3$.

Another way to determine what type of scale we're dealing with is to examine the *variance-covariance* (VCV) matrix of the items, as in Fig. 5.2. A VCV matrix is similar to a correlation matrix, except that we use the raw scores, rather than first converting them to standardized scores. The values along the main diagonal (running from the top left to the bottom right cell) are the variances for each item, and the off-diagonal cells are the covariances. As with a correlation matrix, the VCV matrix is symmetric, in that the covariance in cell$_{1,2}$ is the same as the covariance in cell$_{2,1}$. If a scale has parallel-indicator properties, then all of the variances should be similar in magnitude, as should all of the covariances. In τ-equivalent types of scales, the variances are similar but the covariances are not; and in congeneric scales, neither the variances nor the covariances are similar.

Why is this important? Because the factor loadings are similar in parallel-indicator and τ-equivalent types of scales, it is legitimate to add up the individual items to derive a total score. Strictly speaking, this is not true for congeneric scales, since each item contributes differently to the total score. In practice, though, it probably doesn't matter if there are roughly 10 or more items in the scale. The reason, as we will discuss in greater depth in Chapter 7, is that assigning a greater weight to some items makes less and less of a difference as scales grow longer. However, as we'll discuss later in this chapter in the section on Kuder-Richardson and coefficient alpha, whether or not internal consistency is an accurate measure of a scale's reliability *does* depend on where it sits in this hierarchy.

	X_1	X_2	X_3
X_1	10	4	4
X_2	4	10	4
X_3	4	4	10

(a)

	X_1	X_2	X_3
X_1	10	3	5
X_2	3	10	7
X_3	5	7	10

(b)

	X_1	X_2	X_3
X_1	8	3	5
X_2	3	15	7
X_3	5	7	5

(c)

Fig. 5.2 Variance-covariance matrices for (a) parallel indicators, (b) τ-equivalent, and (c) congeneric scales.

The rationale for measuring homogeneity

Before we begin, some rationale and background for assessing homogeneity are in order. In almost all areas we measure, a simple summing of the scores over the individual items is the most sensible index; this point will be returned to in Chapter 7. However, this 'linear model' approach (Nunnally 1970) works only if all items are measuring the same trait. If the items were measuring different attributes, it would not be logical to add them up to form one total score. On the other hand, if one item were highly correlated with a second one, then the latter question would add little additional information. Hence, there is a need to derive some quantitative measure of the degree to which items are related to each other—i.e. the degree of 'homogeneity' of the scale.

Current thinking in test development holds that there should be a moderate correlation among the items in a scale. If the items were chosen without regard for homogeneity, then the resulting scale could possibly end up tapping a number of traits. If the correlations were too high, there would be much redundancy and a possible loss of content validity. This phenomenon is called the *attenuation paradox* by Loevinger (1954), although it had been recognized earlier by Gulliksen (1945). Up to a point, increasing the homogeneity of a scale (and hence its reliability) increases its validity. Beyond that point, though, too much homogeneity results in a loss of content coverage and thus leads to a *decrease* in validity. At an extreme, if all of the items correlated 1.0 with each other, then a person endorsing one item would endorse all of them; and conversely, a person not endorsing one item would endorse none of them. Thus, the scale would yield only two scores—a perfect score or zero. That is why Cronbach's alpha (α) should not exceed 0.90 (some authors, such as Kline (1979) and Schmitt (1996), say the maximum should be 0.70), and item-total correlations, discussed in the next section, should not exceed 0.70.

It should be noted that this position of taking homogeneity into account, which is most closely identified with Jackson (1970) and Nunnally (1970), is not shared by all psychometricians. Another school of thought is that internal consistency and face validity make sense if the primary aim is to *describe* a trait, behaviour, or disorder, but not necessarily if the goal is to *discriminate* people who have an attribute from those who do not. That is, if we are trying to measure the degree of depression, for example, the scale should *appear* to be measuring it and all of the items should relate to this in a coherent manner. On the other hand, if our aim is to *discriminate* depressed patients from other groups, then it is sufficient to choose items which are answered differently by the depressed group, irrespective of their content. This in fact was the method used in constructing the MMPI, one of the most famous questionnaires for psychological assessment. An item was included in the Depression Scale (D) based on the criterion that depressed patients responded to it in one way significantly more often than did non-depressed people and without regard for the correlation among the individual items. As a result, the D scale has some items which seem to be related to depression, but also many other items which do not. On the other hand, the more recent CES-D (Radloff 1977), which measures depressive symptomatology without diagnosing depression, was constructed following the philosophy of high internal consistency, and its items all appear to be tapping into this domain. If a trend can be detected, it is to-wards scales that are more grounded in theory and are more internally consistent and away from the empiricism that led to the MMPI.

It should also be noted that focusing on internal consistency as a measure of reliability—and Cronbach's α is the most widely used measure of it (Henson 2001)—represents a seismic shift in the understanding of reliability, and not necessarily for the better. As we discuss in Chapter 8, other forms of reliability (e.g. test–retest) examine consistency over time for stable traits. Relying solely on internal consistency, which requires only one administration of the scale, has unfortunately diminished the importance of this attribute of measures.

One last comment is in order before discussing the techniques of item selection. Many inventories, especially those in the realms of psychology and psychiatry, are multidimensional; that is, they are comprised of a number of different scales, with the items intermixed in a random manner. Measures of homogeneity should be applied to the individual scales, as it does not make sense to talk of homogeneity across different subscales. It is important to remember: '*unidimensionality is an assumption that needs to be verified prior to calculating Cronbach's alpha rather than being the focus of what Cronbach's alpha measures*' (McNeish 2018, p. 416; emphasis added).

Item-total correlation

One of the oldest, albeit still widely used, methods for checking the homogeneity of the scale is the *item-total correlation*. As the name implies, it is the correlation of the individual item with the scale total *omitting that item*; hence, the other name for this method is *item-partial total correlation*. If we did not remove the item from the total score, the correlation would be artificially inflated, since it would be based in part on the item correlated with itself. The item can be eliminated in one of two ways: physically or statistically. We can physically remove the item by not including it when calculating the total score. So, for a 5-item scale, Item 1 would be correlated with the sum of Items 2–5; Item 2 with the sum of 1 and 3–5; and so on. One problem with this approach is that for a *k-item* scale, we have to calculate the total score *k* times; this is not a difficult problem, but a laborious one, especially if a computer program to do this is not readily available.

The second method is statistical; the item's contribution to the total score is removed using the formula given by Nunnally (1978):

$$r_{i(t-1)} = \frac{r_{it}\sigma_t - \sigma_i}{\sqrt{\left(\sigma_i^2 + \sigma_t^2 - 2\sigma_i\sigma_t r_{it}\right)}}$$

where $r_{i(t-1)}$ is the correlation of item i with the total, removing the effect of item i; r_{it} is the correlation of item i with the total score; σ_i is the standard deviation of item i; and σ_t is the standard deviation of the total score.

The usual rule of thumb is that an item should correlate with the total score above 0.30. Items with lower correlations should be discarded (Kline 1986). On the other hand, the correlation should not be greater than 0.70; more than this and the scale is likely too narrow and specific, with one question merely a restatement of another (Kline 1979). A negative correlation is a red flag, indicating that either the item was coded incorrectly (e.g. a high value is 'bad', whereas it is 'good' for all of the other items) or the item itself is badly worded and misunderstood.

In almost all instances, the best coefficient to use is the *Pearson product-moment correlation* (Nunnally 1970). If the items are dichotomous, then the usually recommended point-biserial correlation yields identical results; if there are more than two response alternatives, the product-moment correlation is robust enough to produce relatively accurate results, even if the data are not normally distributed (see e.g. Havlicek and Peterson 1977).

Split-half reliability

Another approach to testing the homogeneity of a scale is called *split-half reliability*. Here, the items are randomly divided into two subscales, which are then correlated with each other. This is also referred to as 'odd–even' reliability, since the easiest split is to put all odd-numbered items in one half and even-numbered ones in the other. If the scale is internally consistent, then the two halves should correlate highly.

One problem is that the resulting correlation is an underestimate of the true reliability of the scale, since the reliability of a scale is directly proportional to the number of items in it. Since the subscales being correlated are only half the length of the version that will be used in practice, the resulting correlation will be too low. The Spearman–Brown 'prophesy' formula is used to correct for this occurrence.

The equation for this is as follows:

$$r_{SB} = \frac{kr}{1+(k-1)r}$$

where k is the factor by which the scale is to be increased or decreased and r is the original correlation.

In this case, we want to see the result when there are twice the number of items, so k is set at 2. For example, if we found that splitting a 40-item scale in half yields a correlation of 0.50, we would substitute into the equation as follows:

$$r_{SB} = \frac{2 \times 0.50}{1+(2-1) \times 0.50}$$

Thus, the estimate of the split-half reliability of this scale would be 0.67.

Since there are many ways to divide a test into two parts, there are in fact many possible split-half reliabilities; a 10-item test can be divided 126 ways, a 12-item test 462 different ways, and so on. (These numbers represent the combination of n items taken $n/2$ at a time. This is then divided by 2, since (assuming a 6-item scale) items 1, 2, and 3 in the first half and 4, 5, and 6 in the second half is the same as 4, 5, and 6 in the first part and the remaining items in the second.) These reliability coefficients may differ quite considerably from one split to another.

There are three situations when we should *not* divide a test randomly:

1. Where the score reflects how many items are completed within a certain span of time.

2. If the items are given in order of increasing difficulty.

3. When either the items are serially related or all refer to the same paragraph that must be read.

In the first case, where the major emphasis is on how quickly a person can work, most of the items are fairly easy, and failure is due to not reaching that question before the time limit. Thus, the answers up to the timed cut-off will almost all be correct and those after it all incorrect. Any split-half reliability will yield a very high value, only marginally lower than 1.0.

The second situation, items presented in order of difficulty, is often found in individually administered intelligence and achievement tests as well as some activities of daily living scales. Here, items are presented until they surpass the person's level of ability. Similar to the previous case, the expected pattern of answers is all correct up to that level and all wrong above it (or if partial credits are given, then a number of items with full credit, followed by some with partial credit, and ending with a group given no credit). As with timed tests, it is assumed that people will differ only with regard to the number of items successfully completed and that the pattern of responding will be the same from one person to the next. Again, the split-half reliability will be very close to 1.0.

With related or 'chained' items, failure on the second item could occur in two ways: not being able to answer it correctly; or being able to do it, but getting it wrong because of an erroneous response to the previous item. For example, assume that the two (relatively simple) items were as follows:

A. The organ for pumping blood is:

    the pineal gland

    the heart

    the stomach.

B. It is located in:

    the chest

    the gut

    the skull.

If the answer to A were correct, then a wrong response to B would indicate that the person did not know where the heart is located. However, if A and B were wrong, then the person *may* have known that the heart is located in the chest, but went astray in believing that blood is pumped by the pineal gland. Whenever this can occur, it is best to keep both items in the same half of the scale.

We should also note that in these three types of measures—timed tests, those presented in order of difficulty, and chained questions—the error terms associated with each item are correlated with one another (Green and Yang 2009). This violates one of the key assumptions of classical test theory, that the errors be independent. This is another reason that we should not use split-half reliability, nor any of the other indices described in the section that follows (Kuder–Richardson 20 and coefficient alpha).

Kuder–Richardson 20 and coefficient alpha

There are two problems in using split-half reliability to determine which items to retain. First, as we have just seen, there are many ways to divide a test; and second, it does not tell us which item(s) may be contributing to a low reliability. Both of these problems are addressed with two related techniques: *Kuder–Richardson formula 20* (KR-20; Kuder and Richardson 1937) and *coefficient alpha* (α) (also called Cronbach's alpha; Cronbach 1951).

Both KR-20 and coefficient α make three assumptions of the scale: (1) it is unidimensional; (2) it satisfies the properties of being τ-equivalent; and (3) the errors associated with each of the items do not covary. Coefficient α makes one additional assumption: (4) that the responses are on a continuum and are normally distributed. There is some debate regarding how many response options an item must have to be considered continuous; some have said that five is sufficient (e.g. Rhemtulla et al. 2012), and others have argued for at least seven (Gadermann et al. 2012). The jury is still out, and is likely to be out for quite a while.

KR-20 is appropriate for scales with items which are answered dichotomously, such as 'true–false', 'yes–no', 'present–absent', and so forth. To compute it, the proportion of people answering positively to each of the questions and the standard deviation of the total score must be known, and then these values should be substituted into the following formula:

$$KR\text{-}20 = \frac{k}{k-1}\left(1 - \frac{\sum p_i q_i}{\sigma_T^2}\right)$$

where k is the number of items; p_i is the proportion answering correctly to question i; $q_i = (1-p)$ for each item; and σ_T is the standard deviation of the total score.

Cronbach's α is an extension of KR-20, allowing it to be used when there are more than two response alternatives. If α were used with dichotomous items, the result would be identical to that obtained with KR-20. The formula for α is very similar to KR-20, except that the standard deviation for each item (σ_i) is substituted for $p_i q_i$:

$$\alpha = \frac{k}{k-1}\left(1 - \frac{\sum \sigma_i^2}{\sigma_T^2}\right)$$

Conceptually, both equations give the average of all of the possible split-half reliabilities of a scale. (Actually, this is true only if all of the items have the same variances; that is, it is not true for congeneric or τ-equivalent scales. For these, they are smaller than split-half reliability.) Their advantage in terms of scale development is that, especially with the use of computers, it is possible to do them k times, each time omitting one item. If KR-20 or α increases significantly when a specific item is left out, this would indicate that its exclusion would increase the homogeneity of the scale.

It is nearly impossible these days to see a scale development paper that has not used α, and the implication is usually made that the higher the coefficient, the better. There is an obvious explanation for the ubiquity of the internal consistency coefficient. No repeated administrations are necessary—no multiple observers. You can just administer the scale once to a bunch of people, and then crunch out the alpha. However, there are problems in uncritically accepting high values of α (or KR-20), especially in interpreting them as simply reflecting internal consistency. The first problem is that α is dependent not only on the magnitude of the correlations among the items, but also on the number of items in the scale. A scale can be made to look more 'homogeneous' simply by doubling the number of items, even though the average correlation remains the same. In Fig. 5.3 we have plotted α for a scale with an average inter-item correlation of 0.4. With only two items, α is 0.57. Adding two more items increases α to 0.73. As the scale becomes longer, the increase in length has less effect.

We can see the reason for this by rewriting the formula for α. If all the item variances are equal, then

$$\alpha = \frac{kr_{Avg}}{1 + (k-1)r_{Avg}}$$

where r_{Avg} is the mean inter-item correlation. As k increases, it can swamp a low value of r_{Avg}.

This leads directly to the second problem. If we have two scales which each measure a distinct construct and combine them to form one long scale, α will be high. Cortina (1993) concluded that, 'if a scale has more than 14 items, then it will have an alpha of 0.70 or better even if it consists of two orthogonal dimensions with modest (i.e. 0.30) item correlations. If the dimensions are correlated with each other, as they usually are, then alpha is even greater' (p. 102). Third, if α is too high, then it may suggest a high level of item redundancy—that is, a number of items asking the same question in slightly different ways (Boyle 1991; Hattie 1985). This may indicate that some of the

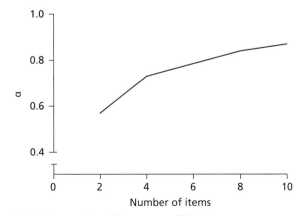

Fig. 5.3 The effect of the number of items on coefficient α.

items are unnecessary and that the scale as a whole may be too narrow in its scope to have much validity. Therefore, what value of α is acceptable? A number of authors say it should be at least 0.70 (e.g. Heppner et al. 1992; Kaplan and Saccuzzo 1997). Nunnally (1978) states that this value should be obtained in the early stages of research, but should be at least 0.80 for basic research (a value also endorsed by Carmines and Zeller (1979), Clark and Watson (1995), and others) and 0.90 for a clinical instrument. A somewhat different approach is taken by Ponterotto and Ruckdeschel (2007). Because, as we have said, α is influenced by the length of the scale and the sample size, they propose a range of values dependent on these factors. Therefore, for example, they would call a value of 0.70 'good' for a scale with fewer than seven items, evaluated with fewer than 100 subjects. However, if the scale has more than 11 items, and the sample size was over 300, α would have to be 0.90 to be called 'good'.

In fact, in our experience, we tend to see alpha coefficients that are *too* high. The situation frequently arises in educational or work settings, where a teacher or supervisor is required to evaluate a student or employees at the end of some period of time. Typically, the evaluation is done on a scale with 5 to 10 items, like 'Responsibility', 'Communication skills', and 'Problem-solving'. It is not uncommon to see alpha greater than 0.9 for such scales even when assessing diverse characteristics. In one recent example (Sherbino et al. 2013), a 7-item scale had an internal consistency of 0.94. Such a high correlation among items suggests, as the authors indicated, that the scale is insensitive to differences among characteristics and should be viewed as evidence for a problem.

As we will see in Chapter 8, there are many different ways of measuring reliability, of which internal consistency (split-half, KR-20, and Cronbach's α) is only one. There has been some debate regarding the relationship between measures of homogeneity and indices based on having the subject repeat the test after some period of time (test–retest reliability) or having two interviewers complete the scale independently (inter-rater reliability). For many years, it was stated that internal consistency provided a *lower* bound of reliability; that is, other types of reliability measures would be higher (e.g. Lord and Novick 1968). However, others have argued that α-type indices are an *upper* bound, and that test–retest and inter-rater reliabilities will be lower (Brennan 2001). This is more than an academic argument. Measures of internal consistency are the most widely used indices of reliability because they are the only ones that can be derived with only one administration of the test. Consequently, many scale development articles report only α and do not go further; therefore, it is important to know if α gives a lower or an upper estimate of reliability.

The answer is that it depends on the nature of the scales. Alpha is an upper estimate of reliability for scales that are parallel or τ-equivalent, but a lower estimate when the scale is congeneric (Graham 2006; Raykov 1997b), and the more the scale deviates from τ-equivalence, the more α underestimates reliability. When all of the items use the same response format (e.g. a 5-point Likert scale), the scale can be considered to be parallel, and thus α is an upper estimate of the scale's reliability (Falk and Savalei 2011). Indeed, it is questionable whether one should use any measure of internal consistency with congeneric scales (Feldt and Charter 2003; Ferketich 1990).

Alpha if item omitted

Many commercially available statistical programs, such as SPSS, SAS, and Stata, report for each item how much α will increase if it is omitted. The implicit message is to remove those items that will result in a higher value. As is the case with much unsoli-cited advice, our unsolicited advice is that it is best if it is ignored for two reasons. First, as we have stressed a number of times, a value of α that is too high may reflect a scale that is too narrow in its focus, sacrificing breadth of coverage for unnecessary internal consistency. Second, 'alpha if deleted' is strongly based on the sample being studied, and the results may change with a different sample (Raykov 1997a, 1997b). That is, the value of α may increase at the level of the sample, but may stay the same or even decrease at the population level. This is especially true for τ-equivalent and congen-eric scales, because the variances for each item are unequal, and the deleted item may contain less error variance than the other items (Dunn et al. 2014).

Confidence interval for KR-20 and coefficient α

Coefficient α and KR-20 are parameters, and, as with all parameters, they should be reported with a confidence interval (CI; for more information about CIs, see Norman and Streiner 2014). Over the years, a number of formulae have been derived. Perhaps the most accurate is that by Duhachek and Iacobucci (2004), but it requires matrix al-gebra (although they provide the code so that the standard error can be calculated by the computer programs SAS and SPSS). More tractable formulae were worked out by Feldt (1965), but reported in a journal rarely read by scale developers; therefore, they were rarely incorporated into text books. They were reintroduced into the psychological literature by Charter (1997). The upper and lower bounds of the CI are calculated by:

$$\text{Lower bound} = 1 - (1 - \alpha)\,\text{FL}$$
$$\text{Upper bound} = 1 - (1 - \alpha)\,\text{FU}$$

where for the 95 per cent CI:

$$F_L = F_{0.975}\left(df_1, df_2\right)$$
$$F_U = \frac{1}{F_{0.975}\left(df_2, df_1\right)}$$
$$df_1 = N - 1$$
$$df_2 = (N - 1)(k - 1)$$

where N is the sample size, and k is the number of items in the scale. For example, if α = 0.80 in a study with 100 subjects completing a 20-item scale, then df_1 = 99 and df_2 = 1,881. We obtain the values for F using a table for critical values of the F-ratio, which is found in the appendices of most statistics books. In this case, we must use df_1 = 100 and df_2 = 1,000 because this is as high as the values in the tables. The value for df_1 is 1.26 and that of df_2 is 1.28 (note that the order of the dfs is reversed for F_U) so that

$$\text{Lower bound} = 1 - (1 - 0.80) \times 1.26 = 0.748$$

$$\text{Upper bound} = 1 - (1 - 0.80) \times (1/1.28) = 0.844$$

Also, note that the CI is not symmetric around α, but is larger for the bound that is closer to 0.5 (i.e. the lower bound when α is above 0.50). It is symmetric only when α = 0.50.

Sample size requirements for KR-20 and coefficient α

Using the CI approach, we can work backwards to determine how many subjects are required to estimate KR-20 and α. We begin by guessing the values of two parameters: the magnitude of the coefficient and how wide or narrow we want the CI to be around this estimate. For example, we may feel that α will be approximately 0.70, and we want the CI to be ± 0.10 (i.e. between 0.60 and 0.80). If we want to be very precise about the sample size, we can follow the formulae given by Bonett (2002). However, the calculations are unnecessarily complex, in our opinion, since we are actually dealing with guesses at each stage of the process. Instead, Fig. 5.4 shows the approximate sample sizes for α = 0.70 and 0.90, and for various values of the CI width (i.e. the upper bound minus the lower bound). As you can see from these graphs, the narrower the CI, the larger the sample size that is needed. Also, as the number of items in the scale increases, the sample size requirements decrease very rapidly until about 10 items and then more slowly. Finally, higher values of α need fewer subjects for the same width of

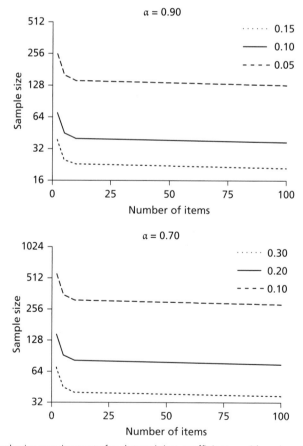

Fig. 5.4 Sample size requirements for determining coefficient α with various CIs.

the CI. What is obvious from these figures is that most studies that report α are woefully small and will result in CIs that are quite broad.

Alternatives to KR-20 and coefficient α

By now it should be obvious that KR-20 and Cronbach's α, despite their ubiquity, are flawed measures, most especially for congeneric scales, but also for parallel indicator and τ-equivalent scales. This raises the question of what should be used in their place. There are a number of alternatives, ranging from the very simple to the computationally complex.

At the simple end of the continuum are the mean inter-item correlation and the mean item-total correlation (which we discussed earlier in this chapter). The mean inter-item correlation should be within the range of 0.15 to 0.20 for scales measuring broad characteristics, such as self-efficacy; and between 0.40 and 0.50 for those tapping more narrow constructs, such as self-efficacy for sports (Clark and Watson 1995). Many statistical packages, such as SPSS, report the item-total correlation for each item, so that it is a simple matter to calculate the mean. In simulations that we have done, we found that the mean item-total correlation is less affected by the length of the scale than the mean inter-item correlation. It is likely good practice to report either or both of these indices in addition to (or in place of) coefficient α.

At the opposite end of the continuum is a coefficient called omega (ω; McDonald 1999). Confusingly, he used the same symbol for two indices, so the one we're interested in here is also referred to as ω_t. The major advantage of ω_t over α is that it yields a higher, and more accurate, value for congeneric scales, and will equal α for parallel and τ-equivalent scales. The major disadvantage, though, is that it is computationally complex and does not appear in most commercial software packages. However, it has been implemented in the R package, and Dunn et al. (2014), McNeish (2018), and Peters (2014) provide tutorials on how to install and use it. There is also a free statistical package called JASP (<https://jasp-stats.org/>) that incorporates omega. It is strongly recommended that, if you have access to any of these, you use McDonald's ω_t rather than Cronbach's α.

Single-item rating scales: are more items always merrier?

In the previous section on 'Alternatives to KR-20 and coefficient α', we pointed out that an increase in the number of items on a scale will, by definition, lead to greater reliability—more is always merrier. If we are simply adding items, this is a straightforward extension of the standard statistics related to the standard error of the mean. As you add more items, the variance due to error of measurement goes down in proportion to the number of items.

However, this is not always the case. The conundrum arises when you consider a contrast between a single global judgement and a multi-item inventory. Consider the following situations:

1. At least 15 studies of OSCEs (Objective Structured Clinical Examinations)—in which students are required to demonstrate some clinical skills at multiple 'stations' each lasting 10 minutes or so—have shown that a single 7-point global rating scale (e.g. 'How good a history was this?') consistently shows higher reliability and

validity than a detailed checklist of yes/no items (e.g. 'Did the student ask the chief complaint?'; Regehr et al. 1998).

2. Rubin et al. (1993), in rating abstracts submitted to a journal, found that the global rating was more reliable than the detailed checklist.

3. Norcini et al. (1990) investigated essay scores with the American Board of Internal Medicine and found that expert physician raters trained for 7 hours in applying detailed criterion checklists had a reliability of 0.36; raters using a single global rating with 3 hours' training had a reliability of 0.63.

4. Assessment of communication skills by standardized patients (people trained to simulate a disease) showed that a single global rating was more reliable than a 17-item checklist (Cohen et al. 1996).

5. The single-item EVGFP (Excellent/Very Good/Good/Fair/Poor) self-report scale correlates highly with longer quality of life instruments, and low scores (F and P) are an excellent predictor of mortality (Diehr et al. 2001).

6. Diener (1984) stated that single-item measures of subjective well-being or life satisfaction had acceptable temporal stability and validity when correlated with multi-item scales.

Why is this the case? Of course, the checklist acts as if behaviours are present or absent, and rates each on a dichotomous scale, which, as we discussed in Chapter 4, leads to loss of information. But while the loss may be severe at an individual item level, by the time 15 or 20 items are used to create a score, the number of items should more than compensate for the loss of reliability at the individual level. A more fundamental problem may be that many global concepts, like health or competence, may not be simply a sum of individual behaviours. As Regehr states regarding the discussion of competence assessment:

> many theorists in the field of competency evaluation are increasingly returning to the recognition that deconstruction of a competency can only proceed so far before the construct itself ceases to be meaningful. For the purposes of evaluating a competency, what is important is not that one performs a behaviour, but why and how one performs the behaviour. Doing the right thing for the wrong reasons or at the wrong time or without understanding its implications is not what we intended by the term 'competent'. And often failing to perform a certain behaviour is not a black mark of incompetence, but rather the hallmark of an expert who has rapidly discerned the nature of the situation and eschews redundancy. In short, competence is not doing everything every time; it is doing the appropriate things at the appropriate time. The evaluation of this cannot be and should not be objective. In fact, it is the very interpretative nature of such activity that makes it an expert performance. (2007, personal communication.)

In areas outside of education, single-item self-reports had the highest test–retest reliabilities when they tapped objective facts (e.g. mother's education, grade point average) and stable traits or behaviours (church attendance, educational goals), but, as would be expected, lower ones for unstable and situational aspects of one's life, such as satisfaction with social life (Dollinger and Malmquist 2009).

When is the global inferior to the sum of the items? Presumably, in circumstances where the overall construct really is defined by the items themselves—the fundamental axiom of classical psychometrics—then no single global item will adequately capture the construct. For example, it is difficult to envision that a single question like 'How intelligent are you?' would yield as valid information as an IQ test. For depression, it may be less clear; perhaps, 'How depressed are you?' really is nearly as good as an inventory of questions like 'How well do you sleep?' and 'Have you thought life is not worth living?' We cannot be definitive and must view this as a 'work in progress' with no immediate resolution. Nevertheless, the pervasive nature of the phenomenon suggests a role for further research.

Subscales

Our discussion so far has focussed on unidimensional scales—ones that measure a single attribute and result in a total score. Indeed, as we have said, unidimensionality is a key assumption underlying the use of KR-20, Cronbach's α, and McDonald's ω_t. It's not unusual, though, to find scales that have two or more subscales. These can arise in one of two ways. First, the author can decide at the design stage that there should be separate components to what is being measured. For example, the Student Alcohol Questionnaire (SAQ; Engs and Hanson 1994) was written to include subscales tapping drinking patterns, problems, knowledge, and attitudes. The other, perhaps more widespread way is for the developer or other researchers to use techniques such as factor analysis (described in Appendix B) to break the scale down into subscales. The 30-item Geriatric Depression Scale (Yesavage et al. 1983), for instance, was later found to consist of the five subscales of sad mood, lack of energy, lack of positive mood, agitation, and social withdrawal (Sheikh et al. 1991). This raises two questions: what is the relationship among the subscales and with the whole scale; and do the subscales add any meaningful information over and above the total score?

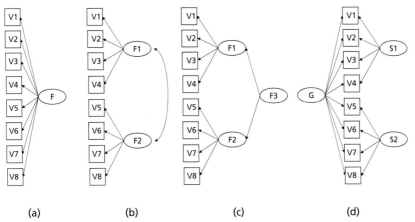

(a) (b) (c) (d)

Fig. 5.5 (a) Unidimensional scale; (b) two factors; (c) second-order model; (d) bifactor model. Note: error variances for each item have been omitted for clarity.

Relationship among the subscales

With regard to the first question, we can differentiate among four different types of scales. Using the notation we introduced in discussing Fig. 5.1, we can illustrate them as in Fig. 5.5, where the error terms associated with each item have been omitted to make the pictures less cluttered. Fig. 5.5(a) depicts a strictly *unidimensional* scale: all of the items are due to the one factor (F) and there are no subscales. Although each item is a reflection of only one common factor, Reise et al. (2010) point out that there are still other random and systematic factors that may also influence the response, such as fatigue, response sets, and reading proficiency. This is the model that many scale developers try to achieve, and that underlies many of the statistics used to assess scales, such as measures of internal consistency and item response theory (described in Chapter 12). However, it is rarely achieved in reality.

In the absence of strict unidimensionality, some other model must be proposed. Fig. 5.5(b) shows a *two-factor* scale. Items 1 through 4 belong to the first factor, and 5 through 8 to the second. In this figure, the two subscales are correlated with each other to some degree, as shown by the curved line between them with arrows at each end. The magnitude of the correlation depends on the type of rotation used in the factor analysis, and the nature of the constructs measured by the factors. If the correlation is low, it may not make sense to add the subscale scores into a total score, and the scale more resembles a multifactor inventory, which we will discuss later in this chapter. Note that in this model, there is no one overarching construct that the scale is measuring. This is most likely the case with the SAQ, where the four subscales are tapping different aspects of problem drinking, and it makes little sense to add the drinking patterns score to the knowledge one.

A more common model is shown in Fig. 5.5(c), called a *second-order* model. Here there is a global construct (F3) which itself is composed of two or more constructs (F1 and F2). For example, the broad construct of anxiety is often seen as consisting of four components: affective, behavioural, cognitive, and physiological. In turn, each of these lead to observable, measurable items (e.g. 'I am so restless that it is hard to keep still'). In this model, there are no direct relationships between the global construct and the individual items; the relationships are mediated through the specific factors. Furthermore, the specific factors are correlated because they all share a common factor.

Finally, a *bifactor* model is shown in Fig. 5.5(d). In this model, there are uncorrelated specific factors (S1 and S2) that give rise to individual items, as with the two-factor and second-order models. However, the global factor (G) also influences all of the items. For more than a century, psychologists have argued about the nature of intelligence. Spearman, who developed the technique of factor analysis, said there was a general factor (g) which underlies all intelligence (Thomson 1947), much like Fig. 5.5(a). In contrast, Thurstone proposed a model similar to Fig. 5.5(d)—specific factors (Ss) influencing individual aspects of intelligence, such as knowledge and fluid intelligence, in addition to the g factor (Deary et al. 2008). Thus, each item is a result of both a general and a specific factor. In other situations, the general factor can be a 'nuisance' one, such as response set or method variance (i.e. all of the measures are self-report scales).

Determining if a scale is unidimensional or has correlated subscales is relatively straightforward for those who are knowledgeable in factor analysis (and knowledgeable means more than simply following the default options in many programs, which are wrong for scale development; see Norman and Streiner 2014). However, deciding if a scale is better modelled with a second-order or bifactor model requires an even greater knowledge of the technique as well as of confirmatory factor analysis (CFA) or specialized software, and is therefore far beyond the scope of this book. For those who are interested, see Reise et al. (2010) and Reise (2012).

The contribution of the subscales

The second question that was raised was whether the subscales contribute any meaningful information over and above the total score. Simply because the scale developer set out to include subscales or a post hoc factor analysis was able to find some does not in and of itself guarantee that they add much (or anything) in their own right. For example, Cook et al. (2021) analysed the Pain Catastrophizing Scale (Sullivan et al. 1995), which was designed to have three subscales: helplessness, magnification, and rumination. However, they concluded that the scale was essentially unidimensional, and that the subscales added little information that the total score did not.

The good news is that there are indices to determine this. One is the Explained Common Variance (ECV; Reise 2012). It is the ratio of the variance explained by the common factor divided by the variance explained by the common factor plus all the specific factors. The closer the value is to 1, the more the variance is due simply to the common factor and the less important are the specific ones. An ECV of 0.5, for example, means that the variance of the scale can be equally divided between the common factor and the specific ones. One problem with the ECV, though, is that it could be high even if the general factor is weak, so neither the total score nor the subscale scores are strong. This problem is resolved with a variation of McDonald's ω, called *omega hierarchical* ω_H (Zinbarg et al. 2005). It, too, estimates the proportion of variance explained by the common factor with a metric that can be interpreted as a reliability coefficient. In a similar manner, the reliability of each subscale can be determined with yet another variant of ω, called *omega subscale* ω_S (Reise et al. 2013).

The bad news, again, is that the necessary parameters are derived from specialized software or CFA. However, those who are familiar with the R package (R Core Team 2020) can get step-by-step instructions for calculating ω, ω_H, and ω_S in Flora (2020).

Multifactor inventories

If the scale is one part of an inventory that has a number of other scales (usually called 'multifactor' or 'multidimensional' inventories), more sophisticated item analytic techniques are possible. The first is an extension of the item-total procedure, in which the item is correlated with its scale total, *and with the totals of all of the other scales*. The item should meet the criteria outlined earlier for a single index; additionally, this correlation should be higher than with any of the scales it is *not* included in.

The second technique is *factor analysis*. A very basic introduction to factor analysis is given in Appendix B. For more details presented in a non-mathematical fashion, see Norman and Streiner (2003); if you are comfortable with introductory statistics, see Norman and Streiner (2014); and if you love matrix algebra, see Harman (1976).

In an analogous manner, each item in a multifactorial test could be treated as an individual 'test'. Ideally, then, there should be as many factors as separate scales in the inventory. The item should 'load on' (that is - be correlated with) the scale it belongs to and not on any other one. If it loads on the 'wrong' factor or on two or more factors, then it is likely that it may be tapping something other than what the developer intended and should be either rewritten or discarded.

More recent developments in factor analysis allow the test-developer to specify beforehand what they think the final structure of the test should look like—called *confirmatory factor analysis*. The results show how closely the observed pattern corresponds (or fits) to this hypothesized pattern (Darton 1980). Although factor analysis has been used quite often with dichotomous items, this practice is highly suspect and can lead to quite anomalous results (Comrey 1978).

Finally, we should mention one practice that we believe should be strongly discouraged. As readers and reviewers of articles, we have often seen papers in which a scale is factor analysed and a number of subscales are identified. The authors then report coefficient α not only for each subscale, but also for the scale as a whole. Often, it is found that α for the entire scale is higher than for each of the subscales. This is totally illogical; if the scale is multidimensional, as the factor analysis would indicate, then its internal consistency should be low, and a high value of α is due solely to the fact that the whole scale, by definition, is longer than the subscales. If the authors truly believe that a high value of α indicates unidimensionality, then the scale should not be factor analysed in the first place.

When homogeneity does not matter

Our discussion of homogeneity of the scale was based on classical test theory. The assumption is that there is a 'universe' of items that tap a given trait or behaviour, and the scale is composed of a random subset of them. Another way to think of this is that the underlying trait (variously called a *hypothetical construct*, or just a *construct* in personality theory, or a *latent trait* in statistics—terms we will return to in Chapter 10) causes a number of observable manifestations, which are captured by the items. For example, anxiety may result in sweatiness, a feeling of impending doom, excessive worrying, irritability, sleep disturbance, difficulty concentrating, and a host of other symptoms, as shown in the left side of Fig. 5.6. Using the drawing conventions of structural equation modelling (Norman and Streiner 2014), the construct is shown as a circle and the observed (or *measured*) variables are shown as rectangles. The observed variables, in this case, are also called *effect indicators* because they reflect the effect of the construct (Bollen and Lennox 1991).

There are a number of implications of this. First, the items should all be correlated with each other to varying degrees. This means that the average inter-item correlation should be in the moderate range; item-total correlations should be between 0.20 and 0.80; and coefficient α should be somewhere between 0.70 and 0.90. Second, in order

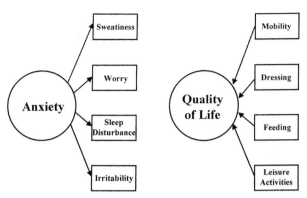

Fig. 5.6 A pictorial representation of effect indicators on the left and causal indicators on the right.

to measure the construct, the specific items do not really matter. That is, it is of little concern if we do not have an item about irritability or discard it because of wording or psychometric issues because there are many other, correlated items that are tapping anxiety (this is referred to as the *interchangeability* of items). We may be unhappy that the scale does not have an item that measures an important aspect of anxiety (an issue of face validity), but from the viewpoint of constructing a scale, the absence of that specific item is of no import. Finally, if we run a factor analysis, we should find a strong first factor, on which all of the items load.

However, there are situations where none of this holds. In the right side of Fig. 5.6, we again have a construct (in this case, quality of life, or QOL), but here the arrows point *to* it rather than *from* it. This reflects the fact that now the measured variables define the construct rather than being defined by it. In this case, the observed variables are referred to as *causal indicators* (Bollen and Lennox 1991), and the one in the circle is a *composite variable*. We encounter this situation in a number of other areas in addition to QOL indices. The most usual is a checklist of phenomena that are not causally re- lated to each other. For example, Holmes and Rahe (1967) constructed a scale of recent stressful life events, including such items as the death of a spouse, receiving a driving ticket, and buying a house. There is no reason to believe that if one event occurred, the others will, too. As another example, Goldberg's General Health Questionnaire (1979) consists of a number of health concerns, drawn from a wide range of disorders. Not only would it not be expected that all of the symptoms would be related to each other, but also some, such as mania and lethargy, may be mutually exclusive.

The implications of this are almost diametrically opposite to the ones we just dis- cussed. First, as the items are not expected to be correlated with each other, it is not appropriate to use the various indices of homogeneity, such as coefficient α, the mean inter-item correlation, and item-total correlations, nor to use statistics that are based on the assumption of homogeneity, such as factor analysis. Second, perhaps more im- portantly, the specific items *do* matter. If the Holmes and Rahe scale omitted divorce, for example, the total score would therefore underestimate a recently divorced person's level of stress. Further, because that item is not expected to be correlated with other ones, its effect will be missed entirely.

Thus, we are concerned with the internal consistency of a scale only when the measured variables are effect indicators, reflecting the effects of an underlying construct, but not when they are causal indicators, that define the construct by their presence. (For more on when α does and does not matter, see Streiner 2003a, 2003b.)

Putting it all together

In outline form, these are the steps involved in the initial selection of items:

1. Pre-test the items to ensure that they:
   a. are comprehensible to the target population
   b. are unambiguous, and
   c. ask only a single question.
2. Eliminate or rewrite any items which do not meet these criteria, and pre-test again.
3. Discard items endorsed by very few (or very many) subjects.
4. Ensure that the scale is unidimensional, using techniques such as factor analysis.
5. Check for the internal consistency of the scale using:

   a. item-total correlation:
      i. correlate each item with the scale total omitting that item
      ii. eliminate or rewrite any with Pearson r less than 0.20
      iii. rank order the remaining ones and select items from the entire range, not just those with the highest correlation, as this will result in too narrow a focus.

   OR

   b. coefficient α, KR-20, or ω :
      i. do not bother to calculate 'α if item eliminated'.
6. For multiscale questionnaires, check that the item is in the 'right' scale by:
   a. correlating it with the totals of all the scales, eliminating items that correlate more highly on scales other than the one it belongs to, or
   b. factor-analysing the questionnaire, eliminating items which load more highly on other factors than the one it should belong to.

Further reading

Writing items

Jackson, D.N. (1970). A sequential system for personality scale development. In *Current topics in clinical and community psychology* (ed. C.D. Spielberger), Vol. 2, pp. 61–96. Academic Press, New York.

Kornhauser, A. and Sheatsley, P.B. (1959). Questionnaire construction and interview procedure. In *Research methods in social relations* (Revised edn) (eds. C. Selltiz, M. Jahoda, M. Deutsch, and S.W. Cook), pp. 546–87. Holt, Rinehart and Winston, New York.

Krause, N. (2002). A comprehensive strategy for developing closed-ended survey items for use in studies of older adults. *Journal of Gerontology: Psychological and Social Sciences*, 57, S263–74.

Woodward, C.A. and Chambers, L.W. (1980). *Guide to questionnaire construction and question writing*. Canadian Public Health Association, Ottawa.

Homogeneity of items

Boyle, G.J. (1991). Does item homogeneity indicate internal consistency or item redundancy in psychometric scales? *Personality and Individual Differences*, **12**, 291–4.

Cortina, J.M. (1993). What is coefficient alpha? An examination of theory and applications. *Journal of Applied Psychology*, **78**, 98–104.

Flora, D.B. (2020). Your coefficient alpha is probably wrong, but which coefficient omega is right? *Advances in Methods and Practices in Psychological Science*, **3**, 484–501.

McNeish, D. (2018). Thanks coefficient alpha: We'll take it from here. *Psychological Methods*, **23**, 412–33.

Sijtsma, K. (2009). On the use, the misuse, and the very limited usefulness of Cronbach's alpha. *Psychometrika*, **74**, 107–20.

Streiner, D.L. (2003a). Starting at the beginning: An introduction of coefficient alpha and internal consistency. *Journal of Personality Assessment*, **80**, 99–103.

Streiner, D.L. (2003b). Being inconsistent about consistency: When coefficient alpha does and does not matter. *Journal of Personality Assessment*, **80**, 217–22.

Subscales

Reise, S.P., Moore, T.M., and Haviland, M.G. (2010). Bifactor models and rotations: Exploring the extent to which multidimensional data yield univocal scale scores. *Journal of Personality Assessment*, **92**, 544–59.

References

Allen, M.J. and Yen, W.M. (1979). *Introduction to measurement theory*. Brooks/Cole, Monterey, CA.

Anastasi, A. (1982). *Psychological testing* (5th edn). Macmillan, New York.

Armstrong, N. and Powell, J. (2009). Patient perspectives on health advice posted on Internet discussion boards: A qualitative study. *Health Expectations*, **12**, 313–20.

Bandalos, D.L. and Enders, C.K. (1996). The effects of non-normality and number of response categories on reliability. *Applied Measurement in Education*, **9**, 151–60.

Barnette J.J. (2000). Effects of stem and Likert response option reversals on survey internal consistency: If you feel the need, there is a better alternative to using those negatively worded stems. *Educational and Psychological Measurement*, **60**, 361–70.

Benson, J. and Hocevar, D. (1985). The impact of item phrasing on the validity of attitude scales for elementary school children. *Journal of Educational Measurement*, **22**, 231–40.

Bollen, K. and Lennox, R. (1991). Conventional wisdom on measurement: A structural equation perspective. *Psychological Bulletin*, **110**, 305–14.

Bonett, D.G. (2002). Sample size requirements for testing and estimating coefficient alpha. *Journal of Educational and Behavioral Statistics*, **27**, 335–40.

Boyle, C.M. (1970). Differences between patients' and doctors' interpretation of some common medical terms. *British Medical Journal*, **2**, 286–9.

Boyle, G.J. (1991). Does item homogeneity indicate internal consistency or item redundancy in psychometric scales? *Personality and Individual Differences*, **12**, 291–4.

Brennan, R.L. (2001). An essay on the history and future of reliability from the perspective of replications. *Journal of Educational Measurement*, **38**, 295–317.

Campbell, E.J.M., Scadding, J.G., and Roberts, R.S. (1979). The concept of disease. *British Medical Journal*, **ii**, 757–62.

Campostrini, S. and McQueen, D.V. (1993). The wording of questions in a CATI-based lifestyle survey: Effects of reversing polarity of AIDS-related questions in continuous data. *Quality & Quantity*, **27**, 157–70.

Carmines, E.G. and Zeller, R.A. (1979). *Reliability and validity assessment*. Sage, Thousand Oaks, CA.

Charter, R.A. (1997). Confidence interval procedures for retest, alternate form, and alpha coefficients. *Perceptual and Motor Skills*, **84**, 1488–90.

Chiavaroli, N. (2017). Negatively-worded multiple choice questions: An avoidable threat to validity. *Practical Assessment, Research, and Evaluation*, **22**, Article 3.

Clark, L.A. and Watson, D. (1995). Constructing validity: Basic issues in objective scale development. *Psychological Assessment*, **7**, 309–19.

Cohen, D.S., Colliver, J.A., Marcy, M.S., Fried, E.D., and Swartz, M.H. (1996). Psychometric properties of a standardized patient checklist and rating-scale form used to assess interpersonal and communication skills. *Academic Medicine*, **71**, S87–9.

Comrey, A.L. (1978). Common methodological problems in factor analysis. *Journal of Consulting and Clinical Psychology*, **46**, 648–59.

Cook, K.F., Mackey, S., Jung, C., and Darnall, B.D. (2021). The factor structure and subscale properties of the pain catastrophizing scale: Are there differences in the distinctions? *Pain Reports*, **6**, e909.

Cortina, J.M. (1993). What is coefficient alpha? An examination of theory and applications. *Journal of Applied Psychology*, **78**, 98–104.

Cronbach, L.J. (1951). Coefficient alpha and the internal structure of tests. *Psychometrika*, **16**, 297–334.

Cutilli, C.C. (2007). Health literacy in geriatric patients: An integrative review of the literature. *Orthopaedic Nursing*, **26**, 43–8.

Dale, E. and Eichholz, G. (1960). *Children's knowledge of words*. Ohio State University, Columbus, OH.

Darton, R.A. (1980). Rotation in factor analysis. *The Statistician*, **29**, 167–94.

Deary, I.J., Lawn, M., and Bartholomew, D.J. (2008). A conversation between Charles Spearman, Godfrey Thomson, and Edward L. Thorndike: The International Examinations Inquiry Meetings 1931–1938. *History of Psychology*, **11**, 122–42.

Diehr, P., Williamson, J., Patrick, D.L., Bild, D.E., and Burke, G.L. (2001). Patterns of self-rated health in older adults before and after sentinel health events. *Journal of the American Geriatric Society*, **49**, 36–44.

Diener, E. (1984). Subjective well-being. *Psychological Bulletin*, **95**, 542–75.

Dollinger, S.J. and Malmquist, D. (2009). Reliability and validity of single-item self-reports: With special relevance to college students' alcohol use, religiosity, study, and social life. *Journal of General Psychology*, **136**, 231–41.

Dowie, J. (2002a). Decision validity should determine whether a generic or condition-specific HRQOL measure is used in health care decisions. *Health Economics*, **11**, 1–8.

Dowie, J. (2002b). 'Decision validity ...': A rejoinder. *Health Economics*, **11**, 21–2.

Duhachek, A. and Iacobucci, D. (2004). Alpha's standard error (ASE): An accurate and precise confidence interval estimate. *Journal of Applied Psychology*, **89**, 792–808.

Dunn, T.J., Baguley, T., and Brunsden, V. (2014). From alpha to omega: A practical solution to the pervasive problem of internal consistency estimation. *British Journal of Psychology*, **105**, 399–412.

Enders, C.K. and Bandalos D.L. (1999). The effects of heterogeneous item distributions on reliability. *Applied Measurement in Education*, **12**, 133–50.

Engs, R.C. and Hanson, D.J. (1994). The Student Alcohol Questionnaire: An updated reliability of the drinking patterns, problems, knowledge, and attitude subscales. *Psychological Reports*, **74**, 12–14.

Fage-Butler, A.M. and Jensen, M.N. (2015). Medical terminology in online patient–patient communication: Evidence of high health literacy? *Health Expectations*, **19**, 643–53.

Falk, C.F. and Savalei, V. (2011). The relationship between unstandardized and standardized alpha, true reliability, and the underlying measurement model. *Journal of Personality Assessment*, **93**, 445–53.

Feldt, L.S. (1965). The approximate sampling distribution of Kuder–Richardson reliability coefficient twenty. *Psychometrika*, **30**, 357–70.

Feldt, L.S. (1993). The relationship between the distribution of item difficulties and test reliability. *Applied Measurement in Education*, **6**, 37–48.

Feldt, L.S. and Charter, R.A. (2003). Estimating the reliability of a test split into two parts of equal or unequal length. *Psychological Methods*, **8**, 102–9.

Ferketich, S. (1990). Focus on psychometrics: Internal consistency estimates of reliability. *Research in Nursing & Health*, **13**, 437–40.

Flemons, W.W. and Reimer, M.A. (1998). Development of a disease-specific health-related quality of life questionnaire for sleep apnea. *American Journal of Respiratory and Critical Care Medicine*, **158**, 494–503.

Flesch, R. (1948). A new readability yardstick. *Journal of Applied Psychology*, **32**, 221–33.

Flora, D.B. (2020). Your coefficient alpha is probably wrong, but which coefficient omega is right? *Advances in Methods and Practices in Psychological Science*, **3**, 484–501.

Fox, M.T., Sidani, S., and Streiner, D.L. (2007). Using standardized survey items with older adults hospitalized for chronic illness. *Research in Nursing and Health*, **30**, 468–81.

Fry, E.A. (1968). A readability formula that saves time. *Journal of Reading*, **11**, 513–16.

Gadermann, A.M., Guhn, M., and Zumbo, B.D. (2012). Estimating ordinal reliability for Likert-type and ordinal item response data: A conceptual, empirical, and practical guide. *Research & Evaluation*, **17**, 1–13.

Goldberg, D.P. (1979). *Manual of the general health questionnaire.* NFER, Windsor.

Graesser, A.C., Cai, Z., Louwerse, M.M., and Daniel, F. (2006). Question Understanding Aid (QUAID): A Web facility that tests question comprehensibility. *Public Opinion Quarterly*, **70**, 3–22.

Graham, J.M. (2006). Congeneric and (essentially) tau-equivalent estimates of score reliability. *Educational and Psychological Measurement*, **66**, 930–44.

Green, S.B. and Yang, Y. (2009). Commentary on coefficient alpha: A cautionary tale. *Psychometrika*, **74**, 121–35.

Gulliksen, H. (1945). The relation of item difficulty and inter-item correlation to test variance and reliability. *Psychometrika*, **10**, 79–91.

Harman, H.H. (1976). *Modern factor analysis* (3rd edn). University of Chicago Press, Chicago, IL.

Hattie, J. (1985). Methodology review: Assessing unidimensionality of tests and items. *Applied Psychological Measurement*, **9**, 139–64.

Havlicek, L.L. and Peterson, N.L. (1977). Effect of the violation of assumptions upon significance levels of the Pearson *r*. *Psychological Bulletin*, **84**, 373–7.

Henson, R.K. (2001). Understanding internal consistency reliability estimates: A conceptual primer on coefficient alpha. *Measurement and Evaluation in Counseling and Development*, **34**, 177–89.

Heppner, P.P., Kivlighan, D.M., and Wampold, B.E. (1992). *Research design in counseling.* Brooks/Cole, Pacific Grove, CA.

Holden, R.R., Fekken, G.C., and Jackson, D.N. (1985). Structured personality test item characteristics and validity. *Journal of Research in Personality*, **19**, 386–94.

Holmes, T.H. and Rahe, R.H. (1967). The Social Readjustment Rating Scale. *Journal of Psychosomatic Research*, **11**, 213–18.

Horan, P.M., DiStefano, C., and Motl, R.W. (2003). Wording effects in self-esteem scales: Methodological artifact or response style? *Structural Equation Modeling*, **10**, 435–55.

Jackson, D.N. (1970). A sequential system for personality scale development. In *Current topics in clinical and community psychology*, Vol. 2 (ed. C.D. Spielberger), pp. 61–96. Academic Press, New York.

Jackson, D.N. (1984). *Personality Research Form manual.* Research Psychologists Press, Port Huron, MI.

Kaplan, R.M. and Saccuzzo, D.P. (1997). *Psychological testing: Principles, applications, and issues* (4th edn). Brooks/Cole, Pacific Grove, CA.

Kline, P. (1979). *Psychometrics and psychology.* Academic Press, London.

Kline, P. (1986). *A handbook of test construction.* Methuen, London.

Kuder, G.F. and Richardson, M.W. (1937). The theory of estimation of test reliability. *Psychometrika*, **2**, 151–60.

Likert, R.A. (1932). A technique for the measurement of attitudes. *Archives of Psychology*, **140**, 44–53.

Lindwall, M., Barkoukis, V., Grano, C., Lucidi, F., Raudsepp, L., Liukkonen, J., et al. (2012). Method effects: the problem with negatively versus positively keyed items. *Journal of Personality Assessment*, **94**, 196–204.

Loevinger, J. (1954). The attenuation paradox in test theory. *Psychological Bulletin*, **51**, 493–504.

Lord, F.M. and Novick, M.R. (1968). *Statistical theory of mental test scores.* Addison-Wesley, Reading, MA.

Mangione, C.M., Lee, P.P., Pitts, J., Gutierrez, P., Berry, S., and Hays, R.D. (1998). Psychometric properties of the National Eye Institute Visual Function Questionnaire (NEI-VFQ). NEI-VFQ field test investigators. *Archives of Ophthalmology*, **116**, 1496–504.

McDonald, R.P. (1999). *Test theory: A unified approach.* Erlbaum: Mahwah, NJ.

McLaughlin, G.H. (1969). SMOG grading: A new readability formula. *Journal of Reading*, **12**, 639–46.

McNeish, D. (2018). Thanks coefficient alpha: We'll take it from here. *Psychological Methods*, **23**, 412–33.

Melnick, S.A. and Gable, R.K. (1990). The use of negative stems: A cautionary note. *Educational Research Quarterly*, **14**(3), 31–6.

Morin, C.M. (1993). *Insomnia: Psychological assessment and management*. Guilford Press, New York.

Nevo, B. (1985). Face validity revisited. *Journal of Educational Measurement*, **22**, 287–93.

Norcini, J.J., Diserens, D., Day, S.C., Cebul, R.D., Schwartz, J.S., Beck, L.H., et al. (1990). The scoring and reproducibility of an essay test of clinical judgment. *Academic Medicine*, **65**, S39–40.

Norman, G.R. and Streiner, D.L. (2003). *PDQ statistics* (3rd edn). B.C. Decker, Toronto.

Norman, G.R. and Streiner, D.L. (2014). *Biostatistics: The bare essentials* (4th edn). PMPH USA, Shelton, CT.

Nunnally, J.C., Jr. (1970). *Introduction to psychological measurement*. McGraw-Hill, New York.

Nunnally, J.C., Jr. (1978). *Psychometric theory* (2nd edn). McGraw-Hill, New York.

Payne, S.L. (1954). *The art of asking questions*. Princeton University Press, Princeton, NJ.

Peters, G.Y. (2014). The alpha and the omega of scale reliability and validity: Why and how to abandon Cronbach's alpha and the route towards more comprehensive assessment of scale quality. *European Health Psychologist*, **16**, 56–69.

Ponterotto, J.G. and Ruckdeschel, D. (2007). An overview of coefficient alpha and a reliability matrix for estimating adequacy of internal consistency coefficients with psychological research measures. *Perceptual and Motor Skills*, **105**, 997–1014.

R Core Team (2020). *R: A language and environment for statistical computing*. R Foundation for Statistical Computing, Vienna, Austria.

Radloff, L.S. (1977). The CES-D scale: A self-report depression scale for research in the general population. *Applied Psychological Measurement*, **1**, 385–401.

Raykov, T. (1997a). Estimation of composite reliability for congeneric measures. *Applied Psychological Measurement*, **21**, 173–84.

Raykov, T. (1997b). Scale reliability, Cronbach's coefficient alpha, and violations of essential tau-equivalence with fixed congeneric components. *Multivariate Behavioral Research*, **32**, 329–53.

Regehr, G., MacRae, H.M., Reznick, R.K., and Szalay, D. (1998). Comparing the psychometric properties of checklists and global rating scales for assessing performance in an OSCE-format examination. *Academic Medicine*, **73**, 993–7.

Reise, S.P. (2012). The rediscovery of bifactor measurement models. *Multivariate Behavioral Research*, **47**, 667–96.

Reise, S.P., Moore, T.M., and Haviland, M.G. (2010). Bifactor models and rotations: Exploring the extent to which multidimensional data yield univocal scale scores. *Journal of Personality Assessment*, **92**, 544–59.

Reise, S.P., Bonifay, W.E., and Haviland, M.G. (2013). Scoring and modeling psychological measures in the presence of multidimensionality. *Journal of Personality Assessment*, **95**, 129–40.

Reiser, M., Wallace, M., and Schuessler, K. (1986). Direction of wording effects in dichotomous social life feeling items. *Sociological Methodology*, **16**, 1–25.

Rhemtulla, M., Brosseau-Liard, P.É., and Savalei, V. (2012). When can categorical variables be treated as continuous? A comparison of robust continuous and categorical SEM estimation methods under suboptimal conditions. *Psychological Methods*, **17**, 354–73.

Rubin, H.R., Redelmeier, D.A., Wu, A.W., and Steinberg, E.P. (1993). How reliable is peer review of scientific abstracts? Looking back at the 1991 annual meeting of the Society of General Internal Medicine. *Journal of General Internal Medicine*, **8**, 255–8.

Samora, J., Saunders, L., and Larson, R.F. (1961). Medical vocabulary knowledge among hospital patients. *Journal of Health and Human Behavior*, **2**, 83–92.

Schmitt, N. (1996). Uses and abuses of coefficient alpha. *Psychological Assessment*, **8**, 350–3.

Schriesheim, C.A. and Hill, K.D. (1981). Controlling acquiescence response bias by item reversals: The effect on questionnaire validity. *Educational and Psychological Measurement*, **41**, 1101–14.

Seligman, A.W., McGrath, N.E., and Pratt, L. (1957). Level of medical information among clinic patients. *Journal of Chronic Diseases*, **6**, 497–509.

Sheikh, J.I., Yesavage, J.A., Brooks, J.O. Friedman, L., Gratzinger, P., Hill, R.D., *et al.* (1991). Proposed factor structure of the Geriatric Depression Scale. *International Psychogeriatrics*, **3**, 23–8.

Sherbino, J., Kulsegaram, K., Worster, A., and Norman, G.R. (2013) The reliability of encounter cards to assess the CanMEDS roles. *Advances in Health Sciences Education: Theory and Practice*, **18**, 987–96.

Sliter, K.A. and Zickar, M.J. (2013). An IRT examination of the psychometric functioning of negatively worded personality items. *Educational and Psychological Measurement*, **74**, 214–26.

Streiner, D.L. (2003a). Starting at the beginning: An introduction of coefficient alpha and internal consistency. *Journal of Personality Assessment*, **80**, 99–103.

Streiner, D.L. (2003b). Being inconsistent about consistency: When coefficient alpha does and does not matter. *Journal of Personality Assessment*, **80**, 217–22.

Sullivan, M.J.L., Bishop, S.R., and Pivik, J. (1995). The Pain Catastrophizing Scale: Development and validation. *Psychological Assessment*, **7**, 524–32.

Tamir, P. (1993). Positive and negative multiple choice items: How different are they? *Studies in Educational Evaluation*, **19**, 311–25.

Taylor, W.L. (1957). 'Cloze' readability scores as indices of individual differences in comprehension and aptitude. *Journal of Applied Psychology*, **41**, 19–26.

Thomson, G. (1947). Charles Spearman, 1863–1945. *Obituary Notices of Fellows of the Royal Society*, **5**, 373–85.

Wiggins, J.S. and Goldberg, L.R. (1965). Interrelationships among MMPI item characteristics. *Educational and Psychological Measurement*, **25**, 381–97.

Yesavage, J.A., Brink, T.L., Rose, T.L., Lum, O., Huang, V., Adey, M.B., *et al.* (1983). Development and validation of a geriatric depression screening scale: A preliminary report. *Journal of Psychiatric Research*, **17**, 37–49.

Zinbarg, R.E., Revelle, W., Yovel, I., and Li, W. (2005). Cronbach's alpha, Revelle's β, and McDonald's ω_H: Their relations with each other and two alternative conceptualizations of reliability. *Psychometrika*, **70**, 123–33.

Chapter 6

Biases in responding

Introduction to biases in responding

When an item is included in a questionnaire or scale, it is usually under the assumption that the respondent will answer honestly. However, there has been considerable research showing that there are numerous factors which may influence a response, making it a less than totally accurate reflection of reality. The magnitude and seriousness of the problem depends very much on the nature of the instrument and the conditions under which it is used. At the extreme, questionnaires may end up over- or underestimating the prevalence of a symptom or disease; or the validity of the scale may be seriously jeopardized.

Some scale developers bypass the entire problem of responder bias by asserting that their instruments are designed merely to differentiate between groups. In this situation, the truth or falsity of the answer is irrelevant, as long as one group responds in one direction more often than does another group. According to this position, responding 'yes' to an item such as 'I like sports magazines' would not be interpreted as accurately reflecting the person's reading preferences. The item's inclusion in the test is predicated solely on the fact that one group of people *says* it likes these magazines more often than do other groups. This purely empirical approach to scale development reached its zenith in the late 1940s and 1950s, but may still be found underlying the construction of some measures.

However, with the gradual trend towards instruments which are more grounded in theory, this approach to scale construction has become less appealing. The objective now is to reduce bias in responding as much as possible. In this chapter, we will examine some of the sources of error, what effects they may have on the scale, and how to minimize them.

The differing perspectives

The people who develop a scale, those who use it in their work, and the ones who are asked to fill it out, all approach scales from different perspectives, for different reasons, and with differing amounts of information about the instrument. For the person administering the instrument, a specific answer to a given question is often of little interest. That item may be just one of many on a scale, where the important information is the total score, and there is little regard for the individual items which have contributed to it. In other situations, the responses may be aggregated across dozens or hundreds of subjects so that the individual person's answers are buried in a mass of those from other anonymous subjects. Further, what the questioner wants is 'truth'—did the person have this symptom or not, ever engage in this behaviour or not, and so forth. The clinician cannot help the patient or the researcher discover important facts, unless honest answers are given. Moreover, the assessment session is perceived, at least in the assessors' minds, as non-judgemental and their attitude as disinterested. This may appear so obvious to scale developers that it never occurs to them that the respondents may perceive the situation from another angle.

The respondents' perspectives, however, are often quite different. They are often unaware that the individual items are ignored in favour of the total score. Consider the situation when a measure is completed by pencil and paper (a situation which today is as rare as hen's teeth). Even when told that their responses will be scored by a computer, it is quite common to find marginal notes explaining or elaborating their answers. Thus, it appears that respondents treat each item as important in its own right and often believe that their answers will be read and evaluated by another person.

Additionally, their motivation may include the very natural tendency to be seen in a good light; or to be done with this intrusion in their lives as quickly as possible; or to ensure that they receive the help they feel they need. As we will discuss, these and other factors may influence the response given.

Nichols et al. (1989) differentiate between two classes of problematic responses: *content responsive faking* and *content nonresponsivity*. In the former, the responses reflect the question but they are not completely accurate, either intentionally (e.g. faking good or faking bad) or unintentionally (social desirability bias). As the name implies, content nonresponsivity means responding without regard to the content of the item (random or careless responding). Irrespective of the cause, these answers have serious implications for scale development. They introduce error variance, which attenuates correlations with other variables; reduces internal consistency; and may result in erroneous conclusions from factor analysis (Meade and Craig 2012).

Answering questions: the cognitive requirements

Asking a simple question, such as 'How strongly do you feel that you should never spank a child?', requires the respondent to undertake a fairly complex cognitive task. Depending on the theory, there are four (e.g. Tourangeau 1984) or five (Schwarz and Oyserman 2001) steps that people must go through, with an opportunity for bias to creep (or storm) in at each step.

1. *Understanding the question.* The issue here is whether the respondent's interpretation of the question is the same as the test designer's. In Chapter 5, we discussed some methods to try to minimize the difference: by avoiding ambiguous terms and double-barrelled questions, using simple language, and pre-testing in order to determine what the respondent thinks is being asked. Even so, other factors may influence the interpretation. For example, one person may interpret 'spank' to mean any physical action that causes the child to cry; while another may feel that it pertains only to punishment and that slapping a child's hand if he puts it too near the stove is done for the child's protection and does not constitute spanking. The item format itself may affect how the person interprets the question (Schwarz 1999). For instance, if an item asks how often the person gets 'really irritated' and one response

alternative is 'less than once a year', the respondent may infer that the question refers only to major annoyances, since it is highly unlikely that minor ones would occur that infrequently. This may or may not be what the questionnaire developer had in mind, though. Similarly, giving the person a long time frame, such as 'over the past year', would lead the respondent to think the item is referring to more serious events than a shorter time frame of 'over the past week' (Winkielman et al. 1998).

2. *Recalling the relevant behaviour, attitude, or belief.* Once the respondents have read and understood (or even misunderstood) the item, they must recall how often they have done a specific action, or how they felt about something. Questionnaire developers vastly overestimate people's ability to recall past events. Study after study has repeatedly shown for example that people are poor at recalling major health events (Allen et al., 1954; Means et al., 1989), including those resulting in hospitalization (Cannell et al. 1965), even as recently in the year following the event. Poor recall is particularly problematic for measures that use time frames, such as 12-months, from which to determine prevalence of disease; for example, psychiatric disorders like depression. For this reason we (and others) have recommended doing away with the concept of lifetime prevalence altogether (Streiner et al. 2009).

A more general issue is whether adults can recall events from the distant past or how they felt as children. Again, the findings are not encouraging. In a large meta-analysis of studies comparing prospective and retrospective measures of child maltreatment, Baldwin et al. (2019) found, in general, very poor agreement. It was highest for childhood separation from parents ($\kappa = 0.83$); low for physical and sexual abuse ($\kappa = 0.17$ and 0.16); and lowest for neglect ($\kappa = 0.09$). Similarly, reports of liking homework changed from 28 per cent as reported when they were 14 years of age to 58 per cent reported by the same men when they were 48 years old; and reports of being physically disciplined dropped from 82 per cent in adolescence to 33 per cent reported in adulthood (Offer et al. 2000). They concluded that recall should be viewed as 'existential reconstructions' rather than as accurate memories of one's past.

Problems with recall can arise in two different ways: forgetting the event occurred at all or allocating the wrong time period to it. *Telescoping*, in which an event that occurred before the time period is remembered as occurring within the period, is a common example of the latter. If a person is asked how many times she saw a doctor in the last 6 months, she may recall visits that happened 7 or 8 months previously (Clarke et al. 2008).

Drawing on cognitive theory (e.g. Linton 1975; Neisser 1986), Means et al. (1989) hypothesized that, especially for chronic conditions which result in recurring events, people have a 'generic memory' for a group of events and medical contacts and therefore have difficulty recalling specific instances. Further, autobiographical memory is not organized by events, such as being ill, drinking too much, or going to the gym. Rather, there is a hierarchy with *extended periods* at the top (e.g. 'when I worked at Company X' or 'during my first marriage'). Under this are *summarized events*, which reflect repeated behaviours (e.g. 'I worked out a lot during that time'), and *specific events* are at the bottom (Schwarz and Oyserman 2001). Thus, asking respondents how often they saw a physician in the last year or to recall how they felt 6 months ago does not correspond to the manner in which these behaviours are stored in memory, and answers to such questions should be viewed with some degree of scepticism. As Schwarz and Oyserman (2001) state, 'Many recall questions would never be asked if researchers first tried to answer them themselves' (p. 141).

The problem with recall is even more acute with disorders whose symptoms fluctuate over time, such as arthritis, depression, or multiple sclerosis. Often, pain questionnaires, for instance, ask the person to indicate the magnitude of the least, worst, and average pain over the past day or week. The problem is that people cannot recall this, and the ratings that are recorded are heavily influenced by the most salient episode (i.e. the worst pain) and the pain experience just prior to completing the scale (e.g. Bryant 1993; Eich et al. 1985; Jamison et al. 1989). When recall of 'average' pain was compared with pain diaries, it was found that the reported intensity correlated more highly with the average levels experienced during episodes of pain than to overall averages (Stone et al. 2000, 2004); that is, patients ignored times when they did not have any pain, thus biasing the average upwards. Complicating the picture even further, while people overestimate their pain when it is fluctuating, they may underestimate it when it is stable (Salovey et al. 1993).

3. *Inference and estimation.* Because questionnaires rarely ask for events to be recalled in the same way that they are stored in memory, respondents must use a number of inference and estimation strategies. One is called *decomposition and extrapolation* (Schwarz and Oyserman 2001). If a person is asked how many times in the last year they saw a dentist, they may remember that they went twice in the last 3 months. Then they would try to determine whether this was unusual or represented a typical pattern. If the latter, then they would multiply the number by four, and report that they went eight times. There are two possible sources of error: the recall over a shorter period and the determination of how usual this was. Most people overestimate how often rare behaviours occur, and underestimate frequent actions (e.g. Sudman et al. 1996), and multiplying the two only compounds the error. Another manifestation of decomposition and extrapolation is that numerical answers are often given in multiples of 5 or 10, and estimates of elapsed time usually correspond to calendar divisions (i.e. multiples of 7 days or 4 weeks). A beautiful example of this end-digit bias comes from an article by Norcross et al. (1997), which looked at, among other things, the publication record of clinical psychologists. The respondents' recall of the number of articles they published is shown in Fig. 6.1.

There is a steep, relatively smooth decline until 9, and then peaks at multiples of 10, and secondary peaks at multiples of 5. By the same token, other end-digits are conspicuous by their absence; mainly 2, 3, and 7, which is fairly universal. Huttenlocher et al. (1990) found that when physicians reported how many times a patient had visited, they use the actual number up to about 5, then round by 5s up to about 20 visits, and then round by 10s. When asked to report on how many cigarettes were smoked each day, there was a very strong tendency to report the numbers in multiples of 5. The most pronounced peak was at 20, which is the number of cigarettes in one pack. It appeared as if the respondents were not recalling the number of cigarettes, but the number of packs consumed daily (Shiffman 2009).

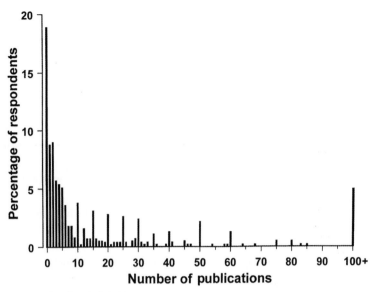

Fig. 6.1 Example of end-digit bias.
Reproduced from Norcross, J.C. et al., Clinical psychologist in the 1990s: II, *The Clinical Psychologist*, Volume 50, Issue 3, pp. 4–11, Copyright © 1997 American Psychological Association, reprinted with permission.

We find a similar phenomenon in demography, known as *age heaping*. When individuals are asked to report their age (or date of birth) in population surveys, it is not unusual to find more ages ending in 0 or 5 than would be expected. Of course, this may be due to rounding based on poor recall or a conscious effort to report one's age in a more favourable light ('I am 43, but I prefer to believe I am 40'). The latter case may be a case of 'faking good' (described in 'Social desirability and faking good'). There is actually a measure—Whipple's index—which can be used to assess the degree to which age heaping is present in a sample (e.g. Spoorenberg 2007). Another inferential strategy, which bedevils researchers and clinicians trying to assess improvement or deterioration, is a person's *subjective theory of stability and change*. A very common question, both on questionnaires and in the clinical interview, is 'How are you feeling now compared to the last time I saw you?' (or '... the last time you filled out this scale?'). The reality is that people do not remember how they felt 3 or 6 months ago. Rather, they use their implicit theory (Ross 1989) of whether or not they have changed or the treatment worked (Schwarz and Oyserman 2001, p. 144):

> Respondents may reconstruct their earlier behaviors as having been more problematic than they were, apparently confirming the intervention's success—provided they believe the intervention was likely to help them (a belief that entails a subject theory of change) ... To assess actual change, we need to rely on before–after, or treatment–control comparisons, and if we have missed asking the right question before the intervention, little can be done after the fact to make up for the oversight.

We discuss this more fully later in this chapter in 'Biases related to the measurement of change'.

4. *Mapping the answer onto the response alternatives.* Having arrived at some estimate of the frequency of a behaviour, or the strength of an attitude, the person now has to translate that to map onto the scale used in the questionnaire. Here we encounter the factors discussed in Chapter 4—how people interpret vague adjectives such as 'very often' or 'frequently', the effects of the numbers placed on the line, the number of response categories, and so forth. The issue is that the response format does not correspond to how respondents originally conceptualized their answer in their own minds. Their response, either orally or by a mark on an answer sheet, represents a 'translation' from their own words into the researcher's; and, as with any translation, something gets lost.

5. *Editing the answer.* What the respondent actually thinks and what they are willing to tell the researcher are not necessarily the same thing. As outlined in the section on The Different Perspectives, the researcher and the respondent have different perspectives and agendas. How and why respondents may edit their answers is the topic for the remainder of this chapter.

Optimizing and satisficing

The hope of the scale developer is that all of the respondents will perform the five steps outlined earlier in a careful and comprehensive manner. Drawing on economic decision-making (Simon 1957), Krosnick (1991; Krosnick and Alwin 1987) uses the term *optimizing* to describe this ideal way of answering. However, as we outlined in the previous section on the different perspectives, the aims of the person who developed the scale and those of the person filling it out are not the same. Especially if the questionnaire is long, the items require considerable cognitive effort to answer them, and the purpose of filling it out is seemingly trivial or irrelevant to the respondents, they may adopt a strategy which allows them to complete the task without much effort. Using another economic decision-making term, Simon calls this *satisficing* (probably a blend of 'satisfy' and 'suffice'): giving an answer which is satisfactory (i.e. a box on the form is filled in), but not optimal. He describes six ways in which satisficing may occur. He refers to the first two as 'weak' forms, in that some cognitive effort is required; whereas the last four are 'strong' types of satisficing, since little or no thought is required.

First, the person may select the first response option that seems reasonable. If the options are presented in written form, the respondent will opt for the one that occurs first, and give only cursory attention to those which appear later. This is referred to as *primacy*. Conversely, if the options are given verbally, it is easier to remember those which came most recently, that is, those towards the end of the list—what is referred to as *recency*. In either case, the choices in the middle get short shrift. Awareness of this phenomenon has led some organizations to minimize its effects in balloting. Recognizing that most voters do not know the people running for office, except for the long and often boring (and unread) position statements they write, and that the task of choosing among them is difficult and seemingly irrelevant for many voters, there is a danger that those whose names are closer to the top of the ballot will receive more votes. Consequently, organizations have adopted the strategy of using multiple forms of the ballot, with the names randomized differently on each version.

A second form of satisficing consists of simply agreeing with every statement, or answering 'true' or 'false' to each item. We will return to this bias later in this chapter, in the section on yea-saying and acquiescence.

Third, the person may endorse the status quo. This is not usually a problem when asking people about their physical or psychological state or about behaviours they may or may not do, but can be an issue when enquiring about their attitudes towards some policy. Having been asked their opinion about, for instance, whether certain procedures should be covered by universal health insurance or if we should allow *in vitro* fertilization for single women, it is easier to say 'keep things as they are' rather than considering the effects of change.

A fourth strategy is to select one answer for the first item, and then to use this response for all of the subsequent questions. This is a particular problem when the response options consist of visual analogue or Likert scales keyed in the same direction so that the person simply has to go down the page in a straight line, putting check marks on each line. The trade-off is that changing the options for each question may minimize this tendency (or at least make it more obvious to the scorer), but it places an additional cognitive demand on the subject, which further fosters satisficing.

Fifth, the person may simply say 'I do not know' or place a mark in a neutral point along a Likert scale. In some circumstances, it may be possible to eliminate these alternatives, such as by using a scale with an even number of boxes, as we described in Chapter 4. However, these may be valid options for some optimizing subjects, and their removal may make their responses less valid.

The last way a person may satisfice is by mentally flipping a coin, that is, to choose a response at random. Krosnick (1991) believes that this is the 'method of last resort', and used only when the previous ones cannot be.

A review of 141 articles found that the most common forms of satisficing were to say 'don't know' or 'no opinion' (27 per cent), followed by selecting the first option (23 per cent), and using the middle alternative (18 per cent). It concluded that primacy, recency, and no-opinion were used most often when the task was difficult, the respondent's ability was low, and motivation was poor (Roberts et al. 2019).

There are two general ways to minimize satisficing. First, the task should be kept as simple as possible. At the most superficial level, this means that the questions should be kept short and the words easy to understand—points covered in Chapter 5. Further, the mental processes required to answer the question should not be overly demanding. For example, it is easier to say how you currently feel about something than how you felt about it in the past; less difficult to remember what you did for the past month than over the past year; and how you feel about one thing rather than comparing two or more, since each requires its own retrieval and evaluation process. Last, the response options should not be overly complex, but must include all possibilities. If there are even a few questions which do not have appropriate answers for some participants, they may stop trying to give the optimal answer and start satisficing.

The second way to decrease satisficing is to maintain the motivation of the respondents. Recognize that motivation is usually higher at the start of a task and begins to flag as the task gets longer and more onerous. Consequently, instruments should be kept as short as possible. (However, as we will see in Chapter 13, 'short' can be up to 100 items or 10 pages.) Another way is to make the respondents accountable for their answers; that is, they feel that they may have to justify what they said. This can be accomplished by asking them to explain why they gave the answer which they did. Last, motivation can be provided externally, by rewarding them for their participation; we will also discuss this further in Chapter 13.

Social desirability and faking good

A person's answer to an item like 'During an average day, how much alcohol do you consume?' or 'I am a shy person' may not correspond to what an outside observer would say about that individual. In many cases, people give a socially desirable answer: the drinker may minimize their daily intake, or the retiring person may deny they are shy, believing it is better to be outgoing. The tension is between how the person wants to be perceived and an honest (accurate) answer—what Austin (1962) described in terms of constative (how things are) and performative (what we desire things to be) language.

As *social desirability* (SD) is commonly conceptualized, the subject is not deliberately trying to deceive or lie; they are unaware of this tendency to put the best foot forward (Edwards 1957). When the person *is* aware and is intentionally attempting to create a false-positive impression, it is called *faking good*. Other terms have been proposed for these phenomena, which are probably more descriptive. SD is sometimes referred to as *self-deception*, reflecting that it is not a conscious attempt to deceive others, but how a person (mis)perceives themself. Faking good, on the other hand, is also called *impression management*, indicating that it deliberately tries to influence how others see the person. Paulhus (2002), one of the leading theoreticians in the area, adds another dimension: whether the self-deception and impression management involves having an inflated view of one's social and intellectual status ('egoistic bias'), or of one's moral qualities ('moralistic bias'). Thus, he postulates four forms of bias: egoistic self-deception and egoistic impression management; and moralistic self-deception and moralistic impression management. Although conceptually different, these various forms of the bias create similar problems for the scale developer, and have similar solutions.

SD depends on many factors: the individual, the person's gender and cultural background, the specific question, and the context in which the item is asked; for example, face-to-face interview versus an anonymous questionnaire. Sudman and Bradburn (1982) derived a list of threatening topics which are prone to SD bias. Among the 'socially desirable' ones apt to lead to over-reporting are being a good citizen (e.g. registering to vote and voting, knowing issues in public debates), being well informed and cultured (e.g. reading newspapers and books, using the library, attending cultural activities), and having fulfilled moral and social responsibilities (e.g. giving to charity, helping friends and relatives). Conversely, there will be under-reporting of 'socially undesirable' topics, such as certain illnesses and disabilities (e.g. cancer, sexually trans-mitted diseases, mental disorders), illegal and non-normative behaviours (e.g. com-mitting a crime, tax evasion, use of drugs and alcohol, non-marital sex), and financial status (income, savings, having expensive possessions).

It is illustrative to give three examples of SD bias. Two of them arose from studies involving self-reported food intake. In the National Diet and Nutrition Survey (Gregory 2005) in the United Kingdom, 48 per cent of women and 29 per cent of men reported low-energy intake—an amount of under-reporting of what they ate that 'causes major problems in the interpretation of dietary data' (Cook et al. 2000, p. 616). The second example comes from the Women's Health Initiative (Anderson et al. 2003), a 15-year study involving over 161,000 women in the United States and costing around $700,000,000. Despite the care taken to pre-test instruments, the dietary data, which were expected to show a relationship between fat intake and disorders such as breast cancer, are useless because of a similar SD bias affecting what was recorded. On average, participants weighed 170 pounds (77 kg) at the start of the study and said they were eating 1,800 calories per day. Fifteen years later, they weighed about 2 pounds (1 kg) less on a reported daily intake of 1,500 calories. Such calorically restricted diets would surely have resulted in a much greater loss of weight. Third, over two-thirds of people with type 1 diabetes over- or under-reported glucose levels, most likely in order to appear to have their levels under tighter control than they actually were (Mazze et al. 1984). In all of these examples, the participants had nothing to gain by falsifying their records, except to appear healthier and more compliant than they actually were.

Another aspect of SD bias is that, as Smith (cited in Berke 1998, p. 1) quipped, 'The average person believes he is a better person than the average person'. This was said in the context of a poll conducted during the President Clinton sex scandal in the late 1990s. People were asked how interested they were in the story, and how interested they felt others were. The results are shown in Fig. 6.2 and speak for themselves—others are much more déclassé than are the respondents.

A debate has raged for many years over whether SD is a trait (whereby the person responds in the desirable direction irrespective of the context) or a state (dependent more on the question and the setting). While the jury is still out, two suggestions have emerged: SD should be minimized whenever possible, and the person's propensity to respond in this manner should be assessed whenever it may affect how they answer (e.g. Anastasi 1982; Jackson 1984).

If answers are affected by SD, the validity of the scale may be jeopardized for two reasons. First, if the object of the questionnaire is to gather factual information, such as the prevalence of a disorder, behaviour, or feeling, then the results obtained may not reflect the true state of affairs. The prime example of this would be items tapping socially sanctioned behaviours relating to sex and abortions; but SD may also affect re-sponses to embarrassing, unpopular, or 'unacceptable' feelings, such as anger towards one's parents, or admitting to voting for the party that lost the last election (or won, depending on recent events). In a similar fashion, the occurrence of positive or socially desired behaviours may be overestimated. For example, Rosse et al. (1998) found that compared to people who were already employed, job applicants scored significantly

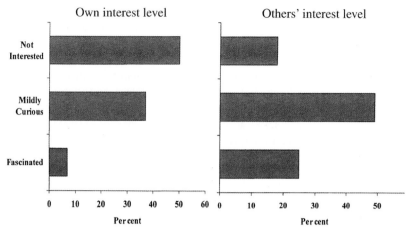

Fig. 6.2 One's own and others' interest in President Clinton's sex life.
Source: data from Keating Holland/CNN, Poll: Clinton scandal has not taught young Americans it's OK to lie, February 17, 1999, Copyright © 1999 Cable News Network, Inc. All Rights Reserved. Available from <http://edition.cnn.com/allpolitics/stories/1999/02/17/poll/>.

higher on desirable traits, such as extroversion, agreeableness, and conscientiousness, and lower on negative ones, such as neuroticism.

The second problem, to which we will return in Chapter 10, involves what is called the 'discriminant validity' of a test. Very briefly, if a scale correlates highly with one factor (e.g. SD), then that limits how highly it can correlate with the factor which the scale was designed to assess. Further, the theoretical rationale of the scale is undermined, since the most parsimonious explanation of what the test is measuring would be 'social desirability', rather than anything else.

The SD of an item can be assessed in a number of ways. One method is to correlate each item on a new instrument with a scale specifically designed to measure SD. Jackson (1970) has developed an index called the *Differential Reliability Index* (DRI), defined as:

$$DRI = \sqrt{\left(r_{is}^2 - r_{id}^2\right)}$$

where r_{is} is the item-scale correlation and r_{id} is the item -SD correlation.

The DRI in essence is the difference between the item -total correlation and the item -SD correlation. Any item which is more highly 'saturated' on SD than with its scale total will result in a DRI approaching zero (note that if r_{id} is ever larger than r_{is}, DRI is undefined). Such an item should be either rewritten or discarded.

A number of scales have been developed to specifically measure the tendency to give socially desirable answers. These include the Crowne and Marlowe (1960) *Social Desirability Scale*, which is perhaps the most widely used such instrument; the *Desirability* (DY) scale on the *Personality Research Form* (Jackson 1984); one developed by Edwards (1957); and most recently, the *Balanced Inventory of Desirable Responding* (BIDR) of Paulhus (1994). These scales most often consist of items that are socially approved, but rarely occur in real life, such as 'I know everything about the candidates before I vote' or 'My manners are as good at home as when I eat out'. These are sometimes given in conjunction with other scales, not so much in order to develop a new instrument, but to see if SD is affecting the subject's responses. If it is not, then there is little to be concerned about; if so, though, there is little that can be done after the fact except to exercise caution in interpreting the results. Unfortunately, the correlations among the SD scales are low. Holden and Fekken (1989) found that the Jackson and Edwards scales correlated 0.71, but the correlation between the Jackson and Crowne–Marlowe scales was only 0.27 and between the Edwards and Crowne–Marlowe scales was 0.26. They interpreted their factor analysis of these three scales to mean that the Jackson and Edwards scales measured 'a sense of one's own general capability', and the Crowne–Marlowe scale tapped 'interpersonal sensitivity'. Similar results were found by Paulhus (1983, 1984). He believes that his factor analysis of various scales indicates that the Edwards scale taps the more covert tendency of SD (what he calls 'self-deception'), while the Crowne–Marlowe scale comprises aspects of both self-deception and faking good (his term is 'impression management'). Despite the negative connotation of the term 'self-deception', there is some evidence that it is a characteristic of well-adjusted people, who are more apt to minimize failures, ignore minor criticisms, and believe they will be successful in undertaking new projects (Paulhus 1986). These findings would explain the relatively low correlations between the Crowne–Marlowe scale and the others.

This leaves the scale constructor in something of a quandary regarding which, if any, SD scale to use. Most people use the Crowne and Marlowe scale, probably more by habit and tradition than because of any superior psychometric qualities. Some have cautioned that because of the content of its items, the Edwards scale is confounded with psychopathology, primarily neuroticism (Crowne and Marlowe 1960; Mick 1996) so that it should be eliminated from the running altogether. The newest scale, the BIDR Version 6 (Paulhus 1994), appears to be the most carefully developed. Although Paulhus recommended scoring the items dichotomously, Stöber et al. (2002) found, not surprisingly, that using a continuous 5- or 7-point Likert scale yielded better results.

The second method to measure and reduce SD, used by McFarlane et al. (1981) in the development of their *Social Relations Scale*, is to administer the scale twice: once using the regular instructions to the subjects regarding its completion, and then asking them to fill it in as they would like things to be, or in the best of all possible worlds. This involved asking them first to list whom they talk to about issues that come up in their lives in various areas. A few weeks later (by this time they should have forgotten their original responses), they were asked to complete it 'according to what you consider to be good or ideal circumstances'. If the scores on any item did not change from the first to the second administration, it was assumed that its original answer was dictated more by SD than by the true state of affairs (or was at the 'ceiling' and could not detect any improvement). In either case, the item failed to satisfy at least one desired psychometric property, and was eliminated.

The term 'faking good' is most often applied to an intentional and deliberate approach by the person in responding to personality inventories. An analogous bias in responding to items on questionnaires is called 'prestige bias' (Oppenheim 1966). To judge from responses on questionnaires, nobody streams reality shows, only educational and cultural programmes. Their only breaks from these activities are to attend concerts, visit museums, and brush their teeth four or five times each day. (One can only wonder why the concert halls are empty and dentists' waiting rooms are full.)

Having said all of this, the question remains how large a problem SD actually is. After more than half a century of research, the issue remains unresolved. On the one hand, some have said that not nearly enough attention is paid to the problems posed by SD bias (e.g. King and Bruner 2000). On the other hand, others maintain that SD is not correlated with other self-report data (e.g. Nolte et al. 2013) and is not predictive of other outcomes (Ones et al. 1996). Some have gone even further, arguing that because SD scales, in particular the Crowne–Marlowe scale, correlate with personality attributes such as neuroticism, they are measuring meaningful traits, and that removing their influence actually decreases the validity of other personality scales (Ellingson et al. 1999; McCrae and Costa 1983).

A recent study has called into question the very validity of SD scales. Lanz et al. (2022) conducted a meta-analysis involving 41 studies and close to 9,000 subjects, to examine the correlation between SD scale scores (including the scales we just listed) and behaviour measured under a very specific condition—an economic game specifically designed to measure prosocial behaviour (e.g. the dictator game; the prisoner's dilemma). If SD scales in fact measure bias (a state), then the correlations between the scales and prosocial behaviour should be negative; if on the other hand, SD scales are measuring a trait, then the correlations across studies should be positive. In fact, the results of the pooled analysis suggested the correlations were closer to zero, suggesting the scales were measuring neither a trait nor a state. Taking into consideration specific scales, or how the game was implemented (e.g. use of incentives or not; online versus lab), did not influence the findings. The authors join a growing chorus of researchers who caution against using these scales at all.

So should we be concerned with SD bias? The answer is probably 'yes, but don't lose too much sleep over it'. Since faking good and the prestige bias are more volitional, they are easier to modify through instructions and careful wording of the items, and it is probably worthwhile to do so. (The success of these tactics, though, is still open to question.) The more unconscious self-deception is less amenable to modification, but is likely less of an issue.

Deviation and faking bad

The opposites of socially desirable responding and faking good are *deviation* and *faking bad*. These latter two phenomena have been less studied than their positive counterparts, and no scales to assess them are in wide use. Deviation is a concept introduced by Berg (1967) to explain (actually, simply to name) the tendency to respond to test items with deviant responses. As is the case for faking good, faking bad occurs primarily within the context of personality assessment, although this may happen any time a person feels they may avoid an unpleasant situation (such as the military draft) by looking bad.

Both SD (or, perhaps, faking good) and deviance (or faking bad) occur together in an interesting phenomenon called the 'hello–goodbye' effect (Hathaway 1948). Before an intervention, a person may present themselves in as bad a light as possible, thereby hoping to qualify for the programme, and impressing the staff with the seriousness of their problems. At termination, they may want to 'please' the staff with their improvement, and so may minimize any problems. The result is to make it appear that there has been improvement when none has occurred, or to magnify any effects that did occur. This effect was originally described in psychotherapy research, but it may arise whenever a subject is assessed on two occasions, with some intervention between the administrations of the scale.

Although SD bias may be a problem, Gough and Bradley (1996) estimate that under non-evaluative testing situations, the incidence of faking good and faking bad are each under 1 per cent.

Detecting problematic responding

Careless responding is unfortunately a fact of life. Moreover, it is likely to get worse as more and more research is conducted online. It has been hypothesized that the reduction in face-to-face contact and personalization as we move from individually administered, paper-and-pencil tests to internet-based instruments results in less accountability and involvement (Johnson 2005). Furthermore, as any parent of teenagers can attest, younger people tend to 'multitask' (Carrier et al. 2009) or more precisely 'task switch' (Kirschner and van Merri ënboer 20 13), despite all the evidence indicating that this leads to poorer performance on all tasks. The effect of these trends is that less attention is paid to filling out the scale, resulting in more random or inaccurate responses.

The issue then becomes how this can be detected. As we mentioned in Chapter 5, some longer inventories take the approach of adding scales composed of items that are highly improbable (e.g. 'I have never touched money') or almost universally endorsed ('I eat on most days'). However, this is impractical if the aim is to develop a single, stand-alone scale. A number of techniques that can be built into such scales have been proposed by Meade and Craig (2012). *Consistency indices* are pairs of items that are either very highly correlated or actual repetitions of the same items, such as 'I exercise every day' and 'I exercise at least seven times a week'. They can also be items that are highly negatively correlated or contradict each other, such as pairing one of the previous items with 'I rarely exercise'. Four or five pairs of such items are usually sufficient. A second approach is to use bogus items, such as 'I was born on February 30th ' or 'I am paid biweekly by leprechauns'.

Finally, respondents can be instructed to give a specific answer : e.g. 'For the next item, circle Strongly Agree'. This is a very powerful method, because the probability of being flagged by this item is $(j - 1)/j$, where j is the number of response options. When k such items are used, the probability of being flagged by any item is $1 - (1/j)^k$. So, if there are three instructed items with five or more response options, there is almost a 100 per cent probability of detecting careless responding. Meade and Craig (2012) recommend one such item for every 50 to 100 real ones, up to a maximum of three.

Minimizing biased responding

A number of techniques have been proposed to minimize the effects of these different biases. One method is to try to disguise the intent of the test, so the subject does not know what is actually being looked for. Rotter's scale to measure locus of control (Rotter 1966), for example, is called the *Personal Reaction Inventory*, a vague title which conveys little about the purpose of the instrument. (But then again, neither does 'locus of control'.)

However, this deception is of little use if the content of the items themselves reveals the objective of the scale. Thus, the second method consists of using 'subtle' items, ones where the respondent is unaware of the specific trait or behaviour being tapped. The item may still have face validity, since the respondent could feel that the question is fair and relevant; however, its actual relevance may be to some trait other than that assumed by the answerer (Holden and Jackson 1979). For example, the item 'I would enjoy racing motorcycles' may appear to measure preferences for spending one's leisure time, while in fact it may be an index of risk-taking. The difficulty with this technique, though, is that the psychometric properties of subtle items are usually poorer than those of obvious ones, and often do not measure the traits for which they were originally intended (Burkhart et al. 1976; Jackson 1971). A third method to reduce the effect of these biases is to ensure anonymity. This is feasible if the scales are mailed to respondents and they can return them in envelopes with no identifying information. Anonymity is less believable when the interview is done over the telephone, or when the person is handed a form to fill out as part of a face-to-face interview. Nederhof (1984) and Wiseman (1972) found some reduction in SD bias with mailed questionnaires, but almost no reduction under the latter two conditions. On the other hand, Web-based questionnaires appear to lead to more reporting of sensitive information and less SD bias (Kreuter et al. 2008). While this may apply to impression management, it likely has much less effect on self-deception.

Random response technique

The preceding methods of minimizing SD bias are only partially effective. Two methods that do seem to work, especially regarding illegal, immoral, or embarrassing behaviours, are called the *random response technique* (RRT; Warner 1965) and the *unmatched count technique* (Raghavarao and Federer 1979). In the most widely used of many variants of the RRT, the respondent is handed a card containing two items: one neutral and one sensitive. For example, the statements can be:

A. I own a DVD.

B. I have used street drugs within the past 6 months.

The respondent is also given a device which randomly selects an A or a B. This can be as simple as a coin, or can be randomly generated using a computer. They are told to flip the coin or touch the computer screen to get a randomly generated response, and truthfully answer whichever item is indicated; the interviewer does not know *which* question was selected, only the response.

In practice, only a portion of the respondents are given these items; the remaining subjects are asked the neutral question ('I own a DVD') directly in order to determine the prevalence of 'true' responses to it in the sample. When two or more such items are used, half of the group will be given the random response technique on half of the questions, and asked about the neutral stems for the remaining items , while this would be reversed for the second half of the sample. An alternative is to use a neutral item where the true prevalence is well known, such as the proportion of families owning two cars or with three children. Of course, the scale developer must be quite sure that the sample is representative of the population on which the prevalence figures were derived.

With this information, the proportion of people answering 'true' to the sensitive item (p_s) can be estimated using the equation:

$$p_s = \left[p_t - (1-p)p_d \right]/P$$

where p_t is the proportion of people who answered 'true', p_d is the proportion saying 'true' to the neutral item on direct questioning, and P is the probability of selecting the sensitive item. The variance of p_s is:

$$Var(p_s) = \frac{p_t(1-p_t)}{nP^2}.$$

and the estimated standard error is the square root of this variance.

The probability of selecting the sensitive item (P) is 50 per cent using a coin toss, but can be modified with other techniques. For example, the computer can be programmed so that A is presented only 30 per cent of the time and B 70 per cent. The closer P is to 1.0, the smaller is the sample size that is needed to obtain an accurate estimate *of* p_s, but then the technique begins to resemble direct questioning and anonymity becomes jeopardized.

Another difficulty with the original Warner technique and its variants is that they are limited to asking questions with only dichotomous answers : 'yes–no' or 'true–false'. Greenberg et al. (1971) modified this technique so that both the sensitive and the neutral questions ask for numerical answers, such as:

A. How many times during the past year have you slept with someone who is not your spouse?

B. How many children do you have?

In this case, the estimated mean of the sensitive item (μ_s) is:

$$\mu_s = \frac{(1-P_1)\bar{z}_1 - (1-P_2)\bar{z}_2}{P_1 - P_2},$$

with variance:

$$Var(\mu_s) = \frac{(1-P_1)\left(\frac{s_1^2}{n_1}\right) + (1-P_2)\left(\frac{s_2^2}{n_2}\right)}{(P_1 - P_2)^2}.$$

where $\bar{z}_1$ is the mean for sample 1, n_1 is its sample size, s_1^2 the variance of $\bar{z}_1$ for sample 1, and P_1 the probability of having chosen question A. The terms with the subscript '2' are for a second sample, which is needed to determine the mean value of question B. Other variations on this theme are discussed by Scheers (1992).

The advantage of the RRT is that it gives a more accurate estimate of the true prevalence of these sensitive behaviours than does direct questioning. For example, nine times as many women reported having had an abortion when asked with the random response method as compared with traditional questioning (Shimizu and Bonham 1978). Lensvelt-Mulders et al. (2005) performed a meta-analysis of six articles that were able to compare responses to actual records and 32 comparative studies in which results from the RRT were compared to prevalence estimates from other studies. The RRT underestimated the prevalence by between 28 and 42 per cent, but this was lower than the underestimates produced by telephone, questionnaire, face-to-face, or computer-assisted methods. Further, the more sensitive the area, the more valid were the results from the random response method.

However, there are some penalties associated with this procedure. First, it is most easily done in face-to-face interviews, although it is possible to conduct using a phone or online conferencing platforms such as Zoom or Teams; it obviously cannot be used in mailed surveys. Second, since it is not known which subjects responded to each stem, the answers cannot be linked to other information from the questionnaire. Third, the calculated prevalence depends upon three estimates: the proportion of subjects responding to the sensitive item; the proportion answering 'true'; and the proportion of people who respond 'true' to the neutral stem. Since each of these is measured with error, a much larger sample size is required to get stable estimates. Formulae for estimating sample size for various RRT methods are given by Ulrich et al. (2012).

Unmatched count technique

The major problem with the RRT, as already mentioned, is that it cannot be used with mailed or online surveys because it requires some form of randomization device; this is overcome with the unmatched count technique (UCT). As with the RRT, the sample is divided in two. The first group gets a list of between two and five statements, such as:

A. I own a cat.

B. I have read the book *The Prince*.

C. I have visited Morocco.

D. I can tell you what 'item response theory' is.

The respondents indicate how many of the statements are true, without indicating which specific items are endorsed. The second group gets the same list and instructions, but with the addition of a sensitive item, such as 'I have stolen from my employer'. The technique's name comes from the fact that the number of statements each group receives is unmatched.

The prevalence of the sensitive question is simply the difference between the mean number of items endorsed by the two groups. For example, if the mean of the first group is 1.8 and that of the second 2.1 (it must be higher because they are given more statements), then the estimated prevalence is 2.1–1.8 = 0.30 = 30 per cent.

The UCT has the same limitation as the RRT: the results apply to the group as a whole, and responses cannot be linked to other information that may have been gathered about individuals. Also, to get accurate estimates, there must be at least 40–50 people in each group (Dalton et al. 1994). Care must also be used in selecting the statements. If all of them would be endorsed by a large proportion of respondents (e.g. 'I can drive a car'), then anonymity would be jeopardized (and worse, seen to be jeopardized) because all 'guilty' people would be easily identified as those who endorsed all items. Although there have not been many studies that have used the UCT, there is some evidence that it may detect even higher rates of illegal or illicit behaviour than even the RRT (Coutts and Jann 2011).

Yea-saying or acquiescence

Yea-saying, also called *acquiescence bias*, is the tendency to give positive responses, such as 'true', 'like', 'often', or 'yes', to a question (Couch and Keniston 1960). At its most extreme, the person responds in this way irrespective of the content of the item so that even mutually contradictory statements are endorsed. Thus, the person may respond 'true' to two items like 'I always take my medication on time' and 'I often forget to take my pills'. At the opposite end of the spectrum are the 'nay-sayers'. It is believed that this tendency is more or less normally distributed so that relatively few people are at the extremes, but that many people exhibit this trait to lesser degrees.

End-aversion, positive skew, and halo

In addition to the distortions already mentioned, scales which are scored on a continuum, such as visual analogue and Likert scales, are prone to other types of biases. These include end-aversion bias, positive skew, and the halo effect.

End-aversion bias

End-aversion bias, which is also called the *central tendency bias*, refers to the reluctance of some people to use the extreme categories of a scale. It is based in part on people's difficulty in making absolute judgements, since situations without mitigating or extenuating circumstances rarely occur. The problem is similar to the one some people have in responding to 'true–false' items; they often want to say, 'It all depends' or 'Most of the time, but not always'. The effect of this bias is to reduce the range of possible responses. Thus, if the extremes of a 5-point Likert scale are labelled 'always' and 'never', an end-aversion bias would render this a 3-point scale, with the resulting loss of sensitivity and reliability.

There are two ways of dealing with the end-aversion bias. The first is to avoid absolute statements at the end-points—using 'almost never' and 'almost always' instead of 'never' and 'always'. The problem with this approach is a restriction in the range of responses ; some people may *want* to respond with absolutes, but not allowing them to dilute their answers with less extreme ones. The advantage is a greater probability that all categories will be used.

The second, and opposite, tack is to include 'throw-away' categories at the ends. If the aim is to have a 7-point scale, then nine alternatives are provided, with the understanding that the extreme boxes at the ends will rarely be checked, but are there primarily to serve as anchors. This more or less ensures that all seven categories of interest will be used, but may lead to the problem of devising more adjectives if each box is labelled.

End-aversion bias may introduce additional problems when translated versions of scales are used to compare cultures. As opposed to the highly individualistic culture found in North America, some African and Asian cultures are described as 'collectivistic', in which people are more concerned with how they fit in and belong to social groups. There is a tendency in such societies for people to avoid the extremes of scales, where they may appear different from others, and to favour the middle (e.g. Cheung and Renswold 2000; Hui and Triandis 1989). On the other hand, people from more emotionally expressive countries (e.g. Latin American countries and Italy) are more likely to use the extremes than are residents of North America or northern Europe (Craig and Douglas 2005), even after they have moved north (Weech-Maldonado et al. 2008). While this will not affect the mean values of groups, it will reduce the variance of the scores and hence the correlations of the score with other scales (e.g. Schmitt and Allik 2005).

Positive skew

It often happens, though, that the responses are not evenly distributed over the range of alternatives, but show a positive *skew* towards the favourable end. (Note that, as we mentioned in Chapter 4, this definition of skew is opposite to that used in statistics.) This situation is most acute when a rating scale is used to evaluate students or staff. For example, Linn (1979) found that the mean score on a 5-point scale was 4.11 rather than 3.00, and the scores ranged between 3.30 and 4.56—the lower half of the scale was never used. Similarly, Cowles and Kubany (1959) asked raters to determine if a student was in the lower one-fifth, top one-fifth, or middle three-fifths of the class. Despite these explicit instructions, 31 per cent were assigned to the top fifth and only 5 per cent to the bottom one-fifth.

This may reflect the feeling that since these students survived the hurdles of admission into university and then into professional school, the 'average' student is really quite exceptional. It is then difficult to shift sets so that 'average' is relative to the other people in the normative group, rather than the general population.

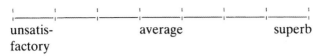

unsatis-   average   superb
factory

Fig. 6.3 Example of a traditional Likert scale.

The effect of skew is to produce a *ceiling effect*: since most of the marks are clustered in only a few boxes at one extreme, the scores are very near the top of the scale. This means that it is almost impossible to detect any improvement, or to distinguish among various grades of excellence.

A few methods have been proposed to counteract this bias, all based on the fact that 'average' need not be in the middle. Since no amount of instruction or training appears to be able to shake an evaluator's belief that the average person under their supervision is far above average, the aim of a scale is then to differentiate among degrees of excellence. Using a traditional Likert scale (Fig. 6.3) will result in most of the scores bunching in the three right-most boxes (or two, if an end-aversion is also present). However, we can shift the centre to look like Fig. 6.4. This gives the evaluator five boxes above average, rather than just three.

Another strategy is to capitalize on the fact that the truly superb students or employees need little feedback, except to continue doing what they have been doing all along, while the unsatisfactory ones are readily apparent to all evaluators even without scales. Rather, we should use the scale to differentiate among the majority of people who fall between these extremes. In this situation, the middle is expanded, at the expense of the ends (see Fig. 6.5).

Note that this version clearly distinguishes the extremes, and offsets 'average'; many other variations on this theme are possible, reflecting the needs and philosophies of the programme.

Halo

Halo is a phenomenon first recognized over a century ago (Wells 1907), whereby judgements made on individual aspects of a person's performance are influenced by the rater's overall impression of the person. Thorndike (1920), who named this effect, gave what is still its best description (p. 447):

> The judge seems intent on reporting his final opinion of the strength, weakness, merit, or demerit of the personality as a whole, rather than on giving as discriminating a rating as possible for each separate characteristic.

He went on to say that 'Obviously a halo of general merit is extended to influence the rating for the special ability and vice versa' (p. 448). For example, if a resident is well

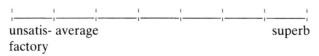

unsatis- average   superb
factory

Fig. 6.4 Example of a modified Likert scale.

out!	below average	average	above average	much above average	excel-lent	great!

Fig. 6.5 Example of an expanded Likert scale.

regarded by a staff physician, then the resident will be evaluated highly in all areas. Conversely, a resident who is felt to be weak in clinical skills, for example, can do no right, and will receive low scores in all categories. To some degree, this reflects reality; people who are good at one thing tend to do well in related areas. Also, many of the individual categories are dependent upon similar traits or behaviours: the ability to establish rapport with patients likely is dependent on the same skills that are involved in working with nurses and other staff. Cooper (1981) refers to this real correlation among categories as 'true halo'. However, the ubiquity of this phenomenon and the very high intercorrelations among many different categories indicate that more is going on: what Cooper calls 'illusory halo', and what we commonly refer to when we speak of the 'halo effect'. In one of the few studies that actually tried to manipulate halo, Keeley et al. (2013) created a series of tapes, manipulating aspects of the lecturer's performance (e.g. confidence, communication style, use of humour) one at a time. In each case, the change affected all of the students' evaluations, so that changes in approachability, for instance, affected ratings of competence, professionalism, and others that were not manipulated.

There have been many theories proposed to explain illusory halo, but many simply boil down to the fact that raters are unable to evaluate people along more than a few dimensions. Very often, one global, summary rating scale about the person conveys as much information as do the individual scales about each aspect of the person's performance (recall the discussion of *single-item rating scales* in Chapter 5).

Many of the techniques proposed to minimize illusory halo involve factors other than the scale itself, such as the training of raters, basing the evaluations on larger samples of behaviour, and using more than one evaluator (e.g. Cooper 1981). The major aspect of scale design, which may reduce this effect, is the use of behaviourally anchored ratings (BARs); instead of simply stating 'below average', for example, concrete examples are used, either as part of the descriptors themselves, or on a separate instruction page (e.g. Streiner 1985). This gives the raters concrete meaning for each level on the scale, reducing the subjective element and increasing agreement among raters. However, the rating scale used by Keeley et al. (2013) did use BARs, with minimal effect.

Framing

Another bias, which particularly affects econometric scaling methods, is called *framing* (Kahneman and Tversky 1984). The name refers to the fact that the person's choice between two alternative states depends on how these states are framed. For example, consider the situation where an outbreak of influenza is expected to kill 600 people in the country. The subject must choose between two programmes:

Programme A: 200 people will be saved.

Programme B: there is a one-third probability that 600 people will be saved, and two-thirds that nobody will be saved.

Nearly 75 per cent of subjects prefer Programme A—assurance that 200 people will be saved—rather than the situation which offers the possibility that everyone could be saved, but at the risk of saving no one. Now consider presenting the same situation, but offering two different programmes:

Programme C: 400 people will die.

Programme D: there is a one-third probability that nobody will die, and two-thirds that 600 will die.

Programmes A and C are actually the same, as are B and D; all that differs is how the situations are presented (or 'framed'). In A, the number of survivors is explicitly stated, and the number who die (400) is implicit; this is reversed in C, where the number who die is given, but not the number who live. From a purely arithmetic point of view, the proportion of people opting for C, then, should be similar to those who choose A. In fact, over 75 per cent select Programme D rather than C, the exact reverse of the first situation.

Kahneman and Tversky explain these seemingly contradictory results by postulating that people are 'risk averse' when gain is involved and 'risk-takers' in loss situations. That is, when offered the possibility of a gain (saving lives, winning a bet, and so on), people tend to take the safer route of being sure they gain something, rather than the riskier alternative of perhaps getting much more but possibly losing everything. In loss situations, though, such as choosing between Programmes C and D, people will gamble on minimizing their losses (although there is the risk that they can lose everything), rather than taking the certain situation that they will lose something.

The problem that this poses for the designer of questionnaires is that the manner in which a question is posed can affect the results that are obtained. For example, if the researchers were interested in physicians' attitudes towards a new operation or drug, they may get very different answers if they said that the incidence of morbidity was 0.1 per cent, as opposed to saying that there was a 99.9 per cent chance that nothing untoward would occur.

In conclusion, the safest strategy for the test developer is to assume that all of these biases are operative and take the necessary steps to minimize them whenever possible.

Biases related to the measurement of change

Earlier in the chapter, in discussing the cognitive demands involved in answering questions, we noted briefly that questions of the form 'Compared to how you were a year ago ...' should be viewed with considerable scepticism, since they require prodigious feats of memory. That is, in answering a question of this form, the respondents are required, self-evidently, to compare their present state to how they were a year ago and subjectively estimate the amount of change that has occurred in the interim. As we indicated, people's memories for events over a period as long as 1 year are extremely fallible.

A moment's reflection will serve to indicate that some memories are fallible over time periods far shorter than 1 year. While you may be able to recall what you had for dinner on your last birthday, it is quite unlikely that you will be able to recall what you ate last Tuesday (unless it was your birthday). As a consequence, it is plausible that measures of change from a previous health state may be vulnerable to possible biases.

Despite these concerns, there has been considerable recent interest in so-called transition measures, which ask the patient to estimate change from a previous state. As one example, a method used to determine the minimally important difference in quality of life (QOL) on a standard questionnaire asks the patient to consider a 4- to 6-week time period and first state whether they are better, the same, or worse, and then indicate on a 7-point scale how much they have changed from *slightly better* to *a great deal better*.

A critical test of whether such estimates are biased is to examine the correlation between the subjective measure of change in health and (1) the present state, or (2) the initial state, as measured by, for example, a standard index of health-related QOL. If the transition measure is unbiased and the variances of the pre-test and post-test are equal, then the correlations with pre-test and post-test should be equal and opposite (Guyatt et al. 2002). That does not turn out to be the case; typically, the correlation with pre-test is much smaller than that with post-test (Guyatt et al. 2002; Norman et al. 1997).

It would appear, then, that transition measures are potentially biased in favour of the present state. But is this simply a reflection of fallible memory for the previous state? Here, the plot thickens. Two theories have emerged to explain this phenomenon— *response shift* (Schwartz and Sprangers 1999) and *implicit theories of change* (Ross 1989). Both specifically address the issue of assessment of a prior health state, which may have occurred days or months earlier. Both also attempt to reconcile the difference which arises between prospective measures, gathered at the time, and retrospective measures, looking back on the previous state. Interestingly, they arrive at opposite conclusions as to the relative validity of prospective and retrospective measures.

Estimates of the prior state—response shift

A disconcerting finding in the measurement of, for example, QOL is that people with very disabling conditions often report that their QOL is as high as or higher than those who are objectively more healthy (e.g. Albrecht and Devlieger 1999; Saigal et al. 2006). Similar paradoxical results include the following:

1. Patients almost always rate their QOL higher than do their families or healthcare providers (Yip et al. 2001).

2. Objective indices of health correlate by only 0.08 with happiness (Okun and George 1984).

3. Couples who have had marital therapy may report that their communication is worse than couples who have not had such treatment.

In brief, across a variety of settings, one's judgement of health, QOL, subjective well-being, happiness, and similar states stays remarkably stable despite large changes in objective measures; or alternatively, judgements may change in situations where there have been no objective changes in the person's state.

One explanation of this phenomenon is called 'response shift' (Schwartz and Sprangers 1999), which refers to the fact that, over time, the meanings of self-reported constructs are subject to change because of the three Rs of recalibration, reprioritization, and reconceptualization. The reason that couples report worse communication after therapy is that they have recalibrated their assessment of how well or poorly they communicate: 'I didn't realize we were doing so badly until we saw the therapist'. Conversely, patients with a traumatic spinal injury or who have developed cancer may state that they have come to realize that their families are more important than work, and that in this regard, they are doing quite well, thank you very much (reprioritization); or modified their conceptualization of 'healthy' from dependence on physical status to using emotional or social criteria. For whatever reason, the standards against which people are evaluating the construct (QOL or communication) have shifted over time, meaning that the ratings done at time 2 based on recall of how they felt at time 1 cannot be trusted.

One way to determine if response shift has occurred is to use 'then' measures (also called 'retrospective pre-tests'). With this design, people complete the scale at time 1; and then at time 2, they fill out the scale twice—once reflecting their current state, and once how they would have filled it out at time 1 (Bray et al. 1984). If there is a larger difference between the then/post-test scores than between the pre-test/post-test ones, and especially if the then scores are lower than the pre-test scores, it can be concluded that response shift has occurred. How much of an issue is response shift? Mayo et al. (2015), using a different methodology, found little evidence for it in a sample of patients with inflammatory bowel disease. However, in a series of studies, Drennan and Hyde (2008) and Howard (1980) concluded that it was a major source of bias that must be controlled.

It is an open question whether retrospective judgement of a health state is more valid because more information is available on the second occasion; or whether the pre- and post-measures cannot be compared because the situational variables are different. The evidence seems to suggest that, when measuring change from a previous state, it would be wise to supplement the pre-test/post-test design with a then/post-test assessment.

Estimates of the prior state—implicit theory of change

An alternative view is that, in fact, people do not remember the previous state. Instead, their judgement is based on an 'implicit theory' of change beginning with their present state and working backwards (Ross 1989). People begin with 'How do I feel today?', then ask themselves, 'How do I think that things have been changing over the past weeks (months, years)?' This implicit theory of change might imply that there has been steady improvement, deterioration, no change, improvement followed by levelling off, or several other possibilities. For example, the person may think, 'My doctor put me on a pill, and I trust my doctor, so I must be doing better'. Sir Peter Medawar (1967, p. 14) perhaps said it best:

> If a person (a) is sick, (b) receives treatment intended to make him better, and (c) gets better, then no power of reasoning known to medical science can convince him that it may not have been the treatment that restored his health.

But it is based on an impression of the time course, not on analysis of health at specific time points. Finally, the respondents work back from their present state, using their 'implicit theory' to infer what their initial state must have been. From this position, the retrospective judgement of the initial state is viewed as biased, and the prospective judgement obtained at the time is more valid.

Reconciling the two positions

Interestingly, these two theories—response shift and implicit theory of change—can examine the same data showing a low correlation between a prospective judgement of a prior health state (or equivalently, a low correlation between a judgement of change and the pre-test) and arrive at opposite conclusions. For the response-shift theorist, a retrospective judgement derives from additional information which was, by definition, not available at the time of the initial assessment; hence the retrospective judgement is more valid. The implicit theorist presumes that the discrepancy does not arise from a conscious adjustment of the initial state at all, but instead begins with the present state and invokes an implicit theory of change, which cannot be externally verified. From the perspective of implicit theory, the retrospective test is based on two information sources which are irrelevant to the initial judgement—the present state and the theory of change. Hence, the prospective assessment is more valid.

At the time of writing, no critical comparative test of these theories has been conducted. Indeed, it is not at all straightforward to determine what might constitute a critical test (Norman 2003). Regardless, one clear conclusion is possible. Retrospective judgements of change based on recall of a previous state are not at all straightforward and unbiased. The uncritical application of 'transition' measures (which, regrettably, is all too common) is fraught with potential problems of interpretation.

In Chapter 11, we will return to the issue of measuring change, but based on changes in test scores, rather than the person's subjective judgement.

Proxy reporting

Ideally, respondents to a scale or questionnaire should be those people from whom we want the information. However, this is not always possible: children who have not yet learned to read, those with limited intelligence, and people with dementia, for example, may not be able to understand the items or accurately report about their status. Also, in many household surveys, one adult in the home is randomly chosen to be the respondent for all people who are living together. The assumption is made that the *proxy reporter* would give the same information that the other person(s) would give. Consequently, we have to question whether proxies are adequate substitutes or whether they introduce biases of their own.

The picture in this regard has both good and bad news. On the positive side, proxies are fairly accurate reporters about objective, observable phenomena, such as smoking history and leisure activities (Debanne et al. 2001), physical mobility, social isolation, and pain (Boyer et al. 2004) for patients with Alzheimer's disease; or social/interpersonal problems of children with epilepsy (Ronen et al. 2003). On the other hand, proxies are relatively poor judges of internal, emotional states, such as QOL or disability. The results of Yip et al. (2001) are typical of what is found when proxies (family members or healthcare providers) estimate attributes such as 'vitality' and 'mental health' in older people: they give significantly lower scores than those given by the patients themselves. A somewhat more complicated picture emerged in a secondary analysis of a very large nationwide community study by Todorov and Kirschner (2000): proxies under-reported disabilities for people with an age range of 18–64 years, but over-reported them for those older than 65 years. They likely assumed that younger people are able to do more than they say they can do and (typically) underestimated the abilities of older people.

A further complication is that the psychological status of the respondent affects their report as a proxy. For example, mothers with poor self-reported health attribute lower health status scores to their children (Waters et al. 2000); and those with anxiety and depression report more distress in their children (Sawyer et al. 1998).

Part of the difficulty is that proxy reporters can assume a number of different roles and perspectives (Ronen and Streiner 2013). As *observer informants*, they may give their own perspectives and opinions about the patient's subjective states. They can also respond the way they think the patient would; that is, they are acting as *surrogate informants*. Putting themselves in the patient's shoes, they would be *substitute informants*; or they could be *advocacy informants*, seeing their role as advocating for the patient. This has a number of implications, the most important of which is that the instructions must be very clear regarding which role the informant should take. Even with this, though, it may be worthwhile using cognitive interviewing after the proxy has completed the scale, to try to determine from which perspective they are answering. Finally, be aware that, even with explicit instructions, proxies may be serving as advocates when asked to be surrogates, or substitutes when asked to be observers, for example. This will always introduce some degree of noise into the outcome.

Testing the items

Having followed all of the rules regarding item writing in Chapter 5, and being aware of the biases mentioned in this chapter, there is still no guarantee that the questions will be interpreted by the respondents as they were intended to be. Belson (1981), for example, found that fewer than 30 per cent of survey questions were correctly interpreted by readers. Unfortunately, these results are typical of findings in this area.

As these two chapters have pointed out, errors can arise from two sources: the items themselves and the task of answering. With regard to the items, Chapter 5 covered some of the problems—double-barrelled or ambiguous questions, vague modifiers, the use of jargon, and items that are so long that they exceed the processing capacity of the respondents. Factors that interfere with accurate reporting include the various biases and less than optimum response strategies (e.g. satisficing). Statistical techniques, such as item- total correlations and examining the distribution of responses to an item, may help identify that respondents are having trouble with a particular item, but they cannot determine *why* an item is causing problems.

Cognitive methods for testing items

A number of methods have been derived from social and cognitive psychology that help explore how people approach the task of answering questions and, along the way, highlight those items that are causing problems. The major methods are *rephrasing*, *double interviewing*, *thinking aloud interviews*, and *probing*. These generally have three aims: to determine (1) if the respondents understand the question; (2) if they do so consistently; and (3) if they do so in the way that the test developer intended (Collins 2003).

Rephrasing was introduced by Nuckols (1953), and involves asking the people to rephrase the question in their own words, trying to keep the meaning as close to the original as possible. The responses, which are written down verbatim, are later coded into one of four categories: fully correct, generally correct (no more than one part altered or omitted), partially wrong (but the person understood the intent), and completely wrong (Foddy 1993). Similarly, problem items are identified if the person says 'I never heard of that', 'I don't understand what you mean', or 'Can you repeat the question?' (Schechter and Herrmann 1997). Needless to say, there is some degree of subjectivity involved in the coding, and it may be best to have two or three independent raters code the rephrased items.

In the double interview, the respondent first completes the entire scale or interview. Then, for each subject, three or four items are selected, and the interviewer asks questions such as, 'What led you to answer …?' or 'Tell me exactly how you came to that answer' (Foddy 1993). The thinking aloud technique is quite similar, except that it usually omits having the person complete the scale first. Rather, for each question, the person is asked to 'think aloud' as they try to answer the question. For example, if the item reads 'I have a lot on my plate and feel overwhelmed', the respondent may say, 'I definitely feel that I have a lot on my plate, but I don't feel overwhelmed, so I'm not sure how to answer'. This would highlight the fact that the question is double-barrelled and needs to be reworded. Similarly, if the item states 'I exercise often', the person may say they aren't sure what 'often' means, indicating a vague descriptor that should be made more explicit. The interviewer may also ask direct questions, such as 'How did you go about answering that question?' or 'You seemed to hesitate before answering that. What were you thinking of?'

Finally, probing is done after each question. The probes may be the same for all items or may vary depending on the content. Similarly, they may be developed beforehand or be spurred by the respondent's answer to the item (Willis et al. 1991). Probes may consist of questions such as 'How hard or easy was it for you to answer the question?', 'How sure are you of your answer?', 'How did you feel about answering this?', 'What does the term *A* mean to you?', 'How did you feel about answering the question?', or 'How sure are you of your answer?' (Collins 2003). These probes tap different aspects involved in answering questions: comprehension, retrieval, the response, and confidence in the response.

Which technique to use depends very much on the nature of the item. For example, if you are concerned that the person may not understand some of the words, then rephrasing or asking probes such as 'What does the term *illness* (or *stomach*, or whatever) mean to you?' may be the best choice. On the other hand, if the person has to recall information, then thinking aloud or the double interview may be preferable. It is not necessary to use the same technique for all of the items or questions; you should be guided by what is the best way to elicit the information you need, rather than maintaining consistency.

Because all of these techniques significantly increase the time required to complete the full scale or interview, it may be too demanding to do a cognitive interview on the entire scale for each person. In that case, each person would respond to only a subset of questions, which reduces the burden on the respondent, but increases it for the investigator, who must find more people. Finally, if a scale or questionnaire consists of subsections, then each person should be given a sampling of items from each.

With all of these techniques, it is important that they be used with people who are similar to the intended respondents, in terms of age, education, and any other background variables that may affect the understanding of and responding to the questions. Using one's colleagues or samples of convenience, which may bear little resemblance to the final user population, will most likely result in underestimating any potential problems. If pre-testing does not uncover any difficulties with the wording of any of the items, it is more likely a sign of problems with the cognitive testing procedure, rather than an indication that everything is fine. It is difficult to say a priori on how many people the scale should be pre-tested. It is probably best to use the criterion used by qualitative researchers of 'sampling to redundancy'. That is, people are interviewed until no new problems are uncovered. In most cases, this occurs somewhere between 8 and 15 interviews.

Limitations of cognitive testing

Cognitive testing is not a panacea. First, as mentioned earlier, it is a qualitative exercise, and the interpretation of the respondent's answers themselves may be open to interpretation (is *gut* an adequate synonym for *stomach*?). Second, people may not be able to verbalize the mental processes they use in formulating an answer. Finally, there may be a Hawthorne effect, in which people may attend to the items more carefully than they would in real life, simply because they know they will be asked to explain their responses (Wilson et al. 1995). Despite these limitations, though, it is highly recommended that there should be cognitive testing of all new scales and questionnaires or when they are used with populations that differ from the original ones.

Rechecking

Even after all of the items have passed these checks and have been incorporated into the scale, it is worthwhile to check them over informally every few years to see if any terms may have taken on new meanings. For example, liking to go to 'gay parties' has a very different connotation now than it did some years ago, when to most people the word 'gay' had no association with homosexuality.

Further reading

Berg, I.A. (ed.) (1967). *Response set in personality assessment*. Aldine, Chicago, IL.

Couch, A. and Keniston, K. (1960). Yeasayers and naysayers: Agreeing response set as a personality variable. *Journal of Abnormal and Social Psychology*, **60**, 151–74.

Edwards, A.L. (1957). *The social desirability variable in personality assessments and research*. Dryden, New York.

Thorndike, E.L. (1920). A constant error in psychological ratings. *Journal of Applied Psychology*, **4**, 25–9.

Warner, S.L. (1965). Randomized response: Survey technique for eliminating evasive answer bias. *Journal of the American Statistical Association*, **60**, 63–9.

References

Albrecht, G.L. and Devlieger, P.J. (1999). The disability paradox: High quality of life against all odds. *Social Science & Medicine*, **48**, 977–88.

Allen, G.I., Breslow, L., Weissman, A., and Nisselson, H. (1954). Interviewing versus diary keeping in eliciting information in a morbidity survey. *American Journal of Public Health*, **44**, 919–27.

Anastasi, A. (1982). *Psychological testing* (5th edn). Macmillan, New York.

Anderson, G.L., Manson, J., Wallace, R., Lund, B., Hall, D., Davis, S., *et al.* (2003). Baseline monograph: Implementation of the WHI Study Design. *Annals of Epidemiology*, **13**, S5– 17.

Austin, J.L. (1962). *How to do things with words*. Oxford University Press, Oxford.

Baldwin, J.R., Reuben, A., Newbury, J.B., and Danese, A. (2019). Agreement between prospective and retrospective measures of childhood maltreatment: A systematic review and meta-analysis. *JAMA Psychiatry*, **76**, 584–93.

Belson, W.A. (1981). *The design and understanding of survey questions*. Gower, Aldershot.

Berg, I.A. (1967). The deviation hypothesis: A broad statement of its assumptions and postulates. In *Response set in personality assessment* (ed. I.A. Berg), pp. 146–90. Aldine, Chicago, IL.

Berke, R.L. (1998). Clinton's O. K. in the polls, right? *New York Times*, 15 February, pp. 1, 5.

Boyer, F., Novella, J.-L., Morrone, I., Jolly, D., and Blanchard, F. (2004). Agreement between dementia patient report and proxy reports using the Nottingham Health Profile. *International Journal of Geriatric Psychiatry*, **19**, 1026–34.

Bray, J.H., Maxwell, S.E., and Howard, G.S. (1984). Methods of analysis with response-shift bias. *Educational and Psychological Measurement*, **44**, 781–804.

Bryant, R.A. (1993). Memory for pain and affect in chronic pain patients. *Pain*, **54**, 347–51.

Burkhart, B.R., Christian, W.L., and Gynther, M.D. (1976). Item subtlety and faking on the MMPI: A paradoxical relationship. *Journal of Personality Assessment*, **42**, 76–80.

Cannell, C.F., Fisher, G., and Bakker, T. (1965). *Reporting on hospitalization in the Health Interview Survey*. Vital and Health Statistics, Series 3, No. 6. Public Health Service, Hyattsville, MD.

Cheung, G.W. and Renswold, R.B. (2000). Assessing extreme and acquiescence response sets in cross-cultural research using structural equation modeling. *Journal of Cross-Cultural Psychology*, **31**, 187–212.

Clarke, P.M., Fiebig, D.G., and Gerdtham, U.-G. (2008). Optimal recall length in survey design. *Journal of Health Economics*, **27**, 1275–84.

Collins, D. (2003). Pretesting survey instruments: An overview of cognitive methods. *Quality of Life Research*, **12**, 229–38.

Cook, A., Pryer, J., and Shetty, P. (2000). The problem of accuracy in dietary surveys. Analysis of the over 65 UK National Diet and Nutrition Survey. *Journal of Epidemiology and Community Health*, **54**, 611–16.

Cooper, W.H. (1981). Ubiquitous halo. *Psychological Bulletin*, **90**, 218–44.

Couch, A. and Keniston, K. (1960). Yeasayers and naysayers: Agreeing response set as a personality variable. *Journal of Abnormal and Social Psychology*, **60**, 151–74.

Coutts, E. and Jann, B. (2011). Sensitive questions in online surveys: Experimental results for the randomized response technique (RRT) and the unmatched count technique (UCT). *Sociological Methods & Research*, **40**, 169–93.

Cowles, J.T. and Kubany, A.J. (1959). Improving the measurement of clinical performance in medical students. *Journal of Clinical Psychology*, **15**, 139–42.

Craig, C.S. and Douglas, S.P. (2005). *International marketing research* (3rd edn). Wiley, Chichester.

Crowne, D.P. and Marlowe, D. (1960). A new scale of social desirability independent of psychopathology. *Journal of Consulting Psychology*, **24**, 349–54.

Dalton, D.R., Wimbush, J.C., and Daily, C.M. (1994). Using the unmatched count technique (UCT) to estimate base rates for sensitive behavior. *Personnel Psychology*, **47**, 817–28.

Debanne, S.M., Petot, G.J., Li, J., Koss, E., Lerner, A.J., Riedel, T.M., *et al.* (2001). On the use of surrogate respondents for controls in a case-control study of Alzheimer's disease. *Journal of the American Geriatric Society*, **49**, 980–4.

Drennan, J. and Hyde, A. (2008). Controlling response shift bias: The use of the retrospective pre-test design in the evaluation of a master's programme. *Assessment & Evaluation in Higher Education*, **33**, 699–709.

Edwards, A.L. (1957). *The social desirability variable in personality assessments and research*. Dryden, New York.

Eich, E., Reeves, J.L., Jaeger, B., and Graff-Radford, S.B. (1985). Memory for pain: Relation between past and present pain intensity. *Pain*, **23**, 375–9.

Ellingson, J.E., Sackett, P.R., and Hough, L.M. (1999). Social desirability corrections in personality measurement: Issues of applicant comparison and construct validity. *Journal of Applied Psychology*, **84**, 155–66.

Foddy, W. (1993). *Constructing questions for interviews and questionnaires*. Cambridge University Press, Cambridge.

Gough, H.G. and Bradley, P. (1996). *CPI manual* (3rd edn). Consulting Psychologists Press, Palo Alto, CA.

Greenberg, B.C., Kuebler, R.R., Abernathy, J.R., and Horvitz, D.G. (1971). Application of the randomized response technique in obtaining quantitative data. *Journal of the American Statistical Association*, **66**, 243–50.

Gregory, J. (2005). *National diet and nutrition survey*. Her Majesty's Stationery Office, London.

Guyatt, G.H., Norman, G.R., and Juniper, E.F. (2002). A critical look at transition ratings. *Journal of Clinical Epidemiology*, **55**, 900–8.

Hathaway, S.R. (1948). Some considerations relative to nondirective counseling as therapy. *Journal of Clinical Psychology*, **4**, 226–31.

Holden, R.R. and Fekken, G.C. (1989). Three common social desirability scales: Friends, acquaintances, or strangers? *Journal of Research in Personality*, **23**, 180–1.

Holden, R.R. and Jackson, D.N. (1979). Item subtlety and face validity in personality assessment. *Journal of Consulting and Clinical Psychology*, **47**, 459–68.

Howard, G.S. (1980). Response-shift bias: A problem in evaluating interventions with pre/post self-reports. *Evaluation Review*, **4**, 93–106.

Hui, C.H. and Triandis, H.C. (1989). Effects of culture and response format on extreme response style. *Journal of Cross-Cultural Psychology*, **20**, 296–309.

Huttenlocher, J., Hedges, L.V., and Bradburn, N.M. (1990). Reports of elapsed time: Bounding and rounding processes in estimation. *Journal of Experimental Psychology: Learning, Memory, and Cognition*, **16**, 196–213.

Jackson, D.N. (1970). A sequential system for personality scale development. In *Current topics in clinical and community psychology*, Vol. 2 (ed. C.D. Spielberger), pp. 61–96. Academic Press, New York.

Jackson, D.N. (1971). The dynamics of structured personality tests: 1971. *Psychological Review*, **78**, 229–48.

Jackson, D.N. (1984). *Personality Research Form manual*. Research Psychologists Press, Port Huron, MI.

Jamison, R.N., Sbrocco, T., and Parris, W.C.V. (1989). The influence of physical and psychosocial factors on accuracy of memory for pain in chronic pain patients. *Pain*, **37**, 289–94.

Johnson, J.A. (2005). Ascertaining the validity of individual protocols from web-based personality inventories. *Journal of Research in Personality*, **39**, 103–29.

Kahneman, D. and Tversky, A. (1984). Choices, values, and frames. *American Psychologist*, **39**, 341–50.

Keeley, J.W., English, T., Irons, J., and Henslee, A. M. (2013). Investigating halo and ceiling effects in student evaluations of instruction. *Educational and Psychological Measurement*, **73**, 440–57.

King, M.F. and Bruner, G.C. (2000). Social desirability bias: A neglected aspect of validity testing. *Psychology & Marketing*, **17**, 79–103.

Kirschner, P.A. and van Merriënboer, J.J. (2013). Do learners really know best? Urban legends in education. *Educational Psychologist*, **48**, 169–83.

Kreuter, F., Presser, S., and Tourangeau, R. (2008). Social desirability bias in CATI, IVR, and Web surveys. *Public Opinion Quarterly*, **72**, 847–65.

Krosnick, J.A. (1991). Response strategies for coping with the cognitive demands of attitude measures in surveys. *Applied Cognitive Psychology*, **5**, 213–16.

Krosnick, J.A. and Alwin, D.F. (1987). An evaluation of a cognitive theory of response order effects in survey measurement. *Public Opinion Quarterly*, **51**, 201–19.

Lanz, L., Thielmann, I., and Gerpott, F.H. (2022). Are social desirability scales desirable? A meta-analytic test of the validity of social desirability scales in the context of prosocial behavior. *Journal of Personality*, **90**, 203–21.

Lensvelt-Mulders, G., Hox, J.J., der Heijden, P., and Mass, C. (2005). Meta-analysis of randomized response research: Thirty-five years of validation. *Sociological Methods & Research*, **33**, 319–48.

Linn, L. (1979). Interns' attitudes and values as antecedents of clinical performance. *Journal of Medical Education*, **54**, 238–40.

Linton, M. (1975). Memory for real world events. In *Explorations in cognition* (eds. D.A. Norman and D.E. Rumelhart), pp. 376–404. Freeman, San Francisco, CA.

Mayo, N.E., Scott, S.C., Bernstein, C.N., and Lix, L.M. (2015). How are you? Do people with inflammatory bowel disease experience response shift on this question? *Health and Quality of Life Outcomes*, **13**, Article 52.

Mazze, R., Shamoon, H., Pasmantier, R., Lucido, D., Murphy, J., Hartmann, K., *et al.* (1984). Reliability of blood glucose monitoring by subjects with diabetes mellitus. *American Journal of Medicine*, **77**, 211–17.

McCrae, R.R. and Costa, P.T., Jr. (1983). Social desirability scales: More substance than style. *Journal of Consulting and Clinical Psychology*, **51**, 882–8.

McFarlane, A.H., Neale, K.A., Norman, G.R., Roy, R.G., and Streiner, D.L. (1981). Methodological issues in developing a scale to measure social support. *Schizophrenia Bulletin*, **1**, 90–100.

Meade, A.W. and Craig, S.B. (2012). Identifying careless responses in survey data. *Psychological Methods*, **17**, 437–55.

Means, B., Nigam, A., Zarrow, M., Loftus, E.F., and Donaldson, M.S. (1989). *Autobiographical memory for health-related events*. Vital and Health Statistics, Series 6, No. 2. Public Health Service, Hyattsville, MD.

Medawar, P.B. (1967). *The art of the soluble.* Methuen & Co., North Yorkshire.

Mick, D.G. (1996). Are studies of dark side variables confounded by socially desirable responding? The case of materialism. *Journal of Consumer Research*, **23**, 106–19.

Nederhof, A.J. (1984). Visibility of response as mediating factor in equity research. *Journal of Social Psychology*, **122**, 211–15.

Neisser, U. (1986). Nested structure in autobiographical memory. In *Autobiographical memory* (ed. D.C. Rubin), pp. 71–81. Cambridge University Press, Cambridge.

Nichols, D.S., Greene, R.L., and Schmolck, P. (1989). Criteria for assessing inconsistent patterns of item endorsement on the MMPI: Rationale, development, and empirical trials. *Journal of Clinical Psychology*, **45**, 239–50.

Nolte, S., Elsworth, G.R., and Osborne, R.H. (2013). Absence of social desirability bias in the evaluation of chronic disease self-management interventions. *Health and Quality of Life Outcomes*, **11**, 114.

Norcross, J.C., Karg, R.S., and Prochaska, J.O. (1997). Clinical psychologist in the 1990s: II. The *Clinical Psychologist*, **50**(3), 4–11.

Norman, G.R. (2003). Hi! How are you? Response shift, implicit theories and differing epistemologies. *Quality of Life Research*, **12**, 239–49.

Norman, G.R., Regehr, G., and Stratford, P.S. (1997). Bias in the retrospective calculation of responsiveness to change: The lesson of Cronbach. *Journal of Clinical Epidemiology*, **8**, 869–79.

Nuckols, R.C. (1953). A note on pre-testing public opinion questions. *Journal of Applied Psychology*, **37**, 119–20.

Offer, D., Katz, M., Howard, K.I., and Bennett, E.S. (2000). The altering of reported experiences. *Journal of the American Academy of Child and Adolescent Psychiatry*, **39**, 735–42.

Okun, M.A. and George, L.K. (1984). Physician- and self-ratings of health, neuroticism, and subjective well-being among men and women. *Personality and Individual Differences*, **5**, 533–9.

Ones, D.S., Viswesvaran, C., and Reiss, A.D. (1996). Role of social desirability in personality testing for personnel selection: The red herring. *Journal of Applied Psychology*, **81**, 660–79.

Oppenheim, A.N. (1966). *Questionnaire design and attitude measurement*. Heinemann, London.

Paulhus, D.L. (1983). Sphere-specific measures of perceived control. *Journal of Personality and Social Psychology*, **44**, 1253–65.

Paulhus, D.L. (1984). Two-component models of socially desirable responding. *Journal of Personality and Social Psychology*, **46**, 598–609.

Paulhus, D.L. (1986). Self deception and impression management in test responses. In *Personality assessment via questionnaire* (eds. A. Angleitner and J.S. Wiggins), pp . 143–65. Springer, New York.

Paulhus, D.L. (1994). *Balanced Inventory of Desirable Responding: Reference manual for BIDR Version 6*. Unpublished manuscript, University of British Columbia, Vancouver, BC.

Paulhus, D.L. (2002). Socially desirable responding: The evolution of a construct. In *The role of constructs in psychological and educational measurement* (eds. H.I. Braun, D.N. Jackson, and D.E. Wiley), pp. 49–69. Lawrence Erlbaum, Mahwah, NJ.

Raghavarao, D. and Federer, W.T. (1979). Block total response as an alternative to the randomized response method in surveys. *Journal of the Royal Statistical Society Series B (Statistical Methodology)*, **41**, 40–5.

Roberts, C., Gilbert, E., Allum, N., and Eisner, L. (2019). Satisficing in surveys: A systematic review of the literature. *Public Opinion Quarterly*, **83**, 598–626.

Ronen, G.M. and Streiner, D.L. (2013). Self- and proxy-rated valuations of outcomes. In *Life quality outcomes in children and young people with neurological and developmental conditions* (eds. G.M Ronen and P.L. Rosenbaum), pp. 234–48. Mac Keith Press, London.

Ronen, G.M., Streiner, D.L., Rosenbaum, P., and the Canadian Pediatric Network (2003). Health-related quality of life in children with epilepsy: Development and validation of self-report and parent proxy measures. *Epilepsia*, **44**, 598–612.

Ross, M. (1989). Relation of implicit theories to the construction of personal histories. *Psychological Review*, **96**, 341–7.

Rosse, J.G., Stecher, M.D., Miller, J.L., and Levin, R.A. (1998). The impact of response distortion on preemployment personality testing and hiring decisions. *Journal of Applied Psychology*, **83**, 634–44.

Rotter, J. (1966). Generalized expectancies for internal versus external control of reinforcement. *Psychological Monographs: General and Applied*, **80** (1), 1–28 .

Saigal S., Stoskopf, B., Pinelli, J., Streiner, D.L., Hoult, L., Paneth, N., *et al.* (2006). Self-perceived health-related quality of life of former extremely low birth weight infants in young adulthood. *Pediatrics*, **118**, 1140–8.

Salovey, P., Smith, A.F., Turk, D.C., Jobe, J.B., and Wills, G.B. (1993). The accuracy of memory for pain: Not so bad most of the time. *APS Journal*, **2**, 184–91.

Sawyer, M.G., Streiner, D.L., and Baghurst, P. (1998). The influence of distress on mothers' and fathers' reports of childhood emotional and behavioral problems. *Journal of Abnormal Child Psychology*, **26**, 407–14.

Schechter, S. and Herrmann, D. (1997). The proper use of self-report questions in effective measurement of health outcomes. *Evaluation & the Health Professions*, **20**, 28–46.

Scheers, N.J. (1992). A review of randomized response techniques. *Measurement and Evaluation in Counseling and Development*, **25**, 27–41.

Schmitt, D.P. and Allik, J. (2005). Simultaneous administration of the Rosenberg Self-Esteem Scale in 53 nations: Exploring the universal and culture-specific features of global self-esteem. *Journal of Personality and Social Psychology*, **89**, 623–42.

Schwartz, C.E. and Sprangers, M.A.G. (1999). Methodological approaches for assessing response shift in longitudinal health related quality of life research. *Social Science & Medicine*, **48**, 1531–48.

Schwarz, N. (1999). Self-reports: How the questions shape the answers. *American Psychologist*, **54**, 93–105.

Schwarz, N. and Oyserman, D. (2001). Asking questions about behavior: Cognition, communication, and questionnaire construction. *American Journal of Education*, **22**, 127–60.

Shiffman, S. (2009). How many cigarettes did you smoke? Assessing cigarette consumption by global report, time-line follow-back, and ecological momentary assessment. *Health Psychology*, **28**, 519 –26.

Shimizu, I.M. and Bonham, G.S. (1978). Randomized response technique in a national survey. *Journal of the American Statistical Association*, **73**, 35–9.

Simon, H.A. (1957). *Models of man*. Wiley, New York.

Spoorenberg, T. (2007). Quality of age reporting: Extension and application of the modified Whipple's index. *Population-E*, **62**, 729–42.

Stöber, J., Dette, D.E., and Musch, J. (2002). Comparing continuous and dichotomous scoring of the Balanced Inventory of Desirable Responding. *Journal of Personality Assessment*, **78**, 370–89.

Stone, A.A., Broderick, J.E., Kaell, A.T., DelesPaul, P.A.E.G., and Poter, L. (2000). Does the peak-end phenomenon observed in laboratory pain studies apply to real-world pain in rheumatoid arthritis? *The Journal of Pain*, **1**, 212–17.

Stone, A.A., Broderick, J.E., Shiffman, S.S., and Schwartz, J.E. (2004). Understanding recall of weekly pain from a momentary assessment perspective: Absolute agreement, between- and within-person consistency, and judged change in weekly pain. *Pain*, **107**, 61–9.

Streiner, D.L. (1985). Global rating scales. In *Assessing clinical competence* (eds. V.R. Neufeld and G.R. Norman), pp. 119–41. Springer, New York.

Streiner, D.L., Patten, S.B., Anthony, J.C., and Cairney, J. (2009). Has "lifetime prevalence" reached the end of its life? An examination of the concept. *International Journal of Methods in Psychiatric Research*, **18**, 221–8.

Sudman, S. and Bradburn, N.M. (1982). *Asking questions: A practical guide to questionnaire design*. Jossey-Bass, San Francisco, CA.

Sudman, S., Bradburn, N.M., and Schwarz, N. (1996). *Thinking about answers: The application of cognitive processes to survey methodology*. Jossey-Bass, San Francisco, CA.

Thorndike, E.L. (1920). A constant error in psychological ratings. *Journal of Applied Psychology*, **4**, 25–9.

Todorov, A. and Kirchner, C. (2000). Bias in proxies' reports of disability: Data from the National Health Interview Survey on Disabilities. *American Journal of Public Health*, **90**, 1248–53.

Tourangeau, R. (1984). Cognitive sciences and survey methods. In *Cognitive aspects of survey methodology: Building a bridge between disciplines* (eds. T. Jabine, M. Straf, J. Tanur, and R. Tourangeau), pp. 73–100. National Academies Press, Washington, DC.

Ulrich, R., Schröter, H., Striegel, H., and Simon, P. (2012). Asking sensitive questions: A statistical power analysis of randomized response models. *Psychological Methods*, **17**, 623–41.

Warner, S.L. (1965). Randomized response: A survey technique for eliminating evasive answer bias. *Journal of the American Statistical Association*, **60**, 63–9.

Waters, E., Doyle, J., Wolfe, R., Wright, M., Wake, M., and Salmon, L. (2000). Influence of parental gender and self-reported health and illness on parent-reported child health. *Pediatrics*, **106**, 1422–8.

Weech-Maldonado, R., Elliott, M. N., Oluwole, A., Schiller, K. C., and Hays, R. D. (2008). Survey response style and differential use of CAHPS rating scales by Hispanics. *Medical Care*, **46**, 963–8.

Wells, F.L. (1907). A statistical study of literary merit. *Archives of Psychology*, **1**(7), 5–30.

Willis, G.B., Royston, P., and Bercini, D. (1991). The use of verbal report methods in the development and testing of survey questionnaires. *Applied Cognitive Psychology*, **5**, 251–67.

Wilson, T.D., LaFleur, S.J., and Anderson, D.A. (1995). The validity and consequences of verbal reports about attitudes. In *Answering questions: Methodology for determining cognitive and communicative processes in survey research* (eds. N. Schwarz and S. Sudman), pp. 91–114. Jossey-Bass, San Francisco, CA.

Winkielman, P., Knäuper, B., and Schwarz, N. (1998). Looking back at anger: Reference periods change the interpretation of (emotion) frequency questions. *Journal of Personality and Social Psychology*, **75**, 719–28.

Wiseman, F. (1972). Methodological bias in public opinion surveys. *Public Opinion Quarterly*, **36**, 105–8.

Yip, J.Y., Wilber, K.H., Myrtle, R.C., and Grazman, D.N. (2001). Comparison of older adult subject and proxy responses on the SF-36 health-related quality of life instrument. *Aging & Mental Health*, **5**, 136–42.

Chapter 7

From items to scales

Introduction to from items to scales

Some scales consist of just one item, such as a visual analogue scale, on which a person may rate their pain on a continuum from 'no pain at all' to 'the worst imaginable pain'. However, the more usual and desirable approach is to have a number of items to assess a single underlying characteristic. This then raises the issue of how we combine the individual items into a scale and then express the final score in the most meaningful way.

By far the easiest solution is to simply add the scores on the individual items and leave it at that. In fact, this is the approach used by many scales. The *Beck Depression Inventory-II* (BDI-II; Beck et al. 1996), for instance, consists of 21 items, each scored on a 0–3 scale, so the final score can range between 0 and 63. This approach is conceptually and arithmetically simple, and makes few assumptions about the individual items; the only implicit assumption is that the items are equally important in contributing to the total score. However, as we saw in Chapter 5, this assumption is true only for parallel and τ-equivalent scales, not for congeneric ones, which, unless proven otherwise, we should assume all scales are.

Since this approach is so simple, there must be something wrong with it. Actually, there are two potential problems. We say 'potential' because, as will be seen later, they may not be problems in certain situations. First, some items may be more important than others, and perhaps should make a larger contribution to the total score. Second, unlike the situation in measuring blood pressure, for example, where it is expected that every blood pressure cuff should, on average, yield the same answer, no one presumes that all scales tapping activities of daily living should give the same number at the end. Under these circumstances, it is difficult, if not impossible, to compare scores on different scales, since each uses a different metric. We shall examine both of these points in some more detail.

Weighting the items

Rather than simply adding up all of the items, a scale or index may be developed which 'weights' each item differently in its contribution to the total score. There are two general approaches to doing this, theoretical and empirical. In the former, a test constructor may feel that, based on their understanding of the field, there are some aspects of a trait that are crucial, and others which are still interesting, but perhaps less germane. It would make at least intuitive sense for the former to be weighted more heavily than the latter. For example, in assessing the recovery of a cardiac patient, their ability to return to work may be seen as more important than resumption of leisure-time activities. In this case, the scale developer may multiply, or weight, the score on items relating to return to work by a factor which would reflect its greater importance. (Perhaps we should mention here that the term 'weight' is preferred by statisticians to the more commonly used 'weigh'.)

The empirical approach comes from the statistical theory of multiple regression. Very briefly, in multiple regression, we try to predict a score (Y) from a number of independent variables (Xs), and it takes the form:

$$Y = \beta_0 + \beta_1 X_1 + \beta_2 X_2 + \ldots + \beta_K X_K,$$

where β_0 is a constant and $\beta_1 \ldots \beta_k$ are the 'beta weights' for k items.

We choose the βs to maximize the predictive accuracy of the equation. There is one optimal set, and any other set of values will result in less accuracy. In the case of a scale, Y is the trait or behaviour we are trying to predict, and the Xs are the individual items. This would indicate that a weighting scheme for each item, empirically derived, would improve the accuracy of the total score (leaving aside for the moment the question of what we mean by 'accuracy').

The question then is whether the benefits outweigh the costs. The answer is that it all depends. Wainer's (1976) conclusion was that if we eliminate items with very small β weights (i.e. those that contribute little to the overall accuracy anyway), then 'it don't make no nevermind' whether the other items are weighted or not.

This was demonstrated empirically by Lei and Skinner (1980), using the Holmes and Rahe (1967) *Social Readjustment Rating Scale* (SRRS). This checklist consists of events that may have occurred in the past 6 months, weighted to reflect how much adjustment would be required to adapt to them. Lei and Skinner looked at four versions of the SRRS:

1. Using the original weights assigned by Holmes and Rahe.

2. Using simply a count of the number of items endorsed, which is the same as using weights of 1 for all items.

3. Using 'perturbed' weights, where they were randomly shuffled from one item to another.

4. Using randomly assigned weights, ranging between 1 and 100.

The life events scale would appear to be an ideal situation for using weights, since there is nearly a 10-fold difference between the lowest (a minor violation of the law, worth 11 points) and highest (death of a spouse, worth 100). On the surface, at least, this differential weighting makes sense, since it seems ridiculous to assign the same weight to the death of a spouse as to receiving a parking ticket. However, they found that the correlations among these four versions were all about 0.97. In other words, it did not matter whether original weights, random weights, or no weights were used; people who scored high on one variant scored high on all of the others, and similarly for people who scored at the low end. Similar results with the SRRS were found by Streiner et al. (1981).

Moreover, this finding is not peculiar to the SRRS; it has been demonstrated with a wide variety of personality and health status measures (e.g. Jenkinson 1991; Streiner et al. 1993). Indeed, Gulliksen (1950) derived an equation to predict how much (or rather, how little) item weighting will affect a scale's correlation with other measures, and hence its validity. The correlation (R) between the weighted and unweighted versions of a test is:

$$R = 1 - \left(\frac{1}{2K\bar{r}} \right) \left(\frac{s}{M} \right)^2$$

where K is the number of items in the scale; $\bar{r}$ is the average correlation among the K items; M is the average of the weights; and s is the standard deviation of the weights. What this equation shows is that the correlation between the weighted and unweighted versions of the test is higher when:

1. there are more items
2. the average inter-item correlation is higher
3. the standard deviation of the weights is lower relative to their mean value.

Empirical testing has shown that actual values are quite close to those predicted by the formula (Retzlaff et al. 1990; Streiner and Miller 1989). This is to be expected with most scales, because they usually have 15–20 items, which are chosen because they all correlate with one another to varying degrees, and the weights are within a narrow range, such as from 1 to 3.

To complicate matters, though, a very different conclusion was reached by Perloff and Persons (1988). They indicated that weighting can significantly increase the predictive ability of an index, and criticize Wainer's work because he limited his discussion to situations where the β weights were evenly distributed over the interval from 0.25 to 0.75, which they feel is an improbable situation.

So, what conclusion can we draw from this argument? The answer is far from clear. It would seem that when there are at least 40 items in a scale, differential weighting contributes relatively little, except added complexity in scoring. With fewer than 40 items (20, according to Nunnally (1970)), weighting *may* have some effect. The other consideration is that if the scale is comprised of relatively homogeneous items, where the β weights will all be within a fairly narrow range, the effect of weighting may be minimal. However, if an index consists of unrelated items, as is sometimes the case with functional status measures ('causal indicators', as we discussed in Chapter 5 under 'When homogeneity does not matter'), then it may be worthwhile to run a multiple regression analysis and determine empirically if this improves the predictive ability of the scale.

There are two forms of weighting that are more subtle than multiplying each item by a number, and are often unintended (and therefore referred to as implicit weighting). The first is having a different number of items for various aspects of the underlying concept being measured, and the second is including items which are highly correlated with one another. To illustrate the first point, assume we are devising a scale to assess childhood behavioural difficulties. In this instrument, we have one item tapping into problems associated with going to bed, and five items looking at disciplinary problems. This implicitly assigns more weight to the latter category, since its potential contribution to the total score can be five times as great as the first area. Even if the parents feel that putting the child to bed is more troublesome to them than the child's lack of discipline, the scale would be weighted in the opposite direction.

There are a few ways around this problem. First, the number of items tapping each component can be equal (which assumes that all aspects contribute equally, as was done in the development of a quality of life scale for children (Ronen et al. 2003)) or proportional to the importance of that area. An item-by-item matrix can be used to verify this, as was discussed in Chapter 3. The second solution is to have subscales, each comprised of items in one area. The total for the subscale would be the number of items endorsed divided by the total number of items within the subscale (and perhaps multiplied by 10 or 100 to eliminate decimals). The scale total is then derived by adding up these transformed subscale scores. In this way, each subscale contributes equally to the total score, even though each subscale may consist of a different number of items.

The second form of implicit weighting is through correlated items. Using the same example of a scale for childhood behavioural problems, assume that the section on school-related difficulties includes the following items:

1. Is often late for school.
2. Talks back to the teacher.
3. Often gets into fights.
4. Does not obey instructions.
5. Ignores the teacher.

If items 2, 4, and 5 are highly correlated, then getting a score on any one of them almost automatically leads to scores on the other two. Thus, these three items are likely measuring the same thing and as such constitute a sub-subscale and lead to problems analogous to those found with the first form of subtle weighting. The same solutions can be used, as well as a third solution: eliminating two of the items. This problem is almost universal, since we expect items tapping the same trait to be correlated (e.g. $r \sim$ 0.50–0.60) , just not *too* correlated (e.g. $r > 0.70$).

Unlike explicit weighting, these two forms are often unintentional. If the effects are unwanted (as they often are), special care and pre-testing the instrument are necessary to ensure that they do not occur.

Missing items

In the majority of cases, the total score on a scale is simply the sum of the scores of the individual items (or of the item scores times their weights, if they exist). A problem arises, though, if some items are omitted by a respondent. There are a few different ways of dealing with this, but none of them is totally satisfactory and each of them depends on making assumptions about the reason for the omissions that are often untestable. Items can be omitted for any one of a number of reasons. The first is that the person skipped it by mistake; for example, they may have intentionally left it out, intending to return to it at the end, but then simply forgot to go back and fill it in. The second reason is that the person found the item objectionable. Although many potentially troublesome items can be caught with adequate pre-testing of the scale, there will always be some people who interpret (or misinterpret) an item to be too intrusive, impolite, or impolitic. Third, the item may be too difficult to understand because of its vocabulary or phraseology. Again, this should be detected in pre-testing, but some items, for some people, may remain troublesome. Fourth, and most commonly, an item is omitted because it does not apply to the person. For example, a question such as 'How hard is it for you to comb your hair?' would be inappropriate for those who are follicularly challenged. Even if the scale developer anticipated this and had a 'Does Not Apply' option, the problem still remains: the question remains unanswered. (Another reason, that the person did not have time to complete the questionnaire, is a problem mainly for timed achievement tests and rarely applies to measures of attitudes, mood, or quality of life. For ways of dealing with this problem, see Ludlow and O'Leary (1999).)

Two of the most common ways of dealing with this problem are to (1) assign a score to the missing item that is the mean of the person's completed items and (2) derive a mean score for the completed items. These two options yield identical results, differing only in that the latter is the total score divided by the number of items. The assumptions are either that the person omitted the item at random , or if the item were deliberately omitted, that it would have been answered with a score consistent with the person's other items. Neither of these assumptions is tenable or testable. Another problem with these approaches is that it underestimates the variance of the total score, because the imputed value is exactly the mean.

The other option is to simply omit the item and base the total score on the items that were completed. This is based on the equally untestable assumption that the person would have given the item a score of zero. But this, too, leads to problems. First, it reduces the total score for that individual, which may underestimate their actual level on the attribute being measured. Second, if the item is scored on a 1–5 scale, a more accurate imputed score may be the lowest possible value, rather than zero. More importantly, though, leaving the item blank plays havoc with most programs that calculate item-based statistics, such as factor analysis or coefficient alpha, where there must be complete data for each subject or the person will be eliminated from the analysis. If items are omitted by a significant proportion of the people, this can result in a drastic reduction in sample size, even if each item is omitted for a small number of people.

As is obvious, there is no ideal solution. If the number of omitted items is small (say 5 per cent or less), then assigning the mean score probably will not distort the results too much, thereby resulting in a complete dataset for subsequent analyses. Once the number of missing items exceeds this, the validity of the results can be questioned. Needless to say, the best strategy is to use items where 'Does Not Apply' does not apply (although this may be difficult with some activities of daily living scales) and to encourage the person to go back and check that every item is answered. Administering the scale by computer, where a response must be entered before advancing to the next item, can minimize the problem of inadvertent omissions. However, the respondent should be offered an option such as 'I prefer not to answer' for each question.

Multiplicative composite scores

The previous section focused on the situation in which each item was given the same weight, and the conclusion was that it is hardly ever worth the effort. In this section, we will discuss a seemingly similar case—where each item is given a different weight by different subjects—and come to a similar recommendation . Do not do it unless it is unavoidable or you are prepared to pay the price in terms of increased sample size and complexity in analysing the results.

Multiplicative composite scores are those in which two values are multiplied together to yield one number. At first glance, this would seem to be a very useful manoeuvre with few drawbacks. Imagine, for example, that supervisors must rate interns on a form that lists a number of components, such as clinical skills, interpersonal skills, self-directed learning, and knowledge base. In any one rotation, the supervisor may have had ample opportunity to observe how the student performs in some of these areas, but may have had a more limited chance to see others. It would seem to make sense that we should ask the supervisor a second question for each component, 'How confident are you in this rating?' Then, when the rating is multiplied by the confidence level, those areas in which the supervisor was more confident would make a greater contribution to the total score, and areas where the supervisor was not as confident would add less. Similarly, if you were devising a quality of life scale, it would seem sensible to multiply people's rating of how well or poorly they could perform some task by some other index which reflects the importance of that task for them. In that way, a person would not be penalized by being unable to do tasks that are done rarely or not at all. Conversely, the total score on the scale would be greatly affected by the important tasks, thus making it easier to detect any changes in quality of life due to some intervention or over time.

The problem arises because multiplying two numbers together (that is, creating a composite measure) affects the resulting total's correlation with another score. More importantly, even if the ratings are kept the same, but simply transformed from one weighting scheme to another (e.g. changed from a −3 to +3 system to a 1- to 7-point scheme), *the scale's correlation with another scale can alter dramatically.*

To illustrate this, imagine that we have an instrument with five items, where each item is scored along a 7-point Likert scale. These are then summed, to form a score (X) for each of five subjects. The items, and their sums, are shown in the second column of Table 7.1, the one labelled Item Score (X). If we correlate these five totals with some other measure, labelled Y in Table 7.1, we find that the correlation is 0.927.

Next assume that each item is weighted for importance on a 7-point scale, with 1 indicating not at all important and 7 extremely important (column 3 in Table 7.1). These scores are then multiplied by X, and the result, along with each subject's total, is shown in column 4. If we correlate these totals with the Ys, we find that the result is 0.681. Now comes the interesting part. Let us keep exactly the same weights for each person but score them on a 7-point scale, where not at all important is −3 and extremely important is + 3; that is, we have done nothing more than subtract four points from each weight. The results of this are shown in the last two columns.

Table 7.1 The effects of changing weighting schemes

Subject	Item score		+1 to +7 weighting		−3 to +3 weighting	
	(X)	Y	Weight	Total	Weight	Total
1	7		1	7	−3	−21
	5		2	10	−2	−10
	7		3	21	−1	−7
	6		4	24	0	0
	3		5	15	1	3
Total	28	25		77		−35
2	1		6	6	2	2
	3		7	21	3	9
	1		1	1	−3	−3
	2		2	4	−2	−4
	4		3	12	−1	−4
Total	11	13		44		0
3	3		4	12	0	0
	4		5	20	1	4
	5		6	30	2	10
	4		7	28	3	12
	3		1	3	−3	−3
Total	19	18		93		23
4	5		2	10	−2	−10
	7		3	21	−1	−7
	6		4	24	0	0
	3		5	15	1	3
	2		6	12	2	4
Total	23	26		82		−10
5	2		7	14	3	6
	3		1	3	−3	−9
	2		2	4	−2	−4
	4		3	12	−1	−4
	5		4	20	0	0
Total	16	15		53		−11

Has this changed anything? Amazingly, the results are drastically different. Instead of a correlation of + 0.681, we now find that the correlation is −0.501. That is, by keeping the weights the same, and simply modifying the numbers assigned to each point on the scale, we have transformed a relatively high positive correlation into an almost equally high negative one. Other linear transformations of the weights can make the correlation almost any value in between (or even more extreme).

Why should this be? The mathematics of it are beyond the scope of this book (the interested reader should look at Evans (1991) for a complete explanation). A brief summary is that the correlation between X and Y, where X is a composite score, depends in part on the variance of the weight, the covariance between X and the weight, and the mean of the weight. Thus, a change that affects any of these factors, but especially the weight's mean, can drastically affect the magnitude and the sign of the correlation.

There is a way to overcome the problem, but it is a costly one in terms of sample size. The method is to use hierarchical (or staged) regression : that is, where the predictor variables are put into the regression equation in stages, under the control of the investigator (see Norman and Streiner (2014) for a fuller explanation). In the first step, any covariates are forced into the model. In step two, the X variable and the weights are added as two additional variables. In the third step, the interaction (that is, the multiplication) of X and the weight is forced in. Any significant increase in the multiple correlation from step 1 to step 2 would indicate that the variables add something to the prediction of Y. Then, the real test of the hypothesis is to see if the multiple correlation increases significantly between the second and the third steps; if so, it would show that the interaction between X and the weight adds something over and above what the variables tell us separately. Of course, we can also break step 2 down, to see if the weights themselves increase the predictive power of the equation.

The cost is that, rather than having one predictor and one dependent variable (ignoring any covariates), we now have three predictors: X, the weighting factor, and the interaction between the two. If we want to maintain a ratio of at least ten subjects for every predictor variable (Norman and Streiner 2014), this triples the required sample size. In the end, unless one's theory demands an interaction term, multiplicative composites should be avoided.

Transforming the final score

The second drawback with simply adding up the items to derive a total score is that each new scale is reported on a different metric, making comparisons among scales difficult. This may not pose a problem if you are working in a brand new area, and do not foresee comparing the results to any other test. However, few such areas exist, and in most cases it is desirable to see how a person did on two different instruments. For example, the BDI-II, as we have said, ranges between a minimum score of 0 and a maximum of 63; while a similar test, the *Self-Rating Depression Scale* (SRDS; Zung 1965), yields a total score between 25 and 100. How can we compare a score of 23 on the former with one of 68 on the latter? It is not easy when the scores are expressed as they are.

The problem is even more evident when a test is comprised of many subscales, each with a different number of items. Many personality tests, like the *Sixteen Personality*

Factor Questionnaire (*16PF*) (Cattell et al. 1970) or the *Personality Research Form* (Jackson 1984), are constructed in such a manner, as are intelligence tests like those developed by Wechsler (1981). The resulting 'profile' of scale scores, comparing their relative elevations, would be uninterpretable if each scale were measured on a different yardstick.

The solution to this problem involves *transforming* the raw score in some way in order to facilitate interpretation. In this section, we discuss three different methods: percentiles, standard and standardized scores, and normalized scores.

Percentiles

A *percentile* is the percentage of people who score (at or) below a certain value. Why is 'at or' in parentheses? Because nobody can agree on a single definition : that is, whether or not it should be there. If we use the definition with the phrase in it, then the lowest score is at the 1st percentile and the highest is at the 100th. If we adopt the definition without that phrase (as we will do in this chapter), then the lowest score is at the 0th percentile, since nobody has a lower one, while the top score is at the 99th percentile. Nobody can be at the 100th percentile, since that implies that everyone, including that person, has a lower score, an obvious impossibility. In medicine, perhaps the most widely used examples of scales expressed in percentiles are developmental height and weight charts. After a child has been measured, their height is plotted on a table for children the same age. If they are at the 50th percentile, that means that they are exactly average for their age; half of all children are taller and half are shorter. Some of the percentiles have special names. The 25th percentile is called the *lower quartile* or Q1. The lower quarter of scores fall below it and three-quarters above it. Analogously, Q3 is the *upper quartile*, with three-quarters of the scores below it and 25 per cent above. The second quartile, Q2, is the *median*; half of the scores are above it and half below. In statistics, the difference between Q3 and Q1 is the *interquartile range* and contains the middle half of the data. It is used as the measure of dispersion for ordinal data, equivalent to the standard deviation used with interval and ratio data.

To show how these are calculated, assume a new test has been given to a large, representative sample, which is called a 'normative' or 'reference' group. If the test is destined to be used commercially, 'large' often means 1,000 or more carefully selected people; for more modest aims, 'large' can mean about 100 or so. The group should be chosen so that their scores span the range you would expect to find when you finally use the test. The next step is to put the scores in *rank order*, ranging from the highest to the lowest. For illustrative purposes, suppose the normative group consists of (a ridiculously small number) 20 people. The results would look something like Table 7.2.

Starting with the highest score, a 37 for Subject 5, 19 of the 20 scores are lower, so a raw score of 37 corresponds to the 95th percentile. Subject 3 has a raw score of 21; since 12 of the 20 scores are lower, Subject 3 is at the 60th percentile (that is, 12/20). A slight problem arises when there are ties, as with Subjects 17 and 8, or 19 and 14. If there are an odd number of ties, as exists for a score of 16, we take the middle person (Subject 20 in this case) and count the number of people below. Since there are six of them, a raw score of 16 is at the 30th percentile, and all three people then get this value.

Table 7.2 Raw scores for 20 subjects on a hypothetical test

Subject	Score	Subject	Score
5	37	19	17
13	32	14	17
2	31	1	16
15	29	20	16
17	26	7	16
8	23	6	15
10	23	11	13
3	21	16	12
12	20	4	10
18	19	9	8

If there is an even number of ties, then you will be dealing with 'halves' of a person. Thus, 8.5 people have scores lower than 17, so it corresponds to the 42.5th percentile. We continue doing this for all scores, and then rewrite the table, putting in the percentiles corresponding to each score, as in Table 7.3.

The major advantage of percentiles is that most people, even those without any training in statistics or scale development, can readily understand them. However, there are a number of difficulties with this approach. One problem is readily apparent in Table 7.3: unless you have many scores, there can be fairly large jumps between the percentile values of adjacent scores. Also, it is possible that in a new sample, some people may have scores higher or lower than those in the normative group, especially if

Table 7.3 The raw scores from Table 7.2 converted to percentiles

Subject	Score	Percentile	Subject	Score	Percentile
5	37	95	19	17	42.5
13	32	90	14	17	42.5
2	31	85	1	16	35
15	29	80	20	16	35
17	26	75	7	16	35
8	23	67.5	6	15	25
10	23	67.5	11	13	20
3	21	60	16	12	10
12	20	55	4	10	5
18	19	50	9	8	0

it was small and not carefully chosen. This makes the interpretation of these more extreme scores problematic at best. Third, since percentiles are ordinal data, they should not be analysed using parametric statistics; means and standard deviations derived from percentiles are not legitimate (strictly speaking anyway).

The fourth difficulty with percentiles is a bit more subtle, but just as insidious. The distribution of percentile scores is rectangular. However, the distribution of raw test scores usually resembles a normal, or bell-shaped, curve, with most of the values clustered around the mean, and progressively fewer ones as we move out to the extremes. As a result, small differences in the middle range become exaggerated and large differences in the tails are truncated. For example, a score of 16 corresponds to the 35th percentile, while a score just 2 points higher is at the 50th percentile. By contrast, a 5-point difference, from 32 to 37, results in just a 5-point spread in the percentiles.

Standard and standardized scores

To get around these problems with percentiles, a more common approach is to use *standard scores*. The formula to transform raw scores to standard scores is:

$$z = \frac{X - \bar{X}}{SD}$$

where X is the total score for an individual, $\bar{X}$ is the mean score of the sample, and SD is the sample's standard deviation.

This 'transforms' the scale to have a mean of 0 and a standard deviation of 1; so, the individual scores are expressed in standard deviation units. Moreover, since the transformation is linear, the distribution of the raw scores (ideally normal) is preserved. (By the same token, if the raw data are skewed, the transformed data will be, too; the z transformation doesn't help us in this regard.) For example, the mean of the 20 scores in the table is 20.0, and the standard deviation is 7.75. We can convert Subject 5's score of 37 into a z-score by putting these numbers into the formula. When we do this, we find:

$$z = \frac{37 - 20}{7.75} = 2.19$$

That is, the Subject's score of 37 is slightly more than two standard deviations above the mean on this scale. Similarly, a raw score of 12 yields a z-score of -1.55, showing that this person's score is about one and a half standard deviations below the group mean.

If all test scores were expressed in this way, then we could compare results across them quite easily. Indeed, we can use this technique on raw scores from different tests, as long as we have the means and standard deviations of the tests. Then, if we received scores on two tests given to a patient at two different times, and purportedly measuring the same thing, we can see if there has been any change by transforming both of them to z-scores. As an example, we can now answer the question, how does a score of 23 on the Beck BDI-II compare with 68 on the Zung SRDS? The mean and SD of the Beck are 11.3 and 7.7, and they are 52.1 and 10.5 for the Zung. Substituting the raw scores into the equation with their respective means and SDs, we find that 23 on the Beck corresponds to a z-score of 1.52, and 65 on the Zung yields a z-score of 1.51. So, although the raw scores are very different, they probably reflect similar degrees of depression.

In real life, though, we are not used to seeing scores ranging from about −3.0 to +3.0; we are more accustomed to positive numbers only, and whole ones at that. Very often, then, we take the second step and transform the z-score into what is called a *standardized* or *T-score* by using the formula:

$$T = \bar{X}' + z\left(SD'\right)$$

where $\bar{X}'$ is the new mean that we want the test to have, SD′ is the desired standard deviation, and z is the original z-score.

We can also go directly from the raw scores to the T-scores by combining this equation with that for the z-score transformation, in which case we obtain:

$$T = \bar{X}' + \frac{\left(SD'\right)\left(X - \bar{X}\right)}{SD}$$

A standardized or T-score is simply a z-score with a new mean and standard deviation. When they were introduced by McCall (1922, 1939; and called T-scores in honour of his famous professor, E.L. Thorndike), T-scores were defined as having a mean of 50 and an SD of 10. This convention is still followed by many personality tests, such as the *Minnesota Multiphasic Personality Inventory* (MMPI) and the *Personality Assessment Inventory*. However, over the years, this convention has been dropped. Many nationwide tests for admission to university, graduate school, or professional programmes use a mean of 500 and an SD of 100. Intelligence tests, for the most part, have a mean of 100 and an SD of 15. If we were developing a new IQ test, we would give it to a large normative sample and then transform each possible total raw score into a z-score. Then, setting $\bar{X}'$ to be 100 and SD′ to be 15, we would translate each z-score into its equivalent T-score. The result would be a new test, whose scores are directly comparable to those from older IQ tests.

Other commonly used transformed scores are the *stanine* and *sten*. Once the raw scores have been transformed into z-scores, then:

$$\text{Stanine} = (z \times 2) + 5 \ (\text{range of scores} = 1 \text{ through } 9)$$
$$\text{Sten} = (z \times 2) + 5.5 \ (\text{range of scores} = 1 \text{ through } 10)$$

The z- and transformed scores do more than simply compare the results on two different tests. Like percentiles, they allow us to see where a person stands in relation to everybody else. If we assume that the scores on the test are fairly normally distributed, then we use the normal curve to determine what proportion of people score higher

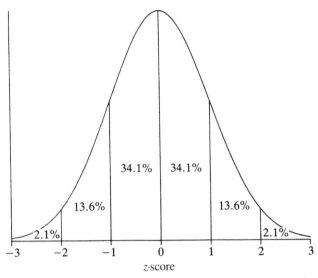

34.1% 34.1%

13.6% 13.6%

2.1% 2.1%

−3 −2 −1 0 1 2 3

z-score

Fig. 7.1 The normal curve.

and lower. As a brief review, a normal curve looks like Fig. 7.1. Most of the scores are clustered around the mean of the test, with progressively fewer scores as we move out to the tails. By definition, 50 per cent of the scores fall below the mean and 50 per cent above , while 68 per cent are between −1 and +1 SD. That means that 84 per cent of scores fall below 1 SD—the 50 per cent below the mean plus 34 per cent between the mean and + 1 SD. To use a concrete example, the MCAT has a mean of 500 and a standard deviation of 100. So, 68 per cent of the people have scores between 400 and 600, and 84 per cent have scores lower than 600 (meaning that 16 per cent have higher scores). We can look up other values in a table of the normal distribution, which can be found in most statistics books (though statistical software packages will generate these values automatically or on request). This is an extremely useful property of z- and T-scores, which is why many widely used tests report their final scores in this way. Another advantage of these scores is that, since they are based on the normal curve, they often more closely meet the assumptions of parametric statistics than do either raw scores or percentiles, although it is not safe to automatically assume that standardized scores *are* normally distributed.

A rough rule of thumb which can be used to check if a scale's T-scores are normally distributed is to look at their range. Because 99.74 per cent of the area of the normal curve lies between ±3 SDs, the range of the T-scores should be similarly constrained. For scales that use $\bar{X} = 50$ and SD = 10, that should mean that T-scores range between 20 and 80. The fact that the MMPI has T-scores that can exceed 120 means that the distribution of raw scores was highly skewed to the right, and should have been transformed to be more normal before the T-scores were derived.

Any clinician who has undergone the painful process of having to relearn normal values of laboratory tests using the SI system must wonder why standard scores are not used in the laboratory. Indeed, the problem is twofold: switching from one measurement system to another; and different values of 'normal' within each system. For example, the normal range for fasting plasma glucose used to be between 70 and 110 mg per cent, and was 1.1–4.1 ng mL^{-1} h^{-1} for plasma renin. In SI units, these same values are 3.9–6.1 mmol L^{-1} for glucose, and 0.30–1.14 ng L^{-1} s^{-1} for renin. Think how much easier life would be if the results of all these diverse tests could be expressed in a common way, such as standard or standardized scores.

Normalized scores

In order to ensure that standard and standardized scores are normally distributed, we can use other transformations which normalize the raw scores. One of the most widely used ones is the *normalized standard score*. Returning to Table 7.3, we take one further step, transforming the percentiles into standard scores from a table of the normal curve which can be found in many textbooks or on the Web. For example, the 95th percentile corresponds to a normalized standard score of 1.65 , the 90th percentile to a score of 1.29, and so on. As with non-normalized standard scores, we can, if we wish, convert these to *standardized*, normalized scores, with any desired mean and standard deviation. In Table 7.4, we have added two more columns : the first showing the transformation from percentiles to normalized standard (z) scores, and then to normalized standardized (T) scores, using a mean of 100 and a standard deviation of 10.

Age and sex norms

Some attributes, especially those assessed in adults like cardiac output, show relatively little change with age and do not differ between males and females. Other factors, such as measures of lung capacity like forced vital capacity, show considerable variation with age or biological sex. It is well known, for example, that females are more prone to admit to depressive symptomatology than are men. The psychometric solution to this problem is relatively easy: separate norms can be developed for each sex, as was done for the MMPI Depression scale and some others on that inventory. However, this may mask a more important and fundamental difficulty: do the sexes differ only in terms of their willingness to endorse depressive items, or does this reflect more actual depression in women? Separate norms assume that the distribution of depression is equivalent for males and females, and it is only the reporting that is different.

The opposite approach was taken by Wechsler (1958) in constructing his intelligence tests. He began with the explicit assumption that males and females do not differ on any of the dimensions that his instruments tap. During the process of developing the tests, he therefore discarded any tasks, such as spatial relations, which did show a systematic bias between the sexes.

These decisions were *theoretically founded* ones, not psychometric ones, based on the developer's conception of how these attributes exist in reality. Deciding whether sex norms should be used (as with the MMPI) or whether more endorsed items means more underlying depression (as in the Beck or Zung scales), or if the sexes *should* differ on some trait such as intelligence reflects a theoretical model. Since these are crucial

Table 7.4 Percentiles from Table 7.3 transformed into normalized standard and normalized standardized scores

Subject	Score	Percentile	Normalized standard score (z)	Normalized standardized score (T)
5	37	95	1.65	116.5
13	32	90	1.29	112.9
2	31	85	1.04	110.4
15	29	80	0.84	108.4
17	26	75	0.67	106.7
8	23	67.5	0.45	104.5
10	23	67.5	0.45	104.5
3	21	60	0.25	102.5
12	20	55	0.13	101.3
18	19	50	0.00	100.0
19	17	42.5	−0.19	98.1
14	17	42.5	−0.19	98.1
1	16	35	−0.39	96.1
20	16	35	−0.39	96.1
7	16	35	−0.39	96.1
6	15	25	−0.67	93.3
11	13	20	−0.84	91.6
16	12	10	−1.29	87.1
4	10	5	−1.65	83.5
9	8	0	−3.00	70.0

in interpreting the results, they should be spelled out explicitly in any manual or paper about the instrument.

Age norms are less contentious, as developmental changes are more objective and verifiable. Some of the many examples of age-related differences are height, weight, and vocabulary. When these exist, separate norms are developed for each age group, and often age-sex group, as boys and girls develop at different rates. The major question facing the test constructor is how large the age span should be in each normative group. The answer depends to a large degree on the speed of maturation of the trait; a child should not change in their percentile level too much in crossing from the upper limit of one age group to the beginning of the next. If this does occur, then it is probable that the age span is too great.

Of course, an additional challenge is that age is imperfectly correlated with biological maturation. Measures of child development that are banded based on calendar age, while convenient, are prone to misclassification errors for this reason (Veldhuizen et al. 2017). This has been described as a problem of relative age effects: a child whose birth date places that child in the upper range of an age band (close to the cut-off for a different (or older age) band) will tend to perform better on tests measuring development (e.g. motor, cognition) than a child whose birth date places the child lower in the age band, simpl y because the former child is relatively older than the latter (Veldhuizen et al. 2014). If the test in question is intended to measure developmental delay, the relatively younger child may appear delayed, when in fact their performance is in the normal range relative to their biological age. Age-banding based on chronological age in others has led to a false positive, which can have significant personal and social costs.

Establishing cut points

Although we have argued throughout this book that continuous measures are preferable to categorical ones, there are times when it is necessary to use a continuous scale in order to predict a dichotomous outcome. For example, we may want to determine for which patients their score on a depression scale is high enough that we will presume they are clinically depressed , or which students have a score on a final exam so low that we could call them failures. Another reason for dichotomizing is that we may want to determine whether the benefit derived from a new treatment is sufficiently large to justify a change in management.

This latter decision has been a preoccupation of measurement in the health sciences, particularly in the assessment of health-related quality of life (HRQL). The goal is laudable, and rests on two points. The first is an explicit recognition that statistical significance reveals nothing about clinical importance, a fact drummed home ad nauseam in statistics books, but promptly forgotten when it comes to publication (e.g. the difference was *highly* significant ($p < 0.0001$)). There are many examples from clinical trials of results that achieved statistical significance, but were of no practical importance, such as streptokinase versus tissue plasminogen activator in the treatment of acute myocardial infarction, where the differences amounted to 7.3 per cent versus 6.3 per cent (Van de Werf 1993). The second point is that, while it is easy to recognize that a difference in mortality of 1 per cent is of little consequence, a difference of 3.1 points on some HRQL instrument is much less comprehensible. Consequently, a literature has emerged that attempts to establish minimum standards for clinically important change (however defined). Conceptually, this is can be seen as an issue of establishing cut points—in this case, between those changes or treatment effects which are beneficial and those which are not.

A number of methods have been worked out in both the educational and clinical domains to approach the problem, and all can be classified roughly as based either on characteristics of the distribution, or on subjective judgements of the cut point, which is more or less independent of the distribution. In education, the distinction is usually referred to as the difference between *norm-referenced* and *criterion-referenced* tests; while in some health measurement areas, such as assessing quality of life, the two broad strategies are called *distribution based* and *anchor based*. As we will see, the distinction ultimately blurs, but it remains a useful starting point.

We will begin by giving a simple (and simplistic) example from each of the approaches:

1. Many lab tests have an established range of normal beyond which the test result is declared to be abnormal (high or low). Not infrequently, the range of normal comes about by simply testing a large number of apparently normal individuals and then establishing a statistical range from the 2.5th to the 97.5th percentile (±2 standard deviations). The problem, of course, is that this strategy ensures that, in any 'normal' population, 5 per cent will always be deemed abnormal. Even if the entire population improves (e.g. everyone starts watching their diet and the mean level of low-density lipoprotein cholesterol drops), by definition 5 per cent will still be abnormal, now including some people who were previously deemed healthy. A more likely occurrence (and one that indeed concerns researchers interested in population rates of obesity) is that as the population grows bigger (in terms of waist size, not numbers of people), cut-offs for obesity based on population norms will increase: What is considered obese today (body mass index >29) will be overweight or may even be normal weight in the future. The solution has been to fix norms, which were derived from a particular historical period (e.g. the 1970s or 1980s), and use this to compare rates today.

2. Most of us went through school and college facing an endless array of final exams, where the pass mark was set at 50 per cent (in Canada) or 65 per cent (in the United States) or some other value, regardless of the actual exam. Occasionally, the results were so bad that the professor was embarrassed into 'bell-curving' the scores, but this was only used in exceptional circumstances. Somehow it never dawned on anyone that 50 per cent, 60 per cent, or whatever the decreed 'pass-mark' was arbitrary, at best. Indeed, the whole necessity of 'bell-curving' comes about because the instructor was presumably unable to anticipate in advance how difficult the test would turn out to be. Such a criterion, however time-honoured, is indefensible, and only withstands assault because individual instructors learn, over time, what kinds of questions can be used in a test to ensure that an acceptable number of students pass and fail around this fixed cut point.

We will now examine the formalized approaches to setting cut points, derived from education and health measurement.

Methods based on characteristics of the distribution

From educational measurement

Perhaps the oldest distribution-based method is the approach called *norm-referenced*. In this method, a fixed percentage of the distribution is set in advance to be below the cut point (i.e. to 'fail'). As one example, for many years, from about 1960 to 1990, the national licensing examinations for medical students in the United States and Canada were norm-referenced. In Canada, the standard was that the failure rate for first-time Canadian graduates would be 4.5 per cent. This criterion, although seemingly as arbitrary as a fixed pass mark of 50 per cent, is actually a bit more rational. When the licensing body went to a multiple choice format from orals and essays, they could no longer rely on examiner judgement for calibration. Consequently, they looked at prior examinations, and found that year by year, about 4–5 per cent of candidates failed. They assumed that this indicated that of all candidates, on average, 4.5 per cent were incompetent (at least, as defined by test performance), and each year the scores were 'bell-curved' to ensure that the failure rate was 4.5 per cent.

The approach is usually assaulted on grounds that 'How can you assume that 5 per cent of the candidates are incompetent? Maybe they're all competent. But you arbitrarily fail some of them. How unfair!' Actually, in the situation where it is used, at a national level, with large numbers of candidates (2,000–20,000) and relatively smaller numbers of questions, it is statistically plausible that the candidate pool changes less from year to year than the question pool. (As a check, examination boards frequently will reuse a small number of questions each year to ensure that there is no drift.)

From health measurement

Historically, the first of distribution-based methods which is usually considered in the quality of life literature is Cohen's effect size (ES; Cohen 1988), defined as the difference between the two means expressed in standard deviation (SD) units (mean difference/SD at baseline). He stated that, in the context of comparing group averages, a small ES is 0.2 (that is, a difference between the means equal to one-fifth of the SD); a medium ES is 0.5; and a large ES is 0.8. His intent in doing so was simply to provide some basis for sample size calculations, not to provide any form of benchmark of clinical importance. However, these criteria have frequently been referred to in the context of deciding on important or unimportant changes. Bear in mind, though, that while some researchers have taken these definitions of small, medium, and large ESs to be holy writ, Cohen himself never intended them to be so. As Thompson (2001) said, 'If people interpreted effect sizes with the same rigidity that $\alpha = 0.05$ has been used in statistical testing, we would merely be being stupid in another metric' (pp. 82– 3).

The second class of distribution-based methods uses a variant on the ES, which divides by the standard error of measurement (SEM), and then establishes cut points based on statistics. There is clearly a relation between the two classes, since , the SEM is related to the test reliability and the baseline SD through the formula:

$$SEM = \sqrt{(1-R)} \times SD_{Baseline}$$

Wyrwich et al. (1999) suggests using a value of 1 SEM, while McHorney and Tarlov (1995) recommend a value of 1.96 SEM, which amounts to a criterion of statistical significance.

Methods based on judgement

From education

Contrasting and borderline groups

The *contrasting groups* and *borderline groups* methods used to set pass/fail standards for examinations are almost completely analogous to the 'minimally important difference' (MID) approach discussed later in this section under 'From health measurement'. The contrasting groups method asks judges to review examinee performance globally (e.g. by reading a whole essay exam, or, in the case of candidates known to the judges, based on ongoing performance), and arrive at a consensus about who should pass or fail. The distributions of scores on the exam for passers and failers are plotted, and the cut score decided subjectively to minimize false positives or negatives. (The receiver operating characteristic (ROC) approach, described later in this section, would be a more objective way to go about this.)

The borderline groups method has been used in Canada to set standards for a national OSCE (Dauphinee et al. 1997; see Chapter 9 for a description of the OSCE). In this method, the examiner at each station completes a checklist indicating which of the actions that were supposed to occur were done by the candidate, so that the sum of these actions performed becomes the score for the station. The examiner also completes a global 7-point scale indicating whether the candidate is a clear fail, borderline fail, borderline pass, clear pass, and so on. The average checklist score for the two 'borderline' groups then becomes the pass mark for the station, and the sum across all stations becomes the overall pass mark.

Absolute methods

Another very complex and time-consuming method has been used almost exclusively for setting standards for multiple choice tests. Indeed, this family of methods is so time-consuming that it is rarely used in contexts other than national, high-stakes, examinations. In the three common approaches, the panel of judges reviews each question and its alternative answers from the perspective of a borderline candidate, and depending on the method, they decide the following:

1. What proportion of the borderline candidates would get it right (Angoff 1971)?
2. Which wrong answers might a borderline candidate choose (Nedelsky 1954)?
3. After grouping all the questions into homogeneous groups based on difficulty, what proportion of the questions in a group would a borderline group answer correctly (Ebel 1972)?

The pass mark then results from summing up these judgements with a method-specific algorithm.

While these methods appear to be fairer than those based on an arbitrary proportion of failures, in fact, unless actual performance data are available, the criterion may be wildly off the mark. A far better approach, and one that is most commonly applied, is to use a judgement approach conducted with performance data on each question, based on previous administrations of the test, available to the judge panel (Shepard 1984).

These absolute methods appear highly specific to multiple choice written examinations, but with some adaptation, might be useful in measuring health. For example, a clinician panel might review a depression inventory, and decide which of the items (e.g. 'I am tired all the time', 'I have lost my appetite') would be endorsed by a 'borderline' patient, at the margin of clinical depression. The sum of these items might become a cut score between normal and depressed.

From health measurement

Although there are a number of anchor-based methods (e.g. Lydick and Epstein 1993), far and away the most common is the minimally important difference (MID; Jaeschke et al. 1989), defined as 'the smallest difference in score in the domain of interest which patients perceive as beneficial and which would mandate in the absence of troublesome side-effects and excessive cost, a change in the patient's management' (p. 408). The approach is directed at determining the difference on an HRQL scale corresponding to a self-reported small but important change on a global scale. To determine this, patients are followed for a period of time, and then asked whether they had got better, stayed about the same, or got worse. If they have improved or worsened, they rate the degree of change from 1 to 7, with 1–3 being a small improvement or worsening, to 6–7 reflecting being very much improved or worsened. The MID is then taken as the mean change on the HRQL scale of the patients who score 1–3.

For decades, there was a contest between proponents of anchor-based and distribution-based methods; however, recently it has become clear that the anchors have won, as evidenced by policy documents from the Food and Drug Administration in the United States (U S FDA 2009). This is not a result of superior psychometric properties. The approaches have some fundamental problems. One serious problem relates to the reliance on a single-item global measure of change. As Coon and Cappeleri (2016) point out, there is something irrational about judging the worth of a multi-item scale against a single global item, notwithstanding some of the anomalies arising from the comparison of multi-item and global scores pointed out earlier. Further, the most common global rating is a 'transition rating' of the form 'Compared to how you felt when you started treatment, how do you feel now?' Such measures tend to be strongly influenced by the present state and only weakly by the initial state; hence, it is unclear what is meant by a 'small' change. Moreover, the method contains a fundamental flaw. Even if the overall treatment effect is zero or negative, there may still be some patients who report positive change, simply from natural variation. And the same variation that defines the MID appears in the denominator of the statistical test of the treatment effect (Norman et al. 1997).

In any case, some evidence suggests that the MID will turn out to be consistently close to about one half a standard deviation, so it may not be worth the effort (Norman et al. 2003).

Summary—approaches to establishing cut points

This has been a very brief and incomplete review of methods used for standard setting. For some comprehensive reviews of standard setting in education, see Norcini and Guelle (2002) and Berk (1986). For discussion of methods to ascertain the minimal difference, see Lydick and Epstein (1993).

However different these classes of methods appear at first glance, the differences may be more illusory than real. In applying the criterion-referenced educational strategies, these yield reliable results only when actual performance data on the test are available, so are hardly as independent of student performance as might be believed.

Indeed, it seems that the main indicator of validity of any criterion-referenced approach is the extent to which it yields failure rates similar to the norm-referenced approach it replaced.

Receiver operating characteristic curves

Another, more objective, approach is used when there is some independent classification dividing people into two groups (as in several of the methods described in the section 'Contrasting and borderline groups').

The technique for establishing the optimal cut point is derived from the early days of radar and sonar detection in the Second World War (Peterson et al. 1954), and the name still reflects that—receiver operating characteristic (ROC). As we increase the sensitivity of the radio (lower the threshold), we pick up both the sound we want to hear as well as background static. Initially, the signal increases faster than the noise. After some point, though, a cross-over is reached, where the noise grows faster than the signal. The optimal setting is where we detect the largest ratio of signal to noise. This technique was later applied to the psychological area of the ability of humans to detect the presence or absence of signals (Tanner and Swets 1954), and then to the ability of diagnostic tests to detect the presence or absence of a state or disease.

In the diagnostic assessment arena, the 'signal' is the number of actual cases of hypertension or depression detected by our scale; the 'noise' is the number of non-cases erroneously labelled as cases; and the analogue of amplification is the cut point of our new scale. If we use something like a quality of life scale, where lower scores indicate more problems, a very low cut-off score (line A in Fig. 7.2) will pick up few true cases, and also make few false positive errors. As we increase the cutting score (line B), we hope we will pick up true cases faster than false ones. Above some optimal value,

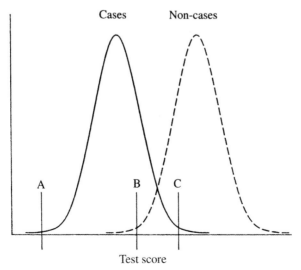

Fig. 7.2 Effects of different cut points.

though, we will continue to detect more true cases, but at the cost of mislabelling many non-cases as cases (line C). The task is to find this optimal value on our scale.

We are assuming that we are dealing with two normal distributions: one based on the scores of people who have the disorder, and one from people who do not. In the vast majority of cases, the two curves overlap, meaning that some cases have quality of life scores that are higher than those of some people who are deemed non-cases; and similarly, some non-cases have lower scores than some cases. No matter where we draw the cut-off, we will misclassify some people.

We begin by drawing up a table, as in Table 7.5, that shows the number of people in each group who receive each score. Based on this, we can construct a series of 2 × 2 tables, each like Table 7.6. Cell A contains the number of actual cases (as determined by the dichotomous gold standard) who are labelled as cases by our new scale (the 'true positives'), while in Cell B are the non-cases erroneously labelled as cases by the test ('false positives'). Similarly, Cell C has the false negatives, and Cell D the true negatives. From this table, we can derive two necessary statistics: the *sensitivity* and the *specificity* of the test. Sensitivity (which is also called the *true positive rate*) is defined as $A/(A + C)$; that is, is the test 'sensitive' in detecting a disorder when it is actually present? Specificity (or the *true negative rate*) is $D/(B + D)$; is the test specific to this disorder, or is it elevated by other ones too?

There are two points to note about sensitivity and specificity. First, the sensitivity at each cut point is derived from only those people who are cases , and the specificity

Table 7.5 The number of cases and non-cases receiving each score

Score	Group		Total
	Cases	**Non-cases**	
<10	0	0	0
10	49	0	49
11	87	5	92
12	92	4	96
13	83	9	92
14	58	30	88
15	68	70	138
16	29	61	90
17	25	56	81
18	4	126	130
19	5	113	118
20	0	26	26
Total	500	500	1,000

Table 7.6 A 2 × 2 table for calculating sensitivity

		Gold standard	
		Case	Non-case
New test	**Case**	A	B
	Non-case	C	D

calculated only from those who are non-cases. As a result, we can derive these numbers, and the ROC curve, without being concerned about the prevalence of the condition in the general population. Second, sensitivity and specificity are like the two arms of an equal-arm balance: if one goes up, the other goes down. Changing the cut point favours one over the other, but it is impossible to increase both without improving the overall performance of the test itself.

To construct an ROC curve, we determine these two values for each possible cut point. Let us assume that we test 500 cases and 500 controls (non-cases) with our new test, which has a total score that could range from 10 to 20. The first row of our first table would contain all the people who had scores of 10, and the second row scores of 11 through 20; the first row of the second table would have scores of 10 and 11, and the second row 12 and higher; and so on, until the last table, where the top row would have all people with scores up to 19, and the bottom row those with a score of 20. (In order to make the graph start and end at one of the axes, we usually add two other tables: one in which everyone has a score above the cut point, and one where they all have scores below it.) The first few tables are shown in the top part of Table 7.7 and a summary of all 12 tables in the lower half. We then make a graph where the X-axis is 1 *minus* the specificity (i.e. the false positive rate) and the Y-axis is the sensitivity (also called the true positive rate), as in Fig. 7.3.

The diagonal line, which runs from point (0, 0) in the lower left-hand corner to (1, 1) in the upper right, reflects the characteristics of a test with no discriminating ability. The better a test is in dividing cases from non-cases, the closer the line will approach the upper left -hand corner. So, Test A in Fig. 7.3 (which is based on the data in Table 7.7) is a better discriminator than Test B. There are a number of criteria for selecting the optimal cut point. The most widely used one minimizes the overall number of errors (false positive and false negative). This is sometimes called the Youden index, or Youden's J, defined as (Sensitivity + Specificity) – 1 (Youden 1950). A better one finds the cut point closest to the upper left (0,1) corner (Perkins and Schisterman 2006). It is called *ER* and is defined as:

$$ER = \sqrt{\left(1 - Sensitivity^2\right) + \left(1 - Specificity^2\right)}$$

An index of the 'goodness' of the test is the *area under the curve*, which is usually abbreviated as D' or AUC. A non-discriminating test (one which falls on the diagonal) has an area of 0.5, and a perfect test has an area of 1.0. (If a test falls below the line and has an area less than 0.5, then it is performing worse than chance; you would do

Table 7.7 Calculations for an ROC curve

Cut-off	Case	Non-case	Cut-off	Case	Non-case	Cut-Off	Case	Non-case
10	49	0	11	136	5	10–12	228	9
11–20	441	500	12–20	364	495	13–20	272	491

Cut point	True positives	False positives	Sensitivity	1 – specificity
<10	0	0	0.000	0.000
10	49	0	0.098	0.000
11	136	5	0.272	0.010
12	228	9	0.456	0.018
13	311	18	0.622	0.036
14	369	48	0.738	0.096
15	437	118	0.874	0.236
16	466	179	0.932	0.358
17	491	235	0.982	0.470
18	495	361	0.990	0.722
19	500	474	1.000	0.948
20	500	500	1.000	1.000

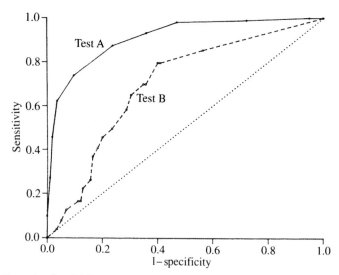

Fig. 7.3 Example of an ROC curve.

better to simply go with the prevalence of the disorder in labelling people, rather than using the test results.) It is difficult to calculate D' by hand, but a number of computer programs are available (e.g. Center and Schwartz 1985; Dorfman and Alf 1969). The standard error of the ROC is given by Hanley and McNeil (1982) as:

$$SE = \left[\frac{D'(1-D') + (N_C - 1)(Q_1 - D'^2) + (N_n - 1)(Q_2 - D'^2)}{N_C N_n} \right]^{\frac{1}{2}}$$

where $Q_1 = D'/(2-D'), Q_2 = 2D'^2/(1-D')$, N_C = number of cases, and N_n = number of non-cases.

The 95 per cent confidence interval (CI) around D' is:

$$CI_{95} = D' \pm 1.96 \times SE$$

Interpreting the area under the curve

In this example, the area under the curve (AUC or D') is 0.911, with an SE of 0.009. This can be interpreted as the probability that the test will yield a score in the abnormal range for a randomly chosen person who is a case that is greater than that for a randomly chosen person who is a non-case (Lasko et al. 2005). So, if we randomly select two people, one who is a case and one who is a non-case, the probability is 91.1 per cent that the former will have a lower score (in this situation, where a lower score is worse) than the former. As a rough guide, AUCs between 0.50 and 0.70 are low; they are moderate between 0.70 and 0.90; and high when the AUC is over 0.90 (Fischer et al. 2003).

Comparing ROC curves

It may seem as if we can compare the performance of two different tests simply by seeing which one has a larger AUC. However, this works only if the two curves do not cross at any point. Figure 7.4 shows two ROC curves with similar AUCs. But, because they cross, the scales have very different properties. Test A is better than B at high levels of specificity (i.e. 1 – Specificity is low), while Test B is better than A when the sensitivity is high. In order to select which one to use, it is necessary to use a variant of the AUC, called the *partial* AUC or pAUC (Lasko et al. 2005; Obuchowski 2003). Instead of calculating the AUC for the entire curve, we focus only on that portion of it that we are interested in when we use the test, such as between a false positive rate of 0.2–0.4, or sensitivities between 0.7 and 0.8. This is almost impossible to calculate by hand, but we can obtain a rough approximation by seeing which test is better at a given false positive rate or sensitivity, rather than looking at a range of false positives or sensitivities.

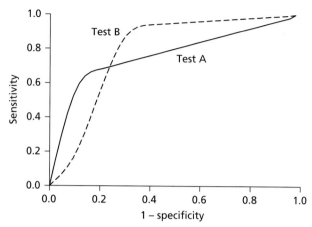

Fig. 7.4 Two ROC curves with equivalent AUCs that cross.

For the sake of completeness, the 95 per cent CI around this AUC is:

$$CI_{95} = 0.911 \pm 1.96 \times 0.009 = 0.893, 0.929$$

There are a few consequences of using the pAUC. First, it is quite possible that we would select a scale that has a smaller AUC, but a larger pAUC within a specific range. Second, a scale that is better within one range of false positives or sensitivities may be worse at a different range. This further illustrates the point that validity is not a fixed property of a test, but depends on the population being assessed and the purpose of the evaluation.

Choosing a cut point

We mentioned previously that the cut point nearest the upper left corner resulted in the smallest overall error rate. There may be some circumstances, though, where it may be preferable to move this point, either up or down, even though the number of false positives may increase faster than the number of true positives. For example, if the consequences of missing a case can be tragic, and second-level tests exist which can weed out the false positives (as with HIV seroconversion), then the cut-off point may be lowered. Conversely, if there are more good applicants than positions, as is the case in admission requests for graduate or professional school, then it makes sense to raise the cut-off. The cost will be an increased number of false negatives (i.e. potentially good students who are denied admission), but relatively few false positives.

Swets (1992), one of the developers of ROC analysis, took costs and benefits into account in selecting the optimal cut point (S_{opt}) with the equation:

$$S_{opt} = \frac{P(neg)}{P(pos)} \times \frac{(B_{TN} - C_{FP})}{(B_{TP} - C_{FN})}$$

where $P(pos)$ is the prior probability, or base rate, of the disorder; $P(neg)$ is $1 - P(pos)$; the Bs and Cs are the benefits and costs; TP is a true positive case; FP a false positive one; and FN a false negative case. The part of the equation to the left of the multiplication sign reflects the slope of the ROC curve at S_{opt}. It says that, in a low-prevalence situation (e.g. detecting hepatitis among all blood donors) and keeping the cost/benefit ratio constant, when $P(neg)$ is much higher than $P(pos)$, the slope is greater than 1, which is the portion of the curve for Test A in Fig. 7.3 on the left where the curve is rising very steeply. When the prevalence is much higher (e.g. hepatitis among intravenous drug users), the ratio of $P(neg)$ to $P(pos)$ becomes smaller. This means the graph is flattening out, as in the right of the graph. So, for highly prevalent conditions, we would use a lenient criterion; whereas for rare ones, the criterion would be much more stringent.

Now let's look at the part of the equation to the right of the multiplication sign and keep the ratio $P(neg)/P(pos)$ constant. When the intervention is effective, S_{opt} is stringent when the cost associated with a false positive diagnosis is high, such as operating on a person who does not have the suspected disease. On the other hand, a more lenient cut point should be set when it's more important to be correct, even when this results in a larger number of false positives. Such would be the case in screening blood donations for HIV or infants for phenylketonuria; missing these would have devastating outcomes.

Needless to say, it is difficult, if not impossible, to attach dollar costs to many outcomes. But even at a subjective level, the equation points to factors that should be considered in setting cut points for diagnostic tests.

Sample size

There are two approaches to determining the sample size needed for an ROC analysis: one is based on the width of the CI around the AUC; and the other is based on testing that the AUC differs significantly from some value (e.g. 0.50, which is the null hypothesis; or from the AUC of a different scale). Unfortunately, neither is easily calculated by hand.

Figuring out the sample size on the width of the CI is based on the fact that the AUC is a parameter and, like any other parameter, such as the mean or a correlation, it is only an estimate of the *true* AUC. We can never know what the true value is, unless we are able to repeat the study an infinite number of times, which is not that feasible given our finite life spans. We begin by guessing what the AUC will be (needless to say, this would be only a rough approximation), and then deciding the maximum width of the CI that we would be willing to tolerate. Based on this, we can use a nomogram (Hanley and McNeil 1982) to determine how many subjects are needed.

The second approach is the more traditional, hypothesis testing way, in which we figure out how large the sample size must be for us to detect a statistically significant difference between the AUC we've obtained and some null hypothesis. The 'null' hypothesis is the one to be nullified; it is not always that the value equals zero (Cohen 1994). When we are looking at a single AUC, the null hypothesis is that it is equal to 0.50; if we are trying to determine if one scale is superior to another, the null value is

Table 7.8 Sample size per group to test the difference between two AUCs with the correlation between the tests of 0.6 (above the main diagonal) and 0.3 (below the main diagonal)

AUC (2)	AUC (1)									
	0.50	0.55	0.60	0.65	0.70	0.75	0.80	0.85	0.90	0.95
0.50	—	404	104	48	28	18	13	9	7	6
0.55	700	—	414	107	49	28	18	12	9	7
0.60	176	700	—	428	110	50	28	17	12	9
0.65	78	175	700	—	440	111	49	28	18	12
0.70	44	78	175	695	—	445	108	49	28	18
0.75	28	44	78	173	680	—	431	110	48	27
0.80	20	28	44	76	168	646	—	421	103	45
0.85	14	19	28	43	74	159	585	—	367	89
0.90	11	14	19	27	41	69	142	486	—	269
0.95	8	11	14	18	25	37	61	115	339	—

Reprinted with permission from Streiner, D.L. and Cairney, J., What's under the ROC? An introduction to receiver operating characteristic curves, *Canadian Journal of Psychiatry*, Volume 52, Issue 2, pp. 121–8, Copyright © 2007 The Canadian Psychiatric Association.

the AUC of that other test. In this latter case, though, we have to take one other factor into account: the correlation between the instruments. Using a computer program for sample size calculation (Hintze 2002), we worked out the approximate sample sizes for an α of 0.05, β of 0.20, and correlations between the scales of 0.3 and 0.6 (Streiner and Cairney 2007); these are given in Table 7.8.

Summary

We have covered four points in this chapter. First, differential weighting of items rarely is worth the trouble. Second, if a test is being developed for local use only, it would probably suffice to simply use the sum of the items. However, for more general use, and to be able to compare the results with other instruments, it is better to transform the scores into percentiles, and best to transform them into z-scores or T-scores. Third, for attributes which differ between males and females, or which show development changes, separate age or age-sex norms can be developed. Fourth, we reviewed a variety of methods for setting cut scores or pass marks.

Further reading

Nunnally, J.C., Jr. (1970). *Introduction to psychological measurement*, chapter 8. McGraw-Hill, New York.

References

Angoff, W.H. (1971). Scales, norms and equivalent scores. In *Educational measurement* (ed. R.L. Thorndike), pp. 508–600. American Council on Education, Washington, DC.

Beck, A.T., Steer, R.A., and Brown, G.K. (1996) *Manual for the Beck Depression Inventory-II*. Psychological Corporation, San Antonio, TX.

Berk, R.A. (1986). A consumer's guide to setting performance standards on criterion-referenced tests. *Review of Educational Research*, **56**, 137–72.

Cattell, R.B., Eber, H.W., and Tatsuoka, M.M. (1970). *Handbook for the Sixteen Personality Factor Questionnaire (16PF)*. Institute for Personality and Ability Testing, Champaign, IL.

Centor, R.M. and Schwartz, J.S. (1985). An evaluation of methods for estimating the error under the receiver operating characteristic (ROC) curve. *Medical Decision Making*, **5**, 149–56.

Cohen, J. (1988). *Statistical power analysis for the behavioral sciences* (2nd edn). Lawrence Erlbaum, Hillsdale, NJ.

Cohen, J. (1994). The earth is round (*p* <.05). *American Psychologist*, **49**, 997–1003.

Coon, C.D. and Cappelleri, J.C. (2016). Interpreting change in scores on patient-reported outcome instruments. *Therapeutic Innovation & Regulatory Science*, **50**, 22–9.

Dauphinee, W.D., Blackmore, D.E., Smee, S., Rothman, A.I., and Reznick, R. (1997). Using the judgments of physician examiners in setting the standards for a national multi-center high stakes OSCE. *Advances in Health Sciences Education: Theory and Practice*, **2**, 201–11.

Dorfman, D.D. and Alf, E. (1969). Maximum likelihood estimation of parameters of signal detection theory and determination of confidence intervals-rating-method data. *Journal of Mathematical Psychology*, **6**, 487–96.

Ebel, R.L. (1972). *Essentials of educational measurement*. Prentice-Hall, Englewood Cliffs, NJ.

Evans, M.G. (1991). The problem of analyzing multiplicative composites: Interactions revisited. *American Psychologist*, **46**, 6–15.

Fischer, J.E., Bachmann, L.M., and Jaeschke, R. (2003). A readers' guide to the interpretation of diagnostic test properties: Clinical example of sepsis. *Intensive Care Medicine*, **29**, 1043–51.

Gulliksen, H.O. (1950). *Theory of mental tests*. Wiley, New York.

Hanley, J.A. and McNeil, B.J. (1982). The meaning and use of the area under a receiver operating characteristic (ROC) curve. *Radiology*, **143**, 29–36.

Hintze, J.L. (2002). *PASS user's guide: II*. NCSS, Kaysville, UT.

Holmes, T.H. and Rahe, R.H. (1967). The social readjustment rating scale. *Journal of Psychosomatic Research*, **11**, 213–18.

Jackson, D.N. (1984). *Personality Research Form manual*. Research Psychologists Press, Port Huron, MI.

Jaeschke, R., Singer, J., and Guyatt, G.H. (1989). Measurement of health status. Ascertaining the minimally important difference. *Controlled Clinical Trials*, **10**, 407–15.

Jenkinson, C. (1991). Why are we weighting? A critical examination of the use of item weights in a health status measure. *Social Science and Medicine*, **32**, 1413–16.

Lasko, T.A., Bhagwat, J.G., Zou, H.H., and Ohno-Machado, L. (2005). The use of receiver operating characteristic curves in biomedical informatics. *Journal of Biomedical Informatics*, **38**, 404–15.

Lei, H. and Skinner, H.A. (1980). A psychometric study of life events and social readjustment. *Journal of Psychosomatic Research*, **24**, 57–65.

Ludlow, L.H. and O'Leary, M. (1999). Scoring omitted and not-reached items: Practical data analysis implications. *Educational and Psychological Measurement*, **59**, 615–30.

Lydick, E. and Epstein, R. S. (1993). Interpretation of quality of life changes. *Quality of Life Research*, **2**, 221–6.

McCall, W.A. (1922). *How to measure in education*. Macmillan, New York.

McCall, W.A. (1939). *Measurement*. Macmillan, New York.

McHorney, C. and Tarlov, A. (1995). Individual-patient monitoring in clinical practice: Are available health status measures adequate? *Quality of Life Research*, **4**, 293–307.

Nedelsky, L. (1954). Absolute grading standards for objective tests. *Educational and Psychological Measurement*, **14**, 3–19

Norcini, J.J. and Guille, R. (2002). Combining tests and setting standards. In *International handbook of research in medical education* (eds. G.R. Norman, C.P.M. van der Vleuten, and D.I. Newble), pp. 810–34. Kluwer, Dordrecht.

Norman, G.R. and Streiner, D.L. (2014). *Biostatistics: The bare essentials* (4th edn). PMPH USA, Shelton, CT.

Norman, G.R., Regehr, G., and Stratford, P.S. (1997). Bias in the retrospective calculation of responsiveness to change: The lesson of Cronbach. *Journal of Clinical Epidemiology*, **8**, 869–79

Norman, G.R., Wyrwich, K.W., and Sloan, J.A. (2003) Interpretation of changes in health-related quality of life: The remarkable universality of half a standard deviation. *Medical Care*, **41**, 582–92.

Nunnally, J.C., Jr. (1970). *Introduction to psychological measurement* . McGraw-Hill, New York.

Obuchowski, N.A. (2003). Receiver operating characteristic curves and their use in radiology. *Radiology*, **229**, 3–8.

Perkins, N.J. and Schisterman, E.F. (2006). The inconsistency of " optimal " cutpoints obtained using two criteria based on the receiver operating characteristic curve. *American Journal of Epidemiology*, **163**, 670–5.

Perloff, J.M. and Persons, J.B. (1988). Biases resulting from the use of indexes: An application to attributional style and depression. *Psychological Bulletin*, **103**, 95–104.

Peterson, W.W., Birdshall, T.G., and Fox, W.C. (1954). The theory of signal detectability. *IRE Transactions: Professional Group on Information Theory*, **4**, 171–212.

Retzlaff, P.D., Sheehan, E.P., and Lorr, M. (1990). MCMI-II scoring: Weighted and unweighted algorithms. *Journal of Personality Assessment*, **55**, 219–23.

Ronen, G.M., Streiner, D.L., Rosenbaum, P., and the Canadian Pediatric Epilepsy Network (2003). Health- related quality of life in children with epilepsy: Development and validations of self-report and parent-proxy measures. *Epilepsia*, **44**, 598–612.

Shepard, L.A. (1984). Setting performance standards. In *A guide to criterion referenced test construction* (ed. R.A. Berk), pp. 169–98. Johns Hopkins Press, Baltimore, MD.

Streiner, D.L. and Cairney, J. (2007). What's under the ROC? An introduction to receiver operating characteristic curves. *Canadian Journal of Psychiatry*, **52**(2), 121–8.

Streiner, D.L. and Miller, H.R. (1989). The MCMI-II: How much better than the MCMI? *Journal of Personality Assessment*, **53**, 81–4.

Streiner, D.L., Norman, G.R., McFarlane, A.H., and Roy, R.G. (1981). Quality of life events and their relationship to strain. *Schizophrenia Bulletin*, **7**, 34–42.

Streiner, D.L., Goldberg, J.O., and Miller, H.R. (1993). MCMI-II weights: Their lack of effectiveness. *Journal of Personality Assessment*, **60**, 471–6.

Swets, J.A. (1992). The science of choosing the right decision threshold in high-stakes diagnostics. *American Psychologist*, **47**, 522–32.

Tanner, W.P., Jr. and Swets, J.A. (1954). A decision-making theory of visual detection. *Psychological Review*, **61**, 401–9.

Thompson, B. (2001). Significance, effect sizes, stepwise methods, and other issues: Strong arguments move the field. *Journal of Experimental Education*, **70**, 80–93.

U S FDA (2009). *U S Department of Health and Human Services Food and Drug Administration Guidance for Industry: Patient-Reported Outcome Measures: Use in Medical Product Development to Support Labeling Claims*. US FDA, Silver Spring, MD .

Van de Werf, F. (1993). Mortality results in GUSTO. *Australian and New Zealand Journal of Medicine*, **23**, 732–4.

Veldhuizen, S., Wade, T.J., Cairney, J., Hay, J.A., and Faught, B.E. (2014) When and for whom are relative age effects important? Evidence from a simple test of cardiorespiratory fitness. *American Journal of Human Biology*, **26**, 476–80.

Veldhuizen, S., Rivard, L., and Cairney, J. (2017). Relative age effects in the Movement Assessment Battery for Children-2: Age banding and scoring errors. *Child Care Health and Development*, **43**, 752–57.

Wainer, H. (1976). Estimating coefficients in linear models: It don't make no nevermind. *Psychological Bulletin*, **83**, 213–17.

Wechsler, D. (1958). *The measurement and appraisal of adult human intelligence* (4th edn). Williams and Wilkins, Baltimore, MD.

Wechsler, D. (1981). *WAIS-R manual: Wechsler Adult Intelligence Scale—Revised* . Psychological Corporation, New York.

Wyrwich, K.W., Nienaber, N.A., Tierney, W.M., and Wolinsky, F.D. (1999). Linking clinical relevance and statistical significance in evaluating intra-individual changes in health-related quality of life. *Medical Care*, **37**, 469–78.

Youden, W.J. (1950). An index for rating diagnostic tests. *Cancer*, **3**, 32–5.

Zung, W.K. (1965). A self-rating depression scale. *Archives of General Psychiatry*, **12**, 63–70.

Chapter 8

Reliability

Introduction to reliability

The concept of *reliability* is a fundamental way to reflect the amount of error, both random and systematic, inherent in any measurement. Yet despite its essential role in judgements of the adequacy of any measurement process, it is devilishly difficult to achieve a real understanding of the psychometric approach to reliability. Some health science researchers also tend to cloud the issue by invoking a long list of possible synonyms, such as 'objectivity', 'reproducibility', 'stability', 'agreement', 'association', 'sensitivity', and 'precision'. Since few of these terms have a formal definition, we will not attempt to show how each differs from the other. Instead, we will concern ourselves with a detailed explanation of the concept of reliability. While some of the terms will be singled out for special treatment later in the chapter, primarily to emphasize their shortcomings, others will be ignored.

Our reasons for this apparently single-minded viewpoint are simple. The technology of reliability assessment was worked out very early in the history of psychological assessment. We once traced its roots back to a textbook written in the 1930s, and the basic definitions were given without reference, indicating that even nine decades ago, the classical definition was viewed as uncontroversial. There is complete consensus within the educational and psychological communities regarding the meaning of the term, and disagreement and debate are confined to a small cadre of biomedical researchers. Moreover, once one understands the basic concept, it appears, in our view, to reflect perfectly the particular requirements of any measurement situation. Although there are some more recent approaches to defining measurement error, such as generalizability theory (see Chapter 9), these represent extensions of the basic approach. Other conflicting views which have arisen in the biomedical research community, such as the treatment of Bland and Altman (1986), offer, in our view, no advantage. This latter method, because of its recent popularity, will be discussed separately.

Basic concepts

What is this elusive concept, and why is it apparently so hard to understand? In order to explore it, we will begin with some common-sense notions of measurement error and eventually link them to the more formal definitions of reliability.

Daily experience constantly reminds us of measurement error. Many of us leap (or crawl) out of bed in the morning and step onto a bathroom scale, hoping to see if avoiding dessert for the past week has resulted in weight loss. We know to disregard any changes less than about 2 lb or 1 kg, since bathroom scales are typically accurate to no better than ±2 lb (±1 kg). If our children are ill, we may measure their temperature with a home thermometer, accurate to about ±0.2°C. Baby's weight gain or loss is measured on a different scale, at home or at the doctor's surgery, accurate to about ±20 g. As we come downstairs, we note the time on our antique longcase (grandfather) clock, and assume that it is accurate to a few minutes. Before donning our coat to leave the house, we check the outside thermometer (±2°F; ±1°C). We leap into our cars and accelerate rapidly up to the speed limit, at least as assessed by our car's speedometer (±5 km/h; ±3 mph) and check the time again as we arrive at work, by looking at our wristwatches (probably quartz, ±15 s). We settle at our desks, pick up the first cup of coffee or tea of the day, and read a new paper on observer error which begins by stating that 'the reliability was calculated with an intraclass correlation, and equalled 0.86'.

Why, for goodness sake, do we have to create some arcane statistic, with no dimension and a range from zero to one, regardless of the measurement situation, in order to express measurement error? To explain, let us review the measurements of the previous paragraph. We begin by assuming that the reader will accept that the measurement errors we cited, while not precisely correct, were at least approximately consistent with our common experience. In the brief 'Day in the Life of ...', we indicated two measurements of time, weight and temperature, each with an approximate error. We are completely comfortable with a bathroom scale accurate to ±1 kg, since we know that individual weights vary over far greater ranges than this, and typical changes from day to day are about the same order of magnitude. Conversely, we recognize that this error of measurement is unacceptable for weighing infants because it exceeds important changes in weight. Similarly, an error of time measurement of several minutes is usually small compared with the anticipated tolerances in daily life (except for European and Japanese trains). Indeed, many people have now reverted back to quartz analogue watches, since they find the extreme accuracy of the digital readouts unnecessary and annoying. Finally, we tolerate an error of measurement of several degrees Celsius for outside air temperature, since we know that it may range from −40° to +40°C in Canada (in the United Kingdom, from −5 to +15), so the measurement error is a small fraction of the true range. The same measurement error is, however, hopeless in a clinical situation since body temperature is restricted to a range of only a few degrees.

In all of these situations, our comfort resides in the knowledge that the error of measurement is a relatively small fraction of the range in the observations. Further, the reason that the measurement error alone provides useful information in the everyday world is that we share a common perception of the expected differences we will encounter. However, such everyday information is conspicuously absent for many measurement scales. To report that the error of measurement on a new depression scale is ±3 is of little value since we do not know the degree of difference among patients, or between patients and non-patients, or how much of a change reflects a clinically important difference. In order to provide useful information about measurement error, it must be contrasted with the expected variation amongst the individuals we may be assessing.

One way to include the information about expected variability between patients would be to cite the ratio of measurement error to total variability between patients.

Since the total variability between patients includes both any systematic variation between patients and measurement error, this would result in a number between zero and one, with zero representing a 'perfect' instrument. Such a ratio would then indicate the ability of the instrument to differentiate among patients. In practice, the ratio is turned around and researchers calculate the ratio *between* patients to the *total* variability (the sum of patient variability and measurement error) so that zero indicates no reliability, and one indicates no measurement error and perfect reliability. Thus the formal definition of reliability is:

$$\text{Reliability} = \frac{\text{Subject Variability}}{\text{Subject Variability} + \text{Measurement Error}}.$$

Since one statistical measure of variability is *variance*, this can be expressed more formally as:

$$Reliability = \frac{\sigma_s^2}{\sigma_s^2 + \sigma_e^2}$$

where subscript 's' stands for 'Subjects' and the subscript 'e' for 'Error'. Because σ_s^2 is always less than $\sigma_s^2 + \sigma_e^2$ the reliability will always be between 0 and 1.0. The only exception to this is Cronbach's α, discussed in Chapter 5. If the scale is multidimensional, or some items are inversely related to others, α can occasionally be negative (Krus and Helmstadter 1993), which is an indication that something is wrong in the construction or scoring of the scale.

Thus, the reliability coefficient expresses the proportion of the total variance in the measurements $\left(\sigma_s^2 + \sigma_e^2\right)$ which is due to 'true' differences between subjects $\left(\sigma_s^2\right)$ As we shall see, 'true' is defined in a very particular way, but this awaits a detailed discussion of the methods of calculation.

This definition of reliability has a very long history. Formally, it is derived from what is commonly referred to as *Classical Test Theory*, which goes back to the turn of the last century and the work of Karl Pearson, of Pearson's correlation fame. Classical test theory simply states that any observation, O_{ij} (the jth observation on object i), is composed of two components—a true score, T_i (for object i), and error associated with the observation, e_{ij}. The formal calculation of the reliability formula, called an *intraclass correlation*, appears in Fisher's 1925 statistics book (Fisher 1925).

Why is it called the *intraclass correlation*? Well, to understand that, you must recognize that the chapter in Fisher's book directly after 'The Intraclass Correlation' is called 'The Interclass Correlation', and in it he describes what the world knows as the Pearson correlation coefficient. *Intra*class means, naturally enough, within a class—two or more replicates of the same variable—whereas *inter*class is between different variables. Fisher could have called it the Pearson correlation, but he did not like Pearson much (or almost anybody else, for that matter).

Philosophical implications

This formulation of reliability has profound consequences for the logic of measurement. At its root, the reliability coefficient reflects the extent to which a measurement instrument can differentiate among individuals, that is, how well it can tell people apart, since the magnitude of the coefficient is directly related to the variability between subjects. The concept seems restrictively Darwinian and even feudal. But this interpretation is a political not a scientific one, and perhaps reflects a focus on the potentially negative use to which the measurement may be put, rather than the measurement itself.

Reflect back again on the everyday use of measurement. The only reason to apply a particular instrument to a situation is because the act of measurement is providing information about the object of observation. We look at the thermometer outside only because it tells us something about how this day differs from all other days. If the thermometer always gave the same reading because every day was the same temperature as every other day, we would soon stop reading it. We suspect, although we lack direct experience, that because of this people living in tropical climates pay little attention to the temperature, and that other factors, such as rain or humidity, are more important.

This intuition applies equally well to clinical and other professional situations. A medical laboratory measurement is useful only to the extent that it reflects true differences among individuals: in particular, diseased and normal individuals. Chromosome count is not a useful genetic property (despite the fact that we can get perfect agreement among observers) because we all usually have 46 chromosomes. Similarly, most clinical supervisors question the value of global rating scales (the bit of paper routinely filled out by the supervisor at the end of an educational experience rating everything from knowledge to responsibility) precisely because everybody, from the best to the worst, gets rated 'above average'.

Again, this view flies in the face of some further intuitions. Reliability is not necessarily related to agreement and in some cases can be inversely related to it. We have just demonstrated one example, where if all students on all occasions are rated above average, the agreement among raters is perfect but the reliability, by definition, is zero. This is also relevant to the 'number of boxes' issue discussed in Chapter 4. As we decrease the number of boxes on a rating scale, the information value of any observation is reduced and the reliability drops, although the agreement among observers will increase. As an everyday example, Canadians now uniformly talk about the weather in degrees Celsius, but still refer to room temperature in degrees Fahrenheit. We think one reason for this phenomenon is that within the range of acceptable room temperature, from say 68° to 72° Fahrenheit or 20° to 21° Celsius (except the United Kingdom where the lower limit, particularly in bathrooms, is more like 32°F or 0°C), the Celsius scale has only two divisions compared to four for the Fahrenheit one, thus introducing a degree of measurement error, even though two thermometers would agree (within one degree) more often in Celsius.

Experimentalists and many statisticians have difficulty with the concept of reliability as well. To the experimentalist, the goal of science is to detect the effects of experimental interventions. This 'main effect', in a comparison between treatment and control groups, for example, is always confounded, to greater or lesser degree, by differences in individual subjects' responses. Nearly all statistical tests make this contrast explicit; the numerator of the test is the experimental effect, assessed as differences between means, differences in proportions cured or dead, and so on, and the denominator is the expected magnitude of the difference by chance *arising from differences among individuals*. Thus, it is precisely true that the psychometrician's (arguably, the clinician's) *signal* is the experimentalist's and statistician's *noise*; or, as one of our professors put it, 'One person's error variance is another person's profession'.

This paradox was first recognized by Cronbach, the inventor of the alpha coefficient (Chapter 5) and generalizability theory (Chapter 9), in a classic paper written in 1957, called 'The two disciplines of scientific psychology' (Cronbach 1957). Perhaps because of the title, few readers outside psychology (and regrettably, few inside as well) are aware of it. The paradox rears its ugly head in many areas of research.

As one example, clinical researchers often go to great lengths to create inclusion and exclusion criteria in order to enrol just the right kind of (homogeneous) patients in their studies. Sometimes they go to extreme lengths, such as one trial of a cholesterol-lowering drug, which screened 300,000 men in order to find 4,000 who fit the criteria. It is often forgotten that the reason for these extreme measures is because the small treatment effects common in cardiovascular research would be obscured by individual differences if all kinds of patients were enrolled.

On the analysis side, although we use standard statistical packages to develop reliability coefficients, it is literally true that every line in the ANOVA table of concern in these calculations is labelled 'ERROR' by most of the standard packages. Conversely, the 'main effects', or differences between means, which are of interest to the statisticians, are frequently (but not always) ignored in the calculations of reliability.

There is one last important consequence of this formulation. The reliability of a measure is intimately linked to the population to which one wants to apply the measure. There is literally no such thing as *the* reliability of a test, unqualified; the coefficient has meaning only when applied to specific populations. Reliability is relative, just as Einstein said about time. Although some researchers (Bland and Altman 1986) have decried this as a failure of conventional methods for assessing reliability, we believe that this is a realistic view of the act of measurement and not a limitation of reliability. In fact, all of the formulae for reliability make this inevitable. The denominator always has a term reflecting the total variance of the scores. Naturally, the variance of, say, a quality of life scale will be very different in a homogeneous group of rheumatoid patients than in a group consisting of them plus disease-free people and those with ankylosing spondylitis; therefore, the reliability of the scale will be very different in the two groups. Although this may seem undesirable, it is an accurate reflection of the measurement situation. It *is* more difficult to tell people apart if they are relatively similar (i.e. homogeneous) than if they are very different. Reasonably, the reliability coefficient reflects this. Returning to the section 'Basic concepts', it makes no sense to speak of the error of measurement of a thermometer without knowledge of the range of temperature to be assessed. Small differences amongst the objects of measurement are more difficult to detect than large differences. The reliability coefficient explicitly recognizes this important characteristic.

At the risk of repeating ourselves, let us reiterate this point more strongly: it is wrong to speak of 'the reliability of a test' (and as we will see in Chapter 10, its validity). Reliability is not an immutable, inherent property of a scale; it is an interaction among the instrument, the specific group of people taking the test, and the situation. As Gronlund and Linn (1990) have written, 'Reliability refers to the *results* obtained with an evaluation instrument and not to the instrument itself' (p. 78). Whether a scale which has been shown to be reliable with one group of individuals in a particular context is reliable with other people and in different situations is an empirical issue that must be formally assessed. Consequently, it is more accurate to speak of the reliability of test *scores*, rather than of tests. Similarly, a study should not state that 'The reliability of the test was *x.xx*'. Rather, it should say, 'The reliability of the test with this sample was *x.xx*' (Helms et al. 2006).

Needless to say, it is impractical, and often unnecessary, to re-evaluate reliability each time a scale is used. If a test has been shown to be reliable with patients who have had a certain disease for 10 years, it can be assumed to have similar reliability with those who have suffered for 11 years. But, it may or may not be reliable among people who have just been diagnosed with the disease, have a different disorder, or who are being seen for a medical-legal evaluation as opposed to a clinical work-up. To some degree, this is an issue of clinical judgement; are the populations 'similar enough?' Later in this chapter, we will look at some ways to determine what factors may affect a scale's reliability.

Terminology

Before we go much further in our discussion, we should deal with the issue of terminology. What we have been calling *reliability* has been given different names in fields outside of psychology and education, such as 'accuracy', 'precision', 'agreement', 'dependability', 'reproducibility', 'repeatability', and 'consistency', among others. For a variety of reasons, we much prefer, and will continue to use, *reliability*. First, proponents of the other terms cannot agree amongst themselves what they mean. For example, some people use 'accuracy' as a synonym for reliability, others for validity (e.g. Gift and Soeken 1988; Lynn 1989). Second, the alternatives are much like the descriptions of an elephant given by three blind men, each of whom feels only one part of it: the one touching the leg thinks it's like a tree; the one at the tail says it's like a snake; and the one at the trunk describes it as a hose. Similarly, 'repeatability', 'reproducibility', 'consistency', and the rest are describing only one aspect of reliability: the part covered by the term 'Measurement Error' in the equation in the section 'Basic concepts'. We have argued (Streiner and Norman 2006) that the other terms ignore the equally important part of the denominator, 'Subject Variability'. As we have just seen, if two raters place all of their students in the 'above average' category, and do so again when asked to re-evaluate the students one week later, their repeatability, reproducibility, consistency, and agreement will all be perfect, but the reliability will be zero, because there is no true difference among those being rated.

Defining reliability

So far, we have described the idea of reliability in general terms. The time has come to determine how to calculate reliability: that is, how to calculate the different variance components that enter into the coefficient. Perhaps not surprisingly, the analytical approach is based on the statistical technique of Analysis of Variance (ANOVA). Specifically, because in order to calculate reliability we require repeated observations on each subject or patient derived from different observers, times, or versions of the test, we use a method called *repeated measures* ANOVA.

Suppose, for example, that three observers assess a total of ten patients for some attribute (e.g. sadness) on a 10-point scale. The scores are shown in Table 8.1.

It is evident that there is some variability in the scores. Those assigned by the three observers to individual patients range from 2 to 10 units on the scale, with mean scores ranging from 2 to 9. The variability among the mean scores of the observers (5.0 vs 6.0 vs 7.0) suggests that there may be some systematic difference among them. Finally, there is as much as 2 units of disagreement in scores assigned to the same patient by different observers.

These three sources of variance—patients, observers, and error—are represented in different ways in the table: the patients, by the differences within the column on the right (their means); the observers, by the differences among their three column means; and 'random', or unsystematic variation, by the difference between an individual score within the table and its 'expected' value. Thus we have adopted a technical estimate of the 'true' score; it is simply the average of all the observed scores, whether applied to the true score of a patient (that is,each patient's mean) or of an observer (their means). 'True' clearly has a technical definition which is somewhat more limited than the common definition. In fact, 'true' is a poor choice of words, but one that we are stuck with. Strictly speaking, it is the average score that would be obtained if the scale

Table 8.1 Degree of sadness of ten patients rated by three observers

Patient	Observer 1	Observer 2	Observer 3	Mean
1	6	7	8	7.0
2	4	5	6	5.0
3	2	2	2	2.0
4	3	4	5	4.0
5	5	4	6	5.0
6	8	9	10	9.0
7	5	7	9	7.0
8	6	7	8	7.0
9	4	6	8	6.0
10	7	9	8	8.0
Mean	5.0	6.0	7.0	6.0

were given an infinite number of times (an obviously difficult task). Moreover, it refers only to the *consistency* of the score, not to its *accuracy*. For example, a person being evaluated for an executive position may deliberately understate the degree to which they mistrust others. If they completed the scale 20 times, each time with the same bias in place, the average would be a good approximation of their true score, but a bad estimate of their actual feelings. Also, a person's true score will change (we hope) if the underlying characteristic changes. If a depressed person, who has a true score of 18 on some test, benefits from therapy, then both their depression and their true score should move closer to the normal range. Stanley (1971), we think, defined it best: 'As used, true score is not the ultimate fact in the book of the recording angel. Rather, it is the score resulting from systematic factors one chooses to aggregate, including any systematic biasing factors that may produce systematic incorrectness in the scores' (p. 361). That is, systematic errors may jeopardize the test's validity, but they do not affect its reliability.

Bearing in mind what is meant by a 'true' score, we can quantify these sources of variance in sums of squares, calculated as follows:

$$Sum\ of\ squares(observers) = 10\left[(5.0-6.0)^2 + (6.0-6.0)^2 + (7.0-6.0)^2\right] = 20.0$$

The factor of 10 is there because ten patients enter into each sum. Similarly:

$$Sum\ of\ squares(patients) = 3\big[(7.0-6.0)^2 + (5.0-6.0)^2 + (2.0-6.0)^2$$
$$+ \ldots + (8.0-6.0)^2\big] = 114.0$$

Again, there is a factor of 3 in the equation because there are three observers contributing to each value.

Finally, the sum of squares (error) is based on the difference between each individual value and its expected value calculated from the row and column means. We will not go into detail about how these expected values are arrived at; any introductory text book in statistics, such as Norman and Streiner (2014), will explain it. For the first three patients and Observer 1, the expected scores are 6.0, 4.0, and 1.0. The sum of squares is then as follows:

$$Sum\ of\ squares(error) = (6.0-6.0)^2 + (4.0-4.0)^2 + (2.0-1.0)^2 + \ldots + (8.0-9.0)^2$$
$$= 10.0.$$

An ANOVA table can then be developed from the sums of squares, as in Table 8.2.

The next step is to break down the total variance in the scores into components of variance due to patients, observers, and error. It would seem that each mean square is a variance and no further work is required, but such is not the case. Both the calculated mean square due to patients and that due to observers contain some contribution due to error variance. The easiest way to understand this concept is to imagine a situation where all patients had the same degree of sadness, as defined by some external gold standard. Would the patients all then obtain the same scores on our sadness scale?

Table 8.2 Analysis of variance summary table

Source of variation	Sum of squares	Degrees of freedom	Mean square	F	Tail probability
Patients	114.00	9	12.67	22.80	0.0001
Observers	20.00	2	10.00	18.00	0.0001
Error	10.00	18	0.56		
Total	144.00	29			

Not at all. There would be variability in the obtained scores directly related to the amount of random error present in the measurements. The relevant equations relating the mean square (MSs) to variances are:

1. Mean square (error) $= \sigma^2_{err}$

2. Mean square (patients) $= 3\sigma^2_{pat} + \sigma^2_{err}$

3. Mean square (observers) $= 10\sigma^2_{obs} + \sigma^2_{err}$

From these we can show, by some algebraic manipulations, that

1. $\sigma^2(error) = MS_{err} = 0.56$

2. $\sigma^2(patients) = (MS_{pat} - MS_{err})/3 = (12.67 - 0.56)/3 = 4.04$

3. $\sigma^2(observers) = (MS_{obs} - MS_{err})/10 = (10.00 - 0.56)/10 = 0.94$

Finally, we define the reliability coefficient as the ratio of variance between patients to error variance:

$$r = \frac{\sigma^2_{patients}}{\sigma^2_{patients} + \sigma^2_{error}} = \frac{4.04}{4.04 + 0.56} = 0.88$$

An alternative way of writing this formula, which does not involve first calculating the variances, is:

$$r = \frac{MS_{patients} - MS_{error}}{MS_{patients} + (k-1)MS_{error}}$$

where k is the number of raters. This is the 'classical' definition of reliability. The interpretation is that 88 per cent of the variance in the scores results from 'true' variance among patients. It is important to note that when we are discussing reliability, it is the reliability coefficient r and not r^2, which is interpreted as the percentage of score variance attributable to different sources.

This coefficient is called an *intraclass correlation coefficient* or ICC. It is not *the* ICC, but only one form of it. As we shall see, there are different versions, depending on various assumptions we make and what we want to look at. To repeat what we said earlier, Fisher (1925) called it the 'intraclass correlation' because it is computed as the relationship among multiple observations of the *same* variable (i.e. within a class of variable), to distinguish it from Pearson's correlation, which is usually between different variables and hence is an *interclass* correlation. We will revisit this distinction a bit later.

Combining Shrout and Fleiss's (1979) and McGraw and Wong's (1996) terminology, we can refer to this version of the ICC as ICC2(C, 1): the 2 reflecting a 'class 2' ICC in which all patients are evaluated by all raters, C because we are looking at *consistency* among the raters rather than *absolute agreement* (a distinction we will discuss in the next section), and 1 because it is the reliability of a single rater.

Other considerations in calculating the reliability of a test: measuring consistency or absolute agreement

What happened to the variance due to the raters or observers? Although it was calculated in the ANOVA table and found to be highly significant, there was no further mention of it. The reason is that σ^2 (observer) or $MS_{observer}$ terms reflect systematic error or bias (as opposed to the σ^2 (error) or MS_{error} terms, which represent random error), and the classical definition of reliability does not take this into account. If Observer A's scores are consistently two points higher than those of Observer B, there is still *relative* consistency between them, in that the position or ranking of the subjects is the same for both sets of scores. Shrout and Fleiss (1979) re-introduced bias in a classic paper, in which they considered situations where bias may or may not be thought of as an aspect of reliability.

Whether or not to include Observer (i.e. bias) is a decision dependent on whether we want to measure *consistency* or *agreement*. We can illustrate the difference with two examples. In the first, three raters (observers) independently evaluate the dossiers of 300 applicants for 50 openings for professional school, rating each applicant on a 100-point scale. The first rater is particularly harsh in their evaluations, while the third is far more lenient than the other two. In other words, none of the observers ever assigns the same value to a student. However, since their job is, in essence, to rank order the applicants in order to choose the top 50, this lack of agreement is of no consequence. What is important is the consistency of their scores—is the rank ordering the same among them (i.e. is the Pearson or Spearman correlation high)? This is also the situation that occurs when tests are *norm referenced*—that is, when passing or failing is judged in relation to how others did (operationalized by the students' question on the first day of class, 'Will we be marked on a curve?').

In the second example, the raters must determine whether or not the applicants pass a licensing examination in which the examinees must attain a score of at least 65. This is referred to as a *criterion referenced* test because there is an external criterion against which people are judged. In this case, numerical differences among the raters *are* important; they should agree not only with respect to the rank ordering of the students, but also with regard to their absolute value. A similar situation exists when students are tested to see how accurately they can measure a patient's blood pressure, where the criterion is the value obtained by an expert. Again, they must not only rank the patients in the same order but also not deviate from the criterion.

Another way of thinking of the distinction between measuring only consistency as opposed to the more stringent measuring of absolute agreement is whether the raters can be considered a *fixed* or a *random* factor—terms that have been borrowed from ANOVA. Again, two examples will illustrate the difference and their relationship to consistency and absolute agreement. If we did a study in which two raters estimated the degree of pain experienced by infants, we would want to know how reliable the ratings were. Our interest is not the reliability of raters in general, but only those who participated in the study. If there was any systematic bias between the raters, such that one tended to give higher values than the other, we could easily compensate for this by adding a constant to the lower rater's scores (or subtracting it from the higher rater's numbers, or using their mean). In this case, the raters are considered to be a *fixed* factor, and this would correspond to measuring of *consistency*.

On the other hand, if we were developing the pain scale and were interested in how reliable any two raters were in using it, then the raters in our study would be considered to be a random sample of all possible raters. Consequently, we would treat observers as a *random* factor. Because we cannot compensate for the difference between raters, they must also have similar *absolute* values.

We presented the formulae for the ICC for consistency in the section 'Defining reliability'. The corresponding equations' absolute agreement for a single score is:

$$ICC2(A,1) = \frac{\sigma^2_{patients}}{\sigma^2_{patients} + \sigma^2_{observers} + \sigma^2_{error}}$$

or

$$ICC2(A,1) = \frac{MS_{patients} - MS_{error}}{MS_{patients} + \frac{k}{n}(MS_{observer} - MS_{error}) + (k-1)MS_{error}}$$

where n is the number of subjects. If we put the numbers from Table 8.2 into the equation, we will get a value of 0.73. This is lower than the value for ICC2(C, 1), which was 0.88. This is a universal truth; reliability based on absolute agreement is always equal to or lower than for consistency—on a conceptual level because we have a more stringent criterion and on a mathematical level because we have added the variance due to observers to the denominator.

The observer nested within subject

One common situation arises when each subject is rated by several different observers, but no observers are common to more than one subject. Some examples would be as follows: students on a course in different tutorial groups rate their tutors' teaching skills; junior residents on different teaching units are rated by chief residents, head nurses, and staff; and patients undergoing physiotherapy are rated by their own and another therapist, but treatment is given by different therapists at different hospitals. The following are common to these situations:

1. All subjects receive more than one observation, but

2. The raters are not necessarily the same across subjects.

At first glance, it would seem impossible to extract a reliability coefficient from these data, since there seems to be no opportunity to actually compare observations. Certainly in the extreme case, where each subject is rated by only one observer, there is no way to separate subject variance, observer variance, and error. But in the situations above, at least a partial separation can be achieved.

The approach is to recognize that the variance of the mean values of the scores of each subject permits an estimate of subject variance, in the usual way. Conversely, variability of the observations around the mean of each subject is a result of within-subject variation, contributed by both systematic differences between observers and error variance. We cannot separate these two sources of variance but we do not really need to, since the denominator of the reliability coefficient contains contributions from both.

To analyse data of this form, we conduct a one-way ANOVA with the subject as a grouping factor and the multiple observations within each subject cell as a 'within-subject' factor. We need not have the same number of observers for each subject, as long as the number of observations per subject exceeds one.

The one-way ANOVA results, eventually, in estimated mean squares between groups and within groups. The former is used to calculate subject variance using the previous formula and the mean square (within) estimates the error variance. The reliability coefficient can then be calculated with these variance estimates, using the formula for $ICC2(C,1)$. In this case, though, the formula would be referred to as $ICC1(C,1)$ because this is Shrout and Fleiss's 'class 1' ICC, in which the subjects are evaluated by different raters. All that is lost is the ability to separate the random error component from observer bias; but since observers are a random effect (using the concepts described in the section on Other considerations in calculating the reliability of a test), this is of no consequence.

Even in those situations where there is partial overlap (e.g. fifteen interview teams of three interviewers conduct ten interviews each), the analysis can be approached assuming no overlap of raters, and still yield an unbiased estimate of reliability.

Multiple observations

Finally, let us re-examine the issue of multiple observations. If each patient is assessed by multiple observers or completes some inventory with a number of items or fills out a pain scale on several occasions, it is intuitively obvious that the average of these observations should have a higher reliability than any single item since the errors are random and those associated with each observation are averaged out. In turn, this should be reflected in the reliability coefficient.

The approach is the essence of simplicity: we simply divide the error variance by the number of observations. The equations for the consistency version are:

$$ICC2(C,k) = \frac{\sigma^2_{subjects}}{\sigma^2_{subjects} + \sigma^2_{error}/k}$$

and

$$ICC2(C,k) = \frac{MS_{subjects} - MS_{error}}{MS_{subjects}}$$

and for the absolute agreement are:

$$ICC2(A,k) = \frac{\sigma^2_{subjects}}{\sigma^2_{subjects} + \left(\sigma^2_{observers} + \sigma^2_{error}\right)/k}$$

and

$$ICC2(A,k) = \frac{MS_{subjects} - MS_{error}}{MS_{subjects} + \left(MS_{observers} - MS_{error}\right)/k}$$

Note that if we set $k = 1$, this equation is the same as the one for $ICC2(A,1)$. We can use this fact to take the results from our actual study and estimate what the reliability would be if we were to use fewer or more raters. With k = the actual number of observers in the study, m = the number of raters we are interested in, and $p = (km)$, we can then modify the equation for $ICC2(A,1)$ slightly as follows:

$$ICC2(A,k,m) = \frac{MS_{subjects} - MS_{error}}{MS_{subjects} + \dfrac{p+1}{n}\left(MS_{subjects} - MS_{error}\right) + p\left(MS_{error}\right)}$$

Having shown you the formulae for multiple observations, we should caution you to use them judiciously. Because the reliability based on two or more observations is always higher than that based on a single score, and because computer programs often give both, the temptation is there to report the larger. But which coefficient is reported in a paper depends on how the scale will be used in the field. If the instrument is to be completed by a single rater, then the ICC based on multiple observers would be misleadingly high. The ICC for many raters should be given only if two or more people will actually make the observations, and their scores are averaged. This is often done, for example, when evaluating candidates for professional or medical school, to increase the reliability of a scale because the reliability of a single rater is unacceptably low.

A methodological note on measuring inter-rater reliability

In many studies, two raters evaluate something (a student, an article) and, if there is a disagreement, a third person is brought in to resolve it. For example, two people may read a series of articles to determine if they meet the criteria for inclusion in a meta-analysis. In cases where they disagree, they call in a third rater and either go with the majority or use this person's evaluation, if they are an expert. The issue is when inter-rater reliability should be calculated—before or after the resolution.

In such cases, the only valid measure of reliability is the one measured before the differences are resolved. As Krippendorff (2013) has said, 'The reliability of the data after this reconciliation effort is merely arguable' (p. 275). The estimate of reliability based on the resolved differences is an overestimate of the actual reliability and provides a false sense of confidence in the measurement instrument (Szafran 2017).

On a practical level, based on measurement theory, the 'best' score would be the average of the three raters, but again, the reliability estimate should be based on the two main raters.

Other types of reliability

Up to this point, we have concerned ourselves with reliability based on examining the effect of different observers on scores. The example we have worked through included only one source of error, that which resulted from different observers' perceptions of the same behaviour. Upon reflection, we can see that there may be other sources of error or contamination in an observation of an individual patient's 'sadness'. For instance, each observer may apply slightly different standards from day to day. This could be tested experimentally by videotaping a group of patients and having the observer do two ratings of the tapes a week or two apart. The resulting reliability is called an *intra-observer reliability* coefficient, since it measures variation that occurs within an observer as a result of multiple exposures to the same stimulus, as opposed to the *inter-observer* reliability we have already calculated.

Note that although many investigators maintain that the demonstration of both inter- and intra-observer reliability is a minimum requirement of a good test, this may be unnecessary. If we recognize that inter-observer reliability contains all the sources of error contributing to intra-observer reliability, plus any differences that may arise between observers, then it is evident that a demonstration of high inter-observer reliability is sufficient; the intra-observer reliability is bound to be higher. However, if the inter-observer reliability is low, we cannot be sure whether this arises from differences within or between observers (or both), and it may then be necessary to continue to an intra-observer reliability study in order to locate the source of unreliability.

Often there are no observers involved in the measurement, as with the many self-rated tests of psychological function, pain, or disease severity (or we might say, there is only one observer, the person completing the scale or test: they are an observer/rater of their own behaviour). Although there are no observers, we are still concerned about the reliability of the scale. The usual approach is to administer it on two occasions separated by a time interval sufficiently short that we can assume that the underlying process is unlikely to have changed. This approach is called *test–retest reliability*. Of course, the trick is to select an appropriate time interval: too long, and things may have changed; too short, and patients may remember their first response and put it down, rather than answering the question *de novo*. Expert opinions regarding the appropriate interval vary from an hour to a year, depending on the task, but generally speaking, a retest interval of 2–14 days is usual. (The section on 'Empirical data on retest reliability', later in this chapter, shows the magnitude of the coefficient expected for various types of tests after different intervals.) Low values of test–retest reliability may indicate one of three things. First, the test may be reliable, but the phenomenon may have changed over time. This may occur with states that can change relatively quickly, such as joint pain or mood. Second, the scale itself may be unreliable (Crocker and Algina 1986). Third, taking the test on one occasion may influence some people's responses on the second administration, because they may have been sensitized to the phenomenon, or may be prompted to think about it more; in other words, the test is 'reactive'. (Note that if everyone is affected to the same degree, this would not adversely affect those definitions of reliability that ignore systematic bias.)

Frequently, measures of internal consistency, as described in Chapter 5, are reported as the reliability of a test. However, since they are based on performance observed in a single sitting, there are many sources of variance, which occur from day to day or between observers, which do not enter into the calculation. Because they can be computed from routine administration of a measure, without the special requirement for two or more administrations, they appear very commonly in the literature but should be interpreted with great caution. Indeed, McCrae et al. (2011), using a very large sample of respondents, have shown a relationship between test–retest reliability and validity, but no relationship between internal consistency and validity. Internal consistency on its own is insufficient to establish its actual reliability; its test–retest and/or inter-rater reliability need also be reported.

In fact, the argument can be made that internal consistency coefficients, as frequently reported, are generally *too* high. For example, if we are considering an observer rating someone's clinical competence, we can anticipate scales assessing history taking, the physical examination, communication skills, management, and the use of tests. But what do we make of it if the internal consistency is 0.8 or 0.9? That suggests all items are measuring pretty well the same thing, which is not the intent of the designer.

Different forms of the reliability coefficient

There has been considerable debate in the literature regarding the most appropriate choice of the reliability coefficient. The coefficients we have derived now are all forms of 'intraclass correlation coefficients'. However, other measures, in particular the Pearson product-moment correlation and Cohen's kappa (Cohen 1960), are frequently used. Altman and Bland (1983; Bland and Altman 1986) have also identified apparent weaknesses in the conventional approach and recommended an alternative.

Accordingly, we will discuss these alternatives and attempt to reconcile the differences among the measures.

Pearson correlation

The Pearson correlation is based on regression analysis and is a measure of the extent to which the relationship between two variables can be described by a straight (regression) line: it is the line of best fit through a set of data points, where the distance between each observation and the line is minimized. In the present context, this is a measure of the extent to which two observations on a group of subjects can be fitted by a straight line. One such relationship is shown in Fig. 8.1. Note that a perfect fit is obtained, thereby resulting in a Pearson correlation of 1.0, despite the fact that the intercept is non-zero and the slope is not equal to 1.0. By contrast, the intraclass correlation will yield a value of 1.0 only if all the observations on each subject are identical, which dictates a slope of 1.0 and an intercept of 0.0. This suggests that the Pearson correlation is an inappropriate and liberal measure of reliability; that is to say, the Pearson coefficient will usually be higher than the true reliability. In practice, however, the predominant source of error is usually due to random variation, and under these circumstances, the Pearson and intraclass correlations will be very close.

There are other reasons to prefer the intraclass correlation over the Pearson correlation. We began this chapter with an example that used three observers and proceeded to calculate a single ICC. If we had used the Pearson correlation, we must use the data pairwise and create one correlation for Observer 1 versus Observer 2, another for Observer 1 versus Observer 3, and a third for Observer 2 versus Observer 3. With

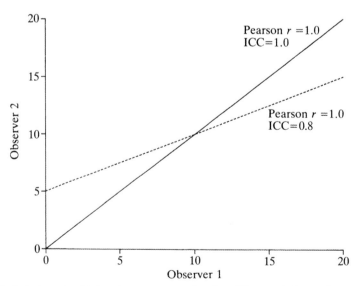

Fig. 8.1 Typical graph of inter-observer scores, showing difference between Pearson correlation and intraclass correlation.

10 observers, we would still have one ICC, but we must now contend with 45 Pearson correlations, and there is no agreed way to average or combine them. Finally, in some studies, the pairs of scores are 'unordered'. For example, if we are looking at the relationship between scores on some measure for identical twins, whether a given twin is assigned to variable 1 or variable 2 is totally arbitrary, but would change the value of Pearson's r. However, because the ICC is based on pooled data for each variable, rather than the difference between pairs, it is unaffected. This makes it ideal for reliability studies where group assignment is arbitrary.

Kappa coefficient

Although this chapter (and most of this book) has dealt at length with situations where there is a supposed underlying continuum, there are many situations in the health sciences which have only two levels—presence or absence, positive or negative, abnormal or normal, dead or alive. A straightforward approach is to calculate a simple agreement: the proportion of responses in which the two observations agreed. Although straightforward, this measure is very strongly influenced by the distribution of positives and negatives. If there is a preponderance of either normal or abnormal cases, there will be a high agreement by chance alone. The kappa coefficient (Cohen 1960) explicitly deals with this situation by examining the proportion of responses in the two agreement cells (yes/yes, no/no) in relation to the proportion of responses in these cells which would be expected by chance, given the marginal distributions.

For example, suppose we were to consider a judgement by two observers of the presence or absence of a Babinski sign (an upgoing toe following the scratching of the bottom of the foot) on a series of neurological patients. The data might be displayed in a contingency table like Table 8.3.

The overall agreement is simply $(20 + 55)/100 = 75$ per cent. However, we would expect that a certain number of agreements would arise by chance alone. Specifically, we can calculate the expected agreement from the marginals; the top left cell would have $(35 \times 30)/100 = 10.5$ expected observations, and the bottom right cell would have $(70 \times 65)/100 = 45.5$ expected ones. Kappa corrects for chance agreement in the following manner:

$$\kappa = \frac{P_o - P_e}{1.0 - P_e}$$

where P_o is the observed proportion of agreements and P_e is the proportion expected by chance. In this case:

$$\kappa = \frac{\left(\dfrac{75}{100}\right) - \left(\dfrac{10.5 + 45.5}{100}\right)}{1.0 - \left(\dfrac{10.5 + 45.5}{100}\right)} = 0.43$$

Table 8.3 Contingency table for two observers

		Observer 2		
		Present	**Absent**	**Total**
	Present	20	15	35
Observer 1	**Absent**	10	55	65
	Total	30	70	100

It is also possible to calculate kappa from the raw data, without first converting to proportions. The formula is:

$$\kappa = \frac{f_o - f_e}{N - f_e}$$

where f_o and f_e are the observed and expected frequencies and N is the total sample size, which in this case would be:

$$\kappa = \frac{75 - 56}{100 - 56} = 0.43$$

For a 2×2 table, we can also calculate the standard error of kappa:

$$SE(\kappa) = \sqrt{\frac{P_o(1 - P_o)}{N(1.0 - P_e)^2}}$$

which in this case equals:

$$\sqrt{\frac{0.75(1 - 0.75)}{100(1.0 - 0.56)^2}} = 0.098$$

Therefore, instead of a raw agreement of 0.75, we end up with a chance corrected agreement of 0.43, with a standard error of about 0.10. In circumstances where the frequency of positive results is very low or very high, it is very easy to obtain impressive figures for agreement, although agreement beyond chance is virtually absent.

In the example we have chosen, the approach to assessment of observer agreement appears to have little in common with our previous examples, where we used ANOVA methods. However, if we considered judgements using multiple categories, the parallel may become more obvious. For example, suppose the same observers were assessing muscle strength, which is conventionally done on a 6-point scale from 0 = flaccid to 5 = normal strength. In this case, a display of agreement would involve a 6 × 6 contingency table.

Since the coefficient we calculated previously considers only total agreement and does not provide partial credit for responses that differ by only one or two categories, it would be inappropriate for scaled responses as in the present example. However, an extension of the approach, called *weighted kappa* (Cohen 1968), does consider partial agreement.

Weighted kappa actually focuses on disagreement, so that the cells of total agreement on the top-left to bottom-right diagonal have weights of zero and two opposite corners have the maximum weights. Weighted kappa is then a sum of the weighted frequencies corrected for chance. The actual formula is:

$$\kappa_w = 1.0 - \frac{\sum w_{ij} \times P_{o_{ij}}}{\sum w_{ij} \times P_{e_{ij}}}$$

where w_{ij} is the weight assigned to the i, j cell, and $P_{o_{ij}}$ and $P_{e_{ij}}$ are the observed and expected proportions in the i, j cell.

As originally formulated, the weights could be assigned arbitrary values between 0 and 1. However, the problem with using your own weights, however sensible they may seem, is that you can no longer compare your kappa with anyone else's. Unless there are strong prior reasons, the most commonly used weighting scheme, called *quadratic weights*, which bases disagreement weights on the square of the amount of discrepancy, should be used.

Let's work through an example. To keep it simpler, we will use only three categories rather than six, and have the two observers rate the Babinski sign as Present, Indeterminate, and Absent; the data are presented in Table 8.4. The numbers in the upper left corner of each cell are the quadratic weights, those in the middle are the

Table 8.4 Contingency table for two observers and three categories

		Observer 2			
		Present	**Indeterminate**	**Absent**	**Total**
Observer 1	**Present**	0	1	4	
		15	3	2	20
		(5)	(3)	(12)	
	Indeterminate	1	0	1	
		8	10	7	25
		(6.25)	(3.75)	(15)	
	Absent	4	1	0	
		2	2	51	55
		(13.75)	(8.25)	(33)	
	Total	25	15	60	100

observations, and the ones in parentheses are the expected frequencies. Then, using frequencies rather than percentages, we obtain:

$$\kappa_w = 1.0 - \frac{(0 \times 15) + (1 \times 3) + (4 \times 12) + \cdots + (0 \times 51)}{(0 \times 5) + (1 \times 3) + (4 \times 12) + \cdots + (0 \times 33)} = 1 - 0.266 = 0.734$$

If this weighting scheme is used, then the weighted kappa is exactly identical to the intraclass correlation coefficient, as long as the sample size is large enough so that $[(N + 1)/N]$ approximates the value of 1 (Fleiss and Cohen 1973). That is, if we coded Present as 1, Indeterminate as 2, and Absent as 3, ran a repeated measures ANOVA on the data with two observations, and then computed the ICC, it would turn out to be identical to kappa using quadratic weights (this equality doesn't hold with other weighting schemes). Similarly, in the first example using the Babinski sign, if we turned the 100 observations into 100 pairs of data points with each positive sign coded 1 and each negative coded 0, then there will be 20 (1–1) pairs, 15 (1–0) pairs, 10 (0–1) pairs, and 70 (0–0) pairs. The repeated measures ANOVA on these 200 observations would yield an unweighted kappa of 0.43.

Different authors, such as Fleiss (1981), Cicchetti and Sparrow (1981), and Landis and Koch (1977), have proposed various criteria for the magnitude of kappa and weighted kappa. These are summarized in Table 8.5. Although they differ with regard to terminology and the exact cut-off values, they can be summarized briefly: don't bother with any value less than 0.60, and even 0.75 is pushing the lower limit.

Kappa coefficient versus the ICC

Having gone through all of this, our recommendation would be to forget about kappa or weighted kappa for any except the most simple 2 × 2 tables, and use the ICC instead.

Table 8.5 Various criteria for kappa

Kappa	Landis and Koch	Cicchetti and Sparrow	Fleiss
<0	Poor	Poor	Poor
0.00–0.20	Slight		
0.21–0.40	Fair		
0.41–0.60	Moderate	Fair	Fair to good
0.61–0.75	Substantial	Excellent	
0.75–0.80			Excellent
0.80–1.00	Almost perfect		

Source: data from Cicchetti, D.V. and Sparrow, S.A., Developing criteria for establishing interrater reliability of specific items: Applications to assessment of adaptive behavior, *American Journal of Mental Deficiency*, Volume 86, Issue 2, pp. 127–37, Copyright © 1981; Landis, J.R. and Koch, G.G., The measurement of observer agreement for categorical data, *Biometrics*, Volume 33, pp. 159–74, Copyright © 1977; and Fleiss, J.L., *Statistical methods for rates and proportions*, Second Edition, Wiley, New York, USA, Copyright © 1981.

Berk (1979) gives 11 reasons why the ICC (and the extension of it, generalizability theory, discussed in Chapter 9) is superior. We won't list all of them, but some of them include: (1) the ability to isolate factors affecting reliability; (2) flexibility, in that it is very simple to analyse reliability studies with more than two observers and more than two response options; (3) we can include or exclude systematic differences between raters (bias) as part of the error term; (4) it can handle missing data; (5) it is able to simulate the effect on reliability of increasing or decreasing the number of raters; (6) it is far easier to let the computer do the calculations; and (7) it provides a unifying framework that ties together different ways of measuring inter-rater agreement—all of the designs are just variations on the theme of the ICC.

Dichotomous-ordinal scales

On the other hand, Cicchetti (1976) states that his weighting scheme for kappa is better suited for *dichotomous-ordinal* (DO) *scales*: ones in which an ordinal scale has a lowest value to indicate the absence of an attribute, and then values to indicate the amount of the attribute if it is present (e.g. 1 = No pathology present; 2 = Slight amount present; 3 = Mild amount present; 4 = Moderate amount present; 5 = Extreme amount present). He argues that a discrepancy between None and Slight is far more serious than a difference between Mild and Moderate, although both reflect a difference of one step. In the first case, the difference indicates that one rater believes the pathology is absent and the other feels it is present; while the latter case is just a discrepancy in the degree of pathology present. In this limited situation, we would agree with him, bearing in mind the proviso that the results may change if a scheme other than Cicchetti's is used.

Cicchetti weighting in DO scales is based on agreement, rather than disagreement. For intermediate values, the linear agreement weights vary depending on the number of points on the scale. For a scale with k points, we begin by calculating W, which is 2 $(k - 1)$. Hence, a 5-point scale has a weight of 8. Then, the linear weights themselves are calculated by:

$$\frac{W-1}{W-1}; \frac{W-2}{W-1}; \frac{W-3}{W-1} \cdots \frac{W-W}{W-1}$$

which, for a 5-point scale would be:

$$\frac{7}{7}; \frac{6}{7}; \frac{5}{7}; \cdots \frac{0}{7} = 1.0; \lfloor 0.86; 0.71 \rfloor; \lfloor 0.57; 0.43 \rfloor; \lfloor 0.29; 0.14 \rfloor; 0.0$$

Notice that after 1.0 (complete agreement), the numbers are paired. The first reflects a difference when both raters say the trait is present, and the second a difference when one rater says present and the other absent. Thus, 0.86 is used when both raters say Present but differ in rating severity by one point (e.g. if one rater says Slight and the other Mild, or Mild versus Moderate, etc.); and 0.71 for a discrepancy between None and one point (which in this case is Slight). The second pairing is for differences of two points: 0.57 when both raters give a rating in the Present zone, and 0.43 for a difference between None and Mild; and so forth. Finally, 0.0 reflects complete disagreement (None versus the highest value of Present).

The method of Bland and Altman

An alternative method of examining agreement was proposed by Altman and Bland (1983; Bland and Altman 1986), which has the apparent virtue of independence of the true variability in the observations. We have discussed earlier in this chapter under Philosophical implications why we would view this independence as a liability, not an asset. However, because this method has achieved considerable prominence in the clinical literature, we will review it in detail.

The method is designed as an absolute measure of agreement between two measuring instruments, which are on the same scale of measurement. As such, it retains the virtue of the intraclass correlation, in contrast to the Pearson correlation, in explicitly separating the bias (or main effect) of the instrument from random error. The approach is used for pairs of observations and begins with a plot of the difference between the two observations against the mean of the pairs of observations. One then calculates the average difference in the observations and the standard deviation of the differences. Finally one calculates the *limits of agreement*, equal to the mean difference ± twice the standard deviation.

However, all this is obtainable from the ICC calculation. The mean difference is analytically related to the observer variance calculated in the ICC (actually, it equals $\sqrt{(2/n \times SS_{obs})}$. The standard deviation of the differences is similarly related to the error variance $\sqrt{MS_{err}}$. A statistical test of the observer bias can be performed and would yield the same significance level as the test in the ANOVA.

While, as we have seen, the parameters of the Altman and Bland method can be derived from the calculated values that go into the ICC, it has the small advantage that these values are reported directly. Further, the graph can potentially alert the researcher to other systematic differences, such as a monotonic drift in the agreement related to the value of the measurement, or a systematic increase in error related to the value of the measurement.

Issues of interpretation

Reliability, the standard error of measurement, and the standard error of estimate

One difficulty with expressing the reliability coefficient as a dimensionless ratio of variances instead of an error of measurement is that it is difficult to interpret a reliability coefficient of 0.7 in terms of an individual score. However, since the reliability coefficient involves two quantities—the error variance and the variance between subjects—it is straightforward to work backwards and express the error of measurement in terms of the other two quantities. The *standard error of measurement* (SEM) is defined in terms of the standard deviation (σ) and the reliability (R) as

$$SEM = \sigma_X \sqrt{1 - R}$$

where σ_X is the standard deviation of the observed scores.

The SEM is expressed in the same unit of measurement as the original scores. This equation tells us that when the reliability of the test is 1.0, then there is no error of measurement and the SEM is zero. At the other extreme, if the reliability is zero, then the SEM equals the standard deviation of the observed scores. This relationship is plotted for some values of reliability in Fig. 8.2. The interpretation of this graph is that if we begin with a sample of known standard deviation, for example, with a reliability of 0.8, the error of measurement associated with any individual score is 45 per cent of the standard deviation. With a reliability of 0.5, the standard error is 70 per cent of a standard deviation; so we have improved the precision of measurement by only 30 per cent over the information we would have prior to doing any assessment of the individual at all.

Although the ICC and the SEM are related, as seen in the formula, they tell us different things about the test. The ICC (or any other index of reliability) reflects the scale's ability to differentiate among *people* (i.e. it is a relative measure of reliability); whereas the SEM is an absolute measure, and quantifies the precision of individual *scores* within the subjects (Weir 2005). Indeed, the latest version of the American Educational Research Association, American Psychological Association, and National Council on Measurement in Education (AERA/APA/NCEM) Standards (2014) states that the '[standard error of measurement] is generally more informative than a reliability or generalizability coefficient' (p. 39). Thus, any study reporting the results of a reliability study should include the SEM.

One reason for calculating the SEM is to allow us to draw a confidence interval (CI) around a score. Although this seems straightforward, there are two problems. The first is that it assumes that the SEM is the same for all scores, and we know this is not the

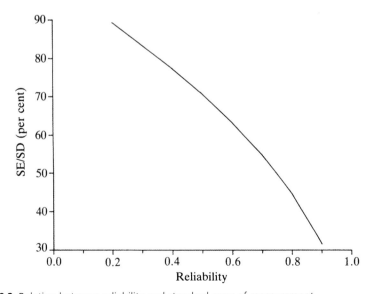

Fig. 8.2 Relation between reliability and standard error of measurement.

case. It is smallest where the observed score is near the test's mean, and increases as the score deviates from it, often being twice as large (Feldt et al. 1985). The CI is centred around the observed score:

$$X_0 \pm Z(SEM)$$

where X_0 is the observed score and Z is the value from the normal curve associated with the desired CI (1.64 for the 90 per cent CI; 1.96 for the 95 per cent CI). If we had a scale with a mean of 50, a standard deviation of 10, and a reliability of 0.8 and a person obtained a score of 65, then the 95 per cent CI would be:

$$SEM = 10\sqrt{1 - 0.8} = 4.47 \quad CI_{95} = 65 \pm 1.96 \times 4.47 = 56.24 - 73.76$$

What this means is that if we tested 1,000 people and used a 95 per cent CI, then 95 per cent of the CIs would capture the true scores. Another way to interpret this is to say that we are 95 per cent confident that the person's true score is somewhere between 56.25 and 73.76.

Expected difference in scores on retesting

If a person takes the same test on two occasions, how big a difference in test scores can be expected? The standard deviation of the difference between two scores is $\sqrt{2} \times SEM$. Modifying the previous example slightly, imagine we have a test where the person's *observed* score was 15 and the SEM was 3. From the normal distribution, the probability is 68 per cent that the true score is between 12 and 18. If the person takes the test a second time, then the probability is 68 per cent that the second score will be somewhere within the interval of $15 - (\sqrt{2} \times SEM)$ and $15 + (\sqrt{2}$ SEM, or between 10.8 and 19.2. The interval is larger because there will be some error in both the first and the second observed scores, whereas in determining the interval in which the true score lies, there is error involved only for the observed score, but not for the true one (Green 1981).

Empirical data on retest reliability

One way of evaluating the adequacy of reliability coefficients obtained from a new instrument is to compare them against tests which are generally assumed to have acceptable levels. Schuerger et al. (1982, 1989) compiled data from a number of personality questionnaires, re-administered over intervals ranging from 2 days to 20 years. Scales which tap relatively stable traits, such as extraversion, have test–retest coefficients in the high 0.70s to low 0.80s when re-administered within the same year, dropping to the mid-0.60s over a 20-year span. Measures of mild and presumably variable pathological states, such as anxiety, have coefficients about 0.10 lower than trait measures. Conversely, IQ tests, especially when administered to adults, have retest reliabilities about 0.10 higher (Schuerger and Witt 1989). Some measures of competence, specifically specialty certification examinations, have been shown to have similar correlations of about 0.70 over a 7- to 10-year interval (Ramsey et al. 1989).

Standards for the magnitude of the reliability coefficient

From the previous sections, it should be evident that reliability cannot be conceived of as a property that a particular instrument does or does not possess; rather, any measure will have a certain degree of reliability when applied to certain populations under certain conditions. The issue which must be addressed is how much reliability is 'good enough'. Authors of textbooks on psychometric theory often make brief recommendations, usually without justification or reference to other recommendations. In fact, there can be no sound basis for such a recommendation, any more than there can be a sound basis for the decision that a certain percentage of candidates sitting an examination will fail.

For what it is worth, here are two authors' opinions for acceptable reliability for tests used to make a decision about individuals: Kelley (1927) recommended a minimum of 0.94, while Weiner and Stewart (1984) suggested 0.85. These standards may be too high, though, to be practical. Only two of the eight subscales of the well-validated SF-36 have reliabilities over 0.90 (Ware and Sherbourne 1992); and the 1-day test–retest reliability of automated systolic blood pressure readings in one study was 0.87 and 0.67 for diastolic blood pressure (Prisant et al. 1992). But as Peterson (1994) has said, 'none of the recommendations have an empirical basis, a theoretical justification, or an analytical rationale. Rather, they appear to reflect either experience or intuition' (p.381).

Fortunately, some authors avoid any such arbitrary judgement. However, the majority of textbooks then make a further distinction, namely, that a test used for individual judgement should be more reliable than one used for group decisions or research purposes. Nunnally (1978), for example, recommended a minimum reliability of 0.70 when the scale is used in research and 0.90 when it is used clinically. Actually, Nunnally said 0.70 may be sufficient in early stages of research in order to save time and energy. In applied settings, even a reliability of 0.80 may not be high enough; and when decisions are made about an individual, the reliability should be above 0.95. There are two possible justifications for this distinction. First, the research will draw conclusions from a mean score averaged across many individuals, and the sample size will serve to reduce the error of measurement in comparison to group differences. Second, rarely will decisions about research findings be made on the basis of a single study; conclusions are usually drawn from a series of replicated studies. But a recommendation of reliability, such as attempted by Weiner and Stewart (1984), remains tenuous since a sample of 1,000 can tolerate a much less reliable instrument than a sample of 10, so that the acceptable reliability is dependent on the sample size used in the research.

Reliability and the probability of misclassification

An additional problem of interpretation arising from the reliability coefficient is that it does not, of itself, indicate just how many wrong decisions (false positives or false negatives) will result from a measure with a particular reliability. There is no straightforward answer to this problem, since the probability of misclassification, when the underlying measure is continuous, relates both to the property of the instrument and to the decision of the location of the cut point. For example, if we had people trained to assess haemoglobin using an office haemoglobinometer and classify patients as normal or anaemic on the basis of a single random blood sample, the number of false positives and false negatives will be dependent on the reliability of the reading of a single sample, but will also depend on two other variables: where we decide to set the boundary between normal and anaemic, and the base rate of anaemia in the population under study.

Sometimes we are dealing with a continuous scale that assigns diagnoses depending on the score. For example, the Beck Depression Inventory-II (Beck et al. 1996) has 21 items, and the score ranges between 0 and 63. Although various cut points have been proposed, one commonly used set calls scores between 0 and 10 'Normal', 11 to 16 is considered to reflect a 'Mild mood disturbance', 17 to 20 as 'Borderline clinical depression', 21 to 30 as 'Moderate depression', and 31 and above as 'Severe depression'. Let's assume a person gets a score of 20, which is at the upper end of the Borderline range. As can be seen in Fig. 8.3, even if the reliability of the scale is 0.95 (top line), then the true score can be in the Mild, Borderline, or Moderate range. If the reliability is 0.70, then the true score can be anywhere from Normal to Severe. While this may be an extreme example, because some of the diagnostic 'bins' are fairly narrow, the message holds for any scale: when the reliability is below 0.95, be very wary of assigning a label to an individual.

Clearly there must be some relationship between the reliability of the scores and the likelihood that the decision will result in a misclassification. Some indication of the relationship between reliability and the probability of misclassification was given

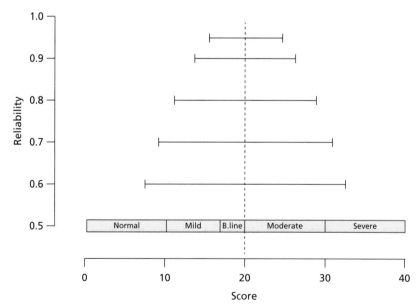

Fig. 8.3 95 per cent confidence intervals around score at different levels of reliability of a scale.

by Thorndike and Hagen (1969), who avoided the 'cut point' problem by examining the ranking of individuals. Imagine 100 people who have been tested and ranked. Consider one individual ranked 25th from the top, and another ranked 50th. If the reliability is 0, there is a 50 per cent chance that the two will reverse order on repeated testing, since the measure conveys no information and the ordering, as a result, is arbitrary. With a reliability of 0.5, there is still a 37 per cent chance of reversal; a reliability of 0.8 will result in 20 per cent reversals; and 0.95 will result in their reversing order 2.2 per cent of the time. From this example, it is evident that reliability of 0.75 is a fairly minimal requirement for a useful instrument.

Reporting reliability coefficients

In our first course in statistics, we are taught that every test must be accompanied by a probability level, and that only those with p levels less than 0.05 are meaningful; results with larger values of p are likely due to chance. The temptation, then, is to report p levels for reliability coefficients. But we are also admonished by religious leaders to avoid temptations and, at least in this regard, they are correct. Performing a test of significance for a reliability coefficient is tantamount to committing a type III error—getting the right answer to a question no one is asking (Streiner 2007).

A test of significance gives the probability that, if the null hypothesis is true, the results could have been due to the effects of chance. However, that is not the important question insofar as reliability is concerned. The issue in reliability (and some validity) testing is the *magnitude* of the coefficient, not the probability that it differs from zero. With a sample size of 50, a correlation of 0.28 is statistically significant, but it would be fatuous to use any scale whose test–retest or inter-rater reliability were this minuscule.

The only time it is legitimate to report a p level for a reliability coefficient is when it is being compared to a minimally acceptable reliability. For example, one may postulate that an instrument should have a reliability greater than 0.70. The null hypothesis, then, is not that reliability is greater than zero, but that it is less than or equal to 0.70. This is the approach taken by Donner and Eliasziw (1987) to calculate sample size requirements for reliability studies, as we explain in more detail below.

A far better approach, and one that is consistent with the recommendations of Wilkinson and the Task Force on Statistical Inference (1999), is to calculate a 95 per cent confidence interval around the reliability coefficient, as we will discuss under 'Standard error of the reliability coefficient and sample size'. The true test is whether the lower bound of the CI is greater than the minimal value of reliability (e.g. 0.70 for a research tool, 0.90 for a clinical one).

Effect of reliability on a study's sample size

If a scale is used as an outcome measure, its reliability has a direct impact on the sample size required to show a statistically significant effect. The reason is that unreliability inflates the variance of the observed scores. More specifically, the observed score variance is σ^2 / R, where σ^2 is the variance of the true score, and R the reliability of the scale. If we need N subjects in order to achieve significance with a perfectly reliable test, then we would need approximately N/R subjects if the reliability coefficient were actually R (Kraemer 1979). A test with a reliability of 0.80 would require a 25 per cent increase in sample size; we would need 43 per cent more subjects with a reliability of 0.70; and a reliability of 0.50 would require a doubling of the sample size. Obviously, the message is to use a scale with a high reliability.

Improving reliability

If we return to the basic definition of reliability as a ratio of subject variance to subject + error variance, we can improve reliability only by increasing the magnitude of the variance between subjects relative to the error variance. This can be accomplished in a number of ways, both legitimate and otherwise.

There are several approaches to reducing error variance. Many authors recommend observer training, although the specific strategies to be used in training raters are usually unspecified. Alternatively, Newble et al. (1980) have suggested that observers have difficulty acquiring new skills. They recommend, as a result, that if consistently extreme observers are discovered, they simply be eliminated from further use. The strategies for improving scale design discussed in Chapter 4 may also contribute to reducing error variance.

Similarly, there are a number of ways of enhancing the true variance. If the majority of individual scores are either very high or very low so that the average score is approaching the maximum or minimum possible (the 'ceiling' or 'floor'), then many of the items are being wasted. The solution is to introduce items that will result in performance nearer the middle of the scale, effectively increasing true variance. One could also modify the descriptions on the scale: for example, by changing 'poor-fair-good-excellent' to 'fair-good-very good-excellent'.

An alternative approach, which is *not* legitimate, is to administer the test to a more heterogeneous group of subjects for the purpose of determining reliability. For example, if a measure of function in arthritis does not reliably discriminate among ambulatory arthritics, administering the test to both normal subjects and bedridden hospitalized arthritics will almost certainly improve reliability. Of course, the resulting reliability no longer yields any information about the ability of the instrument to discriminate among ambulatory patients.

By contrast, it is sometimes the case that a reliability coefficient derived from a homogeneous population is to be applied to a population that is more heterogeneous. It is clear from the above discussion that the reliability in the application envisioned will be larger than that determined in the homogeneous study population. If the standard deviations of the two samples are known, it is possible to calculate a new reliability coefficient, or to *correct for attenuation*, using the following formula:

$$r' = \frac{r \times \sigma^2_{new}}{r \times \sigma^2_{new} + (1-r) \times \sigma^2_{old}}$$

where σ^2_{new} and σ^2_{old} are the variances of the new and original samples, respectively, r is the original reliability, and r' is the corrected reliability.

Perhaps the simplest way to improve reliability is to increase the number of items on the test. It is not self-evident why this should help, but the answer lies in statistical theory. As long as the test items are not perfectly correlated, the true variance will increase as the square of the number of items, whereas the error variance will increase only as the number of items. So, if the test length is tripled, true variance will be nine times as large and error variance three times as large as the original test, as long as the new items are similar psychometrically to the old ones. From the Spearman–Brown formula, which we discussed in Chapter 5, the new reliability will be as follows:

$$r_{SB} = \frac{3 \times r}{1 + 2 \times r}$$

If the original reliability was 0.7, the tripled test will have a reliability of 0.875. The relationship between the number of items and test length is shown in Fig. 8.4.

In practice, the equation tends to overestimate the new reliability, since we tend to think up (or 'borrow') the easier, more obvious items first. When we have to devise new items, they often are not as good as the original ones.

The Spearman–Brown formula can be used in another way. If we know the reliability of a test of a particular length is r and we wish to achieve a reliability of r', then the formula can be modified to indicate the factor by which we must increase the test length, k:

$$k = \frac{r'(1-r)}{r(1-r')}.$$

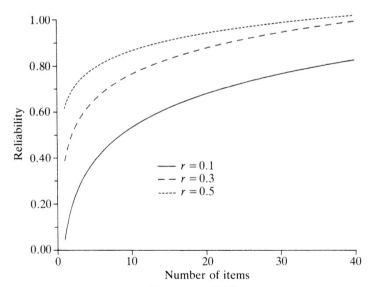

Fig. 8.4 Relation between number of items and reliability.

To improve measures of stability, such as test–retest reliability, one can always shorten the retest interval. However, if the instrument is intended to measure states of duration of weeks or months, the demonstration of retest reliability over hours or days is not useful.

Finally, it is evident from the foregoing discussion that there is not a single reliability associated with a measure. A more useful approach to the issue of reliability is to critically examine the components of variance due to each source of variation in turn and then focus efforts on reducing the larger sources of error variance. This approach, called *generalizability theory*, is covered in Chapter 9.

Standard error of the reliability coefficient and sample size

In conducting a reliability study, we are attempting to estimate the reliability coefficient with as much accuracy as possible; that is, we want to be certain that the true reliability coefficient is reasonably close to the estimate we have determined. This is one form of the *confidence interval* (CI; for further discussion consult one of the recommended statistics books). As we might expect, the larger the sample size, the smaller will be the CI, so that for a given estimate of the CI, we can (in theory) compute the required sample size. Note that this calculation of the CI is for reliability coefficients based on test–retest and inter-rater reliabilities. The CI for coefficient α was discussed in Chapter 5.

To do so, we need to first determine the standard error of the reliability coefficient (which is not the same as the standard error of measurement derived *from* the reliability coefficient). As it turns out, this is quite complex. It leans heavily on the Fisher z_R transformation of the intraclass correlation, given in Fisher's book (1925), which removes skewness in the standard error:

$$z_R = \frac{1}{2} \log_e \left[\frac{1 + (k-1)R}{1-R} \right]$$

where R is the value of the intraclass correlation and k is the number of observations per subject. From this, Fisher derived the formula of the standard error of the z_R transform:

$$SE(z_R) = \sqrt{\frac{k}{2(k-1)(n-2)}}$$

where n is the number of subjects.

So, for any calculated reliability R and a given sample size, we can determine the standard error of the reliability coefficient. For example, if we had conducted a study with 102 observations and five raters and the reliability had turned out to be 0.75, we can then compute the standard error as follows:

(1) The z-transformed reliability is:

$$z_R = \frac{1}{2}log_e \left[\frac{1+(4\times0.75)}{1-0.75} \right] = \frac{1}{2}log_e(16) = 1.386$$

(2) The standard error of the z-transformed R is:

$$SE = \sqrt{\frac{5}{2(4)(100)}} = 0.079$$

(3) So, the upper and lower limits of the z-transformed R are now:

$$1.386 \pm 0.079 = 1.307 \ to \ 1.465$$

(4) Now, we have to work backwards, transforming these limits back to correlations, which we will show just for the lower limit, which is 1.307. From it, we subtract $1/2 \log_e (k-1)$ so that:

$$z'' = 1.307 - \frac{1}{2}log_e(k-1) = 1.307 - 0.6931 = 0.6139$$

and change z'' to r' using the formula:

$$r' = \frac{e^{(2z'')} - 1}{e^{(2z'')} + 1} = \frac{e^{(1.2278)} - 1}{e^{(1.2278)} + 1} = \frac{2.4137}{4.4137} = 0.5469$$

This is multiplied by k; we add $(k-2)$; and divide by $2 (k-1)$:

$$\frac{(r' \times k) + (k-2)}{2(k-1)} = \frac{(0.5469 \times 5) + 3}{2 \times 4} = 0.717$$

Doing the same for the upper limit gives us 0.780.

(5) Therefore, finally, we can say that the estimated reliability is 0.75, with a range (±SE) of 0.717 to 0.780. Because of the properties of the distribution, this is not quite symmetrical about the estimate.

To compute the required sample size, we begin with an estimate of the likely intraclass correlation, R. We then estimate the likely certainty we want in this estimate (±SE). For example, if we think that the reliability computed from the study is 0.80, and we want to have sufficient sample size to be 95 per cent certain that it is definitely above 0.70, this amounts to setting the 95 per cent confidence interval around the reliability of 0.10 (0.80 minus 0.70). The SE, then, is half this confidence interval, or 0.05.

We also have to know in advance the number of observations we are going to use in the study: for example, five. The derivation of sample size proceeds as follows.

First, compute $R^- = R - SE$. (We use $R - SE$ rather than $R + SE$ because it is more conservative, resulting in a somewhat larger sample size.) Then from the above formula:

$$z_R = \frac{1}{2} log_e \left[\frac{1 + (k-1)R}{1-R} \right] \quad and \quad z = \frac{1}{2} log_e \left[\frac{1 + (k-1)R^-}{1-R^-} \right]$$

We can now compute the SE of the z scores as follows:

$$SE = z_R - z_{R^-}$$

but from the previous equation:

$$SE(z_R) = \sqrt{\frac{k}{2(k-1)(n-2)}}$$

Finally, squaring and cross-multiplying we get:

$$n = 2 + \frac{k}{2(k-1)\left(z_R - z_{R^-}\right)^2}$$

In our previous example, then, we began with a hypothesized reliability R of 0.80, a standard error of 0.05, and five observations per subject:

(1) The log transformed values of R and R^- are:

$$z_R = \frac{1}{2} log_e (4.2 / 0.2) = 1.522$$

and

$$z_{R^-} = \frac{1}{2} log_e (4.0 / 0.25) = 1.386$$

(2) So, the SE is:

$$z_R - z_{R^-} = 1.522 - 1.386 = 0.136$$

(3) Then, the sample size, n (rounding up), is:

$$n = 2 + \frac{5}{(2)(4)(0.136)^2} = 36$$

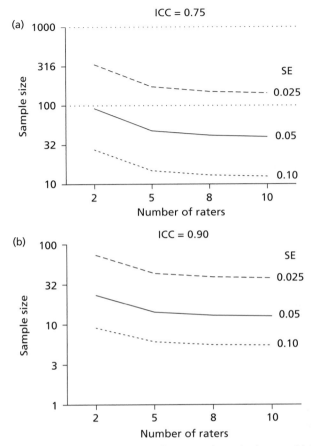

Fig. 8.5 Sample sizes for different numbers of raters and standard errors: (a) ICC = 0.75; and (b) ICC = 0.90.

It is possible to determine all this graphically; however, since the sample size depends on three estimates—R, k, and the confidence interval—multiple graphs are required to display the results. Two such graphs, for ICC = 0.75 and 0.90, are shown in Fig. 8.5.

A somewhat different approach, based on hypothesis testing, is taken by Donner and Eliasziw (1987). In their approach, H_0 (null hypothesis) is that the observed ICC is less than some minimum value. Their exact solution is computationally intense (translation: you don't want to try this at home), but Walter, Eliasziw, and Donner (1998) worked out an approximation that is easier to calculate (yes, these are the simpler formulae) and yields comparable sample size estimates. The number of cases, k, is:

$$k = 1 + \frac{2 \times \left(z_\alpha + z_\beta\right)^2 \times n}{\left(\ln C_0\right)^2 \left(n - 1\right)}$$

where

$$C_o = \frac{1 + \dfrac{np_o}{1-p_o}}{1 + \dfrac{np_1}{1-p_1}}$$

p_0 is the minimally acceptable value; p_1 the hypothesized value of the ICC; n the number of observations (e.g. raters, test administrations); z_α the value of the normal curve for the desired one-tailed α level (e.g. 1.6449 for 0.05); and z_β the value for the β level (e.g. 0.8416 for 0.20). Because in most cases $n = 2$ (e.g. test–retest reliability or two raters) and we use α and β levels of 0.05 and 0.20 respectively, we can simplify the formula even further to be:

$$k = \frac{24.7307}{\left(lnC_O\right)^2}$$

and in Table 8.6 we have given sample sizes for the more usual values of p_0 and p_1. A more complete table, with other values for p_0, p_1, and n, is given in the article by Walter et al. (1998).

Still another approach to estimating sample size is to use a fixed number, but the widely varying estimates found in the literature—from as little as 20 to over 1,000—is a testament to the lack of consensus on this approach (see Charter 1999, 2003b; Feldt and Ankenmann 1999; Guilford 1956; Kline 1986). Cicchetti and Fleiss (1977) argue that in most situations with two raters, a sample size of $2k^2$, where k is the number of points on the scale, should be sufficient. This yields a sample size of about 20 for a 3-point scale; 30 for a 4-point scale; 50 for a 5-point scale; 75 for a 6-point scale; and about 100 for a 7-point scale (Cicchetti 1976).

Table 8.6 Sample sizes for the ICC for two raters or occasions, and for various values of p_0 and p_1

$p0$	$p1$					
	0.70	**0.75**	**0.80**	**0.85**	**0.90**	**0.95**
0.60	204	79	38	20	11	5
0.65	870	189	71	32	16	7
0.70		554	116	41	17	7
0.75			391	78	25	9
0.80				249	45	12
0.85					133	19
0.90						105

Note: all values have been rounded up. $\alpha = 0.05$, $\beta = 0.20$.

So, where does that leave us? Obviously, as Fig. 8.4 shows, we need to take the number of raters and the desired standard error (or equivalently, the confidence interval) into account; and the more subjects the better. But, going above 50 subjects (or using Cicchetti and Fleiss's value of $2k^2$) in many situations is probably statistical overkill.

Reliability generalization

As already mentioned, reliability is not a fixed property of a test; it can vary depending on the characteristics of the group completing it, and the circumstances under which it is filled out. This raises four questions: (1) Is it possible to determine the 'typical' reliability of an instrument? (2) Can we describe the variability in reliability estimates? (3) Can we determine what the reliability would be if we had the raw data from all of the studies? and (4) Is it possible to determine what factors influence the reliability of scores? The answer to all four questions is Yes, and the method of answering them is called *reliability generalization* (RG).

RG was introduced in 1998 by Vacha-Haase, who based it on techniques developed for the meta-analysis of intervention studies (Hunter and Schmidt 2004). Consequently, the steps to be followed in conducting an RG study are closely parallel to those of doing a meta-analysis (Streiner 1991); therefore, they will only be highlighted and not be spelled out in detail. The first step, collecting all the relevant studies, both published and unpublished, presents a different set of challenges in RG studies as compared with traditional meta-analyses. In the latter, almost every retrieved article that meets the inclusion and exclusion criteria will provide some useful information about the phenomenon being investigated. However, most studies that use a scale will not have assessed its reliability, but will report estimates derived from other studies, or in the case of published scales, the test manual (e.g. Wilson 1980). This is most often the case when the focus of the study is not on the psychometric properties of the scale itself, but when the scale is used as an outcome variable (e.g. Caruso et al. 2001; Vacha-Haase 1998). The result is that there are far fewer estimates of reliability than retrieved articles. For example, Yin and Fan (2000) found that fewer than eight per cent of articles that used the *Beck Depression Inventory* reported reliability estimates based on their data.

The next step is to develop a coding form to abstract and record the relevant information from each study. The information that is extracted will likely vary from one RG study to the next, depending on one's hypotheses about the factors that may affect reliability. At the very least, it would include the type of coefficient (that is, internal consistency, test–retest, inter-rater), the sample size, the gender of the respondents, and the key characteristics of the people (e.g. clinical versus non-clinical; age; ethnicity). Henson and Thompson (2002) list a number of other variables that may or may not be considered, and Hunter and Schmidt (2004) give an example of an abstraction form.

The average value of *r* and α

When the mean of a number of correlations is calculated, the first step, according to some authors, is to transform them to Fisher's z' scores in order to normalize their distribution. There is a debate whether this is necessary or desirable in generalization studies. Some argue that it is a necessary step (e.g. Beretvas and Pastor 2003; Hedges and Vevea 1998). The opposite position is based on the fact that, even though they are expressed as rs, reliability coefficients are actually estimates of the variance accounted for (i.e. an r^2 type of statistic; Lord and Novick 1968). Consequently, Thompson and Vacha-Haase (2000) and Henson and Thompson (2002) recommend not using the transformation. The jury is still out, but simulations indicate that more accurate results are obtained when the transformation is not used (Hall and Brannick 2002). However, Cronbach's α is different; it is not normally distributed, and the value from each study (α_i) needs to be transformed, using the formula proposed by Hakstian and Whalen (1976):

$$T_i = \left(1 - \alpha_i\right)^{1/3}$$

Now the first two questions—the typical reliability and the variability in estimates— are quite simple to answer: they would be the mean and standard deviation (SD) of the reliability estimates, and the values of r for test–retest and inter-rater reliabilities, and of T_i for Cronbach's α.

However, this should not be done blindly. It often does not make sense to combine different types of reliability coefficients to derive an 'average' index. Test–retest reliability usually varies with the time between testings; inter-rater reliability may depend on the amount of training given to the raters; and coefficient α is a function, in part, of the number of items (Cortina 1993; Streiner 2003). In any case, it certainly makes no sense to average test–retest, inter-rater, and internal consistency reliability coefficients; they are estimates of different characteristics and cannot be presumed to be equal. This means that when numbers allow, each type of reliability should be analysed separately (Beretvas and Pastor 2003).

There is some debate whether the estimates should be weighted in some way before determining the mean and SD. Some people use the analogy of meta-analysis, where the effect size of a study is weighted by either the sample size or the inverse of the variance so that larger studies or more precise estimates have a greater influence (e.g. Hunter and Schmidt 2004). Others take the position that in RG studies, the sample size may be one of the factors influencing the estimate and should be examined as part of the fourth question so that the unweighted reliabilities should be used. However, the consensus is that the best estimate of the population reliability is one based on the reliability estimate of each study (r_i) weighted by its sample size (n_i). The actual mathematics of combining the reliability coefficients can become somewhat laborious and we won't go into them here. For those who are interested, see Charter (2003a).

Factors affecting the reliability

The fourth issue—determining what affects the magnitude of the reliability—can be addressed in a number of ways. The easiest is to perform a series of univariate analyses between the predictor variables and the reliability estimates, such as correlating the reliabilities with the sample size; doing a *t*-test or one-way ANOVA with gender as the grouping variable; and so on. The most common method is to use linear regression, with the reliabilities as the dependent variable and the predictors as the independent variables. Examination of the standardized regression weights (β) and the structure coefficients (Norman and Streiner 2008) will allow you to see the relative contribution of each factor.

Until relatively recently, the type of regression used in RG studies was the usual one found in most statistics books, called 'fixed-effects' regression. The underlying assumption is that there is one 'true' reliability, and that all of the studies are estimating this one value; differences among the studies are due simply to random variation. In meta-analyses, there has been a gradual shift to using a more complex form of regression, called 'mixed-effects' or 'random-effects' (see Norman and Streiner (2008) for a discussion of this), and now RG studies have begun to adopt the same approach (Beretvas and Pastor 2003). These models allow the 'true', or population value to differ from one study to the next.

The disadvantages of mixed-effects models are that they are more difficult to run and result in lower estimates of the reliability. However, this is counterbalanced by the advantages, which are (1) that it more accurately reflects the real world, and especially (2), it allows one to generalize the findings beyond the specific articles in the RG study. We would strongly recommend that anyone doing an RG study use a mixed-models approach.

Summary

The discussion regarding appropriate measures of reliability is easily resolved. The Pearson correlation is theoretically incorrect but usually fairly close. The method of Altman and Bland is analogous (actually isomorphic) to the calculation of error variance in the ICC and does not explicitly relate this to the range of observations. Thus we are left with kappa and the intraclass correlation, which yield identical results; so the choice can be dictated by ease of calculation, nothing else.

Further reading

Anastasi, A. and Urbina, S. (1996). *Psychological testing* (7th edn). Pearson, New York.

Cronbach, L.J. (1984). *Essentials of psychological testing* (4th edn). Harper and Row, New York.

Nunnally, J.C., Jr. (1970). *Introduction to psychological measurement*. McGraw-Hill, New York.

References

Altman, D.G. and Bland, J.M. (1983). Measurement in medicine: The analysis of method comparison studies. *Statistician*, **32**, 307–17.

American Educational Research Association, American Psychological Association, and National Council on Measurement in Education (2014). *Standards for educational and psychological testing*. American Psychological Association, Washington, DC.

Beck, A.T., Steer, R.A., and Brown, G.K. (1996). *Beck Depression Inventory—Second edition manual.* The Psychological Corporation, San Antonio, TX.

Beretvas, S.N. and Pastor, D.A. (2003). Using mixed-effects models in reliability generalization studies. *Educational and Psychological Measurement*, **63**, 75–95.

Berk, R.A. (1979). Generalizability of behavioral observations: A clarification of interobserver agreement and interobserver reliability. *American Journal of Mental Deficiency*, **83**, 460–72.

Bland, J.M. and Altman, D.G. (1986). Statistical methods for assessing agreement between two methods of clinical measurement. *Lancet*, **i**, 307–10.

Caruso, J.C., Witkiewitz, K., Belcourt-Dittlof, A., and Gottlieb, J.D. (2001). Reliability of scores from the Eysenck Personality Questionnaire: A reliability generalization study. *Educational and Psychological Measurement*, **61**, 675–89.

Charter, R.A. (1999). Sample size requirements for precise estimates of reliability, generalizability, and validity coefficients. *Journal of Clinical and Experimental Neuropsychology*, **21**, 559–66.

Charter, R.A. (2003a). Combining reliability coefficients: Possible application to meta-analysis and reliability generalization. *Psychological Reports*, **93**, 643–7.

Charter, R.A. (2003b). Study samples are too small to produce sufficiently precise reliability coefficients. *Journal of General Psychology*, **130**, 117–29.

Cicchetti, D.V. (1976). Assessing inter-rater reliability for rating scales: Resolving some basic issues. *British Journal of Psychiatry*, **129**, 452–6.

Cicchetti, D.V. (2001). The precision of reliability and validity estimates re-visited: Distinguishing between clinical and statistical significance of sample size requirements. *Journal of Clinical and Experimental Neuropsychology*, **23**, 695–700.

Cicchetti, D.V. and Fleiss, J.L. (1977). Comparison of the null distributions of weighted kappa and the C ordinal statistic. *Applied Psychological Measurement*, **1**, 195–201.

Cicchetti, D.V. and Sparrow, S.A. (1981). Developing criteria for establishing interrater reliability of specific items: Applications to assessment of adaptive behavior. *American Journal of Mental Deficiency*, **86**, 127–37.

Cohen, J. (1960). A coefficient of agreement for nominal scales. *Educational and Psychological Measurement*, **20**, 37–46.

Cohen, J. (1968). Weighted kappa: Nominal scale agreement with provision for scaled disagreement or partial credit. *Psychological Bulletin*, **70**, 213–20.

Cortina, J.M. (1993). What is coefficient alpha? An examination of theory and applications. *Journal of Applied Psychology*, **78**, 98–104.

Crocker, L. and Algina, J. (1986). *Introduction to classical and modern test theory.* Holt, Rinehart and Winston, New York.

Cronbach, L.J. (1957). The two disciplines of scientific psychology. *American Psychologist*, **12**, 671–84.

Donner, A. and Eliasziw, M. (1987). Sample size requirements for reliability studies. *Statistics in Medicine*, **6**, 441–8.

Feldt, L.S. and Ankenmann, R.D. (1999). Determining sample size for a test of the equality of alpha coefficients when the number of part-tests is small. *Psychological Methods*, **4**, 366–77.

Feldt, L.S., Steffan, M., and Gupta, N.C. (1985). A comparison of five methods for estimating the standard error of measurement at specific score levels. *Applied Psychological Measurement*, **9**, 351–61.

Fisher, R.A. (1925). *Statistical methods for research workers.* Oliver and Boyd, Edinburgh.

Fleiss, J.L. (1981). *Statistical methods for rates and proportions* (2nd edn). Wiley, New York.

Fleiss, J.L. and Cohen, J. (1973). The equivalence of weighted kappa and the intraclass correlation coefficient as measures of reliability. *Educational and Psychological Measurement*, **33**, 613–19.

Gift, A.G. and Soeken, K.L. (1988). Assessment of physiologic instruments. *Heart & Lung*, **17**, 128–33.

Green, B.E. (1981). A primer of testing. *American Psychologist*, **36**, 1001–11.

Gronlund, N.E. and Linn, R.L. (1990). *Measurement and evaluation in teaching* (6th edn). Macmillan, New York.

Guilford, J.P. (1956). *Psychometric methods* (2nd edn). McGraw Hill, New York.

Hakstian, A.R. and Whalen, T.E. (1976). A k-sample significance test for independent alpha coefficients. *Psychometrika*, **41**, 219–31.

Hall, S.M. and Brannick, M.T. (2002). Comparison of two random-effects methods of meta-analysis. *Journal of Applied Psychology*, **87**, 377–89.

Hedges, L.V. and Vevea, J.L. (1998). Fixed- and random-effects models in meta-analysis. *Psychological Methods*, **3**, 486–504.

Helms, J.E., Henze, K.T., Sass, T.L., and Mifsud, V.A. (2006). Treating Cronbach's alpha reliability coefficients as data in counseling research. *The Counseling Psychologist*, **34**, 630–60.

Henson, R.K. and Thompson, B. (2002). Characterizing measurement error in scores across studies: Some recommendations for conducting "reliability generalization" studies. *Measurement and Evaluation in Counseling and Development*, **35**, 113–26.

Hunter, J.E. and Schmidt, F.L. (2004). *Methods of meta-analysis: Correcting error and bias in research findings* (2nd edn). Sage, Newbury Park, CA.

Kelley, T.L. (1927). *Interpretation of educational measurements*. World Books, Yonkers, NY.

Kline, P. (1986). *A handbook of test construction*. Methuen, London.

Kraemer, H.C. (1979). Ramifications of a population model for k as a coefficient of reliability. *Psychometrika*, **44**, 461–72.

Krippendorff, K. (2013). *Content analysis: An introduction to its methodology* (3rd edn). Sage, Thousand Oaks, CA.

Krus, D.J. and Helmstadter, G.C. (1993). The probabilities of negative reliabilities. *Educational and Psychological Measurement*, **53**, 643–50.

Landis, J.R. and Koch, G.G. (1977). The measurement of agreement for categorical data. *Biometrics*, **33**, 159–74.

Lord, F.M. and Novick, M.R. (1968). *Statistical theory of mental test scores*. Addison-Wesley, Reading, MA.

Lynn, M.R. (1989). Instrument reliability and validity: How much needs to be published? *Heart & Lung*, **18**, 421–3.

McCrae, R.R., Kurtz, J.E., Yamagata, S., and Terracciano, A. (2011). Internal consistency, retest reliability, and their implications for personality scale validation. *Personality and Social Psychology Review*, **15**, 28–50.

McGraw, K.O. and Wong, S.P. (1996). Forming inferences about some intraclass correlation coefficients. *Psychological Methods*, **1**, 30–46.

Newble, D.I., Hoare, J., and Sheldrake, P.F. (1980). The selection and training of examiners for clinical examinations. *Medical Education*, **4**, 345–9.

Norman, G.R. and Streiner, D.L. (2008). *Biostatistics: The bare essentials* (3rd edn). B.C. Decker, Toronto.

Norman, G.R. and Streiner, D.L. (2014). *Biostatistics: The bare essentials* (4th edn). PMPH USA, Shelton, CT.

Nunnally, J.C. (1978). *Psychometric theory*. McGraw-Hill, New York.

Peterson, R.A. (1994). A meta-analysis of Cronbach's coefficient alpha. *Journal of Consumer Research*, **21**, 381–91.

Prisant, L.M., Carr, A.A., Bottini, P.B., Thompson, W.O., and Rhoades, R.B. (1992). Repeatability of automated ambulatory blood pressure measurements. *Journal of Family Practice*, **34**, 569–74.

Ramsey, P.G., Carline, J.D., Inui, T.S., Larson, E.B., LoGerfo, J.P., and Weinrich, M.D. (1989). Predictive validity of certification by the American Board of Internal Medicine. *Annals of Internal Medicine*, **110**, 719–26.

Schuerger, J.M. and Witt, A.C. (1989). The temporal stability of individually tested intelligence. *Journal of Clinical Psychology*, **45**, 294–302.

Schuerger, J.M., Tait, E., and Tavernelli, M. (1982). Temporal stability of personality by questionnaire. *Journal of Personality and Social Psychology*, **43**, 176–82.

Schuerger, J.M., Zarella, K.L., and Hotz, A.S. (1989). Factors that influence the temporal stability of personality by questionnaire. *Journal of Personality and Social Psychology*, **56**, 777–83.

Shrout, P.E. and Fleiss, J.L. (1979). Intraclass correlations: Uses in assessing rater reliability. *Psychological Bulletin*, **86**, 420–8.

Stanley, J.C. (1971). Reliability. In *Educational measurement* (ed. R. Thorndike) (2nd edn), pp. 356–442. American Council on Education, Washington, DC.

Streiner, D.L. (1991). Using meta-analysis in psychiatric research. *Canadian Journal of Psychiatry*, **36**, 357–62.

Streiner, D.L. (2003). Starting at the beginning: An introduction to coefficient alpha and internal consistency. *Journal of Personality Assessment*, **80**, 99–103.

Streiner, D.L. (2007). A shortcut to rejection: How not to write the results section of a paper. *Canadian Journal of Psychiatry*, **52**, 385–9.

Streiner, D.L. and Norman, G.R. (2006). "Precision" and "accuracy": Two terms that are neither. *Journal of Clinical Epidemiology*, **59**, 327–30.

Szafran, R.F. (2017). The miscalculation of interrater reliability: A case study involving the AAC&U VALUE rubrics. *Practical Assessment, Research & Evaluation*, **22**(11), 1–7.

Thompson, B. and Vacha-Haase, T. (2000). Psychometrics *is* datametrics: The test is not reliable. *Educational and Psychological Measurement*, **60**, 174–95.

Thorndike, R.L. and Hagen, E. (1969). *Measurement and evaluation in education and psychology*. Wiley, New York.

Vacha-Haase, T. (1998). Reliability generalization: Exploring variance in measurement error affecting score reliability across studies. *Educational and Psychological Measurement*, **58**, 6–20.

Walter, S.D., Eliasziw, M., and Donner, A. (1998). Sample size and optimal designs for reliability studies. *Statistics in Medicine*, **17**, 101–10.

Ware, J.E. and Sherbourne, C.D. (1992). The MOS 36-Item Short-Form Survey (SF-36): I. Conceptual framework and item selection. *Medical Care*, **30**, 473–83.

Weiner, E.A. and Stewart, B.J. (1984). *Assessing individuals*. Little Brown, Boston, MA.

Weir, J.P. (2005). Quantifying the test–retest reliability using the intraclass correlation coefficient and the *SEM. Journal of Strength and Conditioning Research*, **19**, 231–40.

Wilkinson, L. and Task Force on Statistical Inference (1999). Statistical methods in psychology journals: Guidelines and explanations. *American Psychologist*, **54**, 594–604.

Wilson, V.L. (1980). Research techniques in *AERJ* articles: 1969 to 1978. *Educational Researcher*, **9**(6), 5–10.

Yin, P. and Fan, X. (2000). Assessing the reliability of Beck Depression Inventory scores: Reliability generalization across studies. *Educational and Psychological Measurement*, **60**, 201–23.

Chapter 9

Generalizability theory

Introduction to generalizability theory

Classical test theory (CTT), upon which the reliability coefficient is based, begins with a simple assumption—that an observed test score can be decomposed into two parts: a 'true' score (which no one really knows) and an 'error' score (that is $Score_{Observed} = Score_{True} + error$). As we discussed in Chapter 8, this assumption then leads directly to the formulation of the reliability coefficient as the ratio of true variance to (true + error) variance.

We saw that there are many approaches to estimating reliability, each of which generates a different coefficient (and often relies on a different study design). One can examine scores from the same observer on two viewings of the same stimulus (intra-observer), different observers of the same stimulus (inter-observer), different occasions separated by a short time interval (test–retest), different items (internal consistency), different forms of the scale (parallel forms), and so on. Further, these standard measures do not exhaust the possible sources of variance. For example, some measures, such as bone density or tenderness, might be expected to be equal on both sides of the body (left–right reliability?), and skin colour might be expected to be the same on the soles of hands and feet (top–bottom reliability?).

It is worth noting something that might be self-evident. There is no such thing as *the* reliability of a test. Not only are there different reliability coefficients depending on what source of error you are studying, but also *there is no direct relation among them*. Each depends on the error variance attributable to the factor. Typically, internal consistency estimates, which are based on the correlations across items, are high—too high, in fact (Norman 2010; Streiner 2003), reflecting the fact that raters cannot really distinguish different characteristics (Park et al. 2014) or that there is unnecessary redundancy among the items of a scale. On the other hand, in a test involving different stations like an OSCE (Objective Structured Clinical Exam), correlations across stations is very low—typically 0.1 to 0.3, a phenomenon called 'content specificity' (Eva et al. 1998). We have observed situations where investigators have substituted one kind of reliability (where they have data) for another (where they don't), which is completely senseless.

Clearly, the assumption that all variance in scores can be neatly divided into true and error variance is simplistic. Instead, for each person we have measured there are, in addition to the 'true' score of that individual, multiple potential sources of error attributed to different factors that can contribute error. Our goal is to obtain the most precise estimate we can of the score that person should have, and we want to identify the various sources of error so we can minimize them.

Conceptually at least, we could consider a long series of studies, each of which determined one source of error variance. We could, perhaps, then put all of these error variances together to arrive at the appropriate reliability coefficients (a meta-analysis of errors estimates if you will). This may not, of itself, be problematic.

Unfortunately, even though it may appear that this would give us the information we need to make some intelligent decisions about the relative contributions of various sources of error, it is not quite that simple. Expanding on our earlier comment arguing against the notion of *the* reliability of a test, we can really only judge the reliability of the test as applied to a particular measurement situation. What this means, among other things, is that a test applied to a relatively homogeneous sample will look worse than when given to a heterogeneous one. So, when different studies yield different reliability coefficients for, say, inter-rater reliability in one study and test–retest in another, it is nearly impossible to determine whether the differences arise from different magnitudes of error from the two situations or different degrees of homogeneity in the two samples. How can you compare a study of test–retest reliability of joint counts in arthritis that involved following a group of hospitalized patients and re-measuring them at 2-day intervals, with a second study of inter-rater reliability of joint counts using a sample of patients from a family practice teaching unit measured every 6 months? One could conjecture that the latter sample was certainly healthier than the hospital patients. Were they more or less homogeneous? Is the error larger or smaller? It's difficult to say.

Furthermore, it is often the case that we need to simultaneously examine more than one source of error variance at a time, just to make sense of the situation. As one example, many studies have been reported of measures of health utility using the standard gamble, as described in Chapter 4. Typically, a group of patients, or non-patients, is asked to rate a series of written health state descriptions twice, a week or two apart. While it may not be obvious (and indeed has eluded some researchers , e.g. Torrance 1976), the 'subject variance' in this situation is the difference among health states, not between raters. But what can be done with the other two variables? We could calculate inter-rater reliability, across the n raters, but need to do this twice—for the two times. Then we could compute test–retest reliability, but must do this for every rater in the sample, for a total of n coefficients, each based on only a small fraction of the data, with predictably wide variation among the individual estimates.

What we really want is some way to use *all* the data to estimate both test–retest reliability and inter-rater reliability: in short, to compute simultaneously the error variance resulting from different raters, from different occasions, and from some potential interaction between the two factors, and then to combine these with a single estimate of subject variance (in this case, variance between health states) to arrive at an overall estimate of test–retest and inter-rater reliability. That is precisely how generalizability (G) theory approaches the situation.

Such subtleties may appear to be the stuff that only statisticians might care about; after all, does it really matter if I calculate a bunch of individual test–retest reliability coefficients and then average them, perhaps by using reliability generalization, as we discussed in Chapter 8? Perhaps not, but that is not the real power of G theory. By calculating all the plausible sources of error simultaneously, so that we can have some confidence that they really are directly comparable with each other, we can make a very powerful statement about the relative contribution of each.

We can then optimally combine observations to arrive at a desired level of reliability. The Spearman–Brown formula (Chapter 8) is a way to relate the number of observations to the overall reliability, one factor at a time. But when we start to recognize multiple sources of error (in the previous example, raters and occasions) we really want to address questions of the form 'If I can get a total of 100 repeated observations on each health state, am I better off to get 100 patients to rate states once, 50 patients twice, 25 patients 4 times, 10 patients 10 times, etc.?' Obviously, if patients contribute a lot of error and occasions relatively less, we should average over more patients and fewer occasions.

Both of these goals can be achieved by G theory, as originally devised by Cronbach et al. (1972). The essence of the theory is the recognition that in any measurement situation there are multiple (in fact, infinite) sources of error variance. An important goal of measurement is to attempt to identify, measure, and thereby find strategies to reduce the influence of these sources on the measurement in question. Although the theory is now over 50 years old, it is only within the last few decades that it has become a routine approach to measurement in the health sciences. A few review articles appeared in the 1980s which elaborated on, or utilized, the concepts of G theory (Boodoo and O'Sullivan 1982; Evans et al. 1981; Shavelson et al. 1989; van der Vleuten and Swanson 1990). However, by far the most authoritative source is Brennan's *Generalizability Theory* (2001). Regrettably, like many authorities, it can on occasion drift into the opaque. Nevertheless, what follows relies heavily on his theoretical developments.

There appears to be recent interest in G theory in the medical, medical education, and health care communities. A Pub Med search on 'generalizability theory' yielded 525 articles. In addition, a number of review articles have appeared (Cor and Peeters 2015; Monteiro et al. 2019; Prion et al. 2016; Vispoel et al. 2018) and at least one systematic review (Anders en et al. 2021), many directed at helping researchers navigate their way through the arcane details of G theory (Bloch and Norman 2012). Still, there are not all that many studies using G theory. We also think that one impediment to the more widespread use of G theory is the paucity of analytical software. While existing general purpose software like SPSS or R can do analysis of variance (ANOVA), this is only the first step in analysing G theory, as we will see. Moreover, for reasons we do not understand, SPSS and SAS are very inefficient in calculation of variance components. Some special purpose software does exist; Brennan wrote the most widely used, urGENOVA, decades ago—in fact, so long ago that it remains structured around command lines.

These concerns led one of us (GN) to collaborate with Ralph Bloch on creating a shell program around urGENOVA called G_String. Over two decades it has become more versatile and now includes features far beyond urGENOVA including handling missing values, estimating G coefficients for complex designs, and simulating data sets with predetermined variance components.

G_String, now in its sixth version, has gradually amassed a following of users. Four recent review articles (Bloch and Norman 2012; Cor and Peeters 2015; Monteiro 2021; Vispoel et al. 2018) have mentioned it, and a systematic review by Anders en et al.

(2021) pointed out that over half the studies reviewed used either G_String (36 per cent) or urGENOVA (18 per cent). Because G_String has emerged as a standard approach to G theory analysis, and is now sufficiently sophisticated to automatically calculate many of the aspects of the analysis such as coefficients for unbalanced designs that previously involved many manual computations, we have changed the format of this chapter from previous versions that featured a detailed derivation of formulae to a step-by-step approach to using G_String, which will do it all for you . The algebraic derivations have been moved into an appendix (Appendix C) for those with PhDs in mathematics or masochistic tendencies.

Generalizability theory fundamentals

G studies typically have three basic components. The initial analysis of the design is called a *generalizability study or G study* and uses ANOVA methods to compute variance components. These, in turn, are used to compute *generalizability coefficients*, which have a similar form to the classical reliability coefficient of Chapter 8. Then, through the second part of generalizability theory (the Decision or *D study*), we are able to derive G coefficients corresponding to each facet of generalization or combination of facets (a term we will define in the next paragraph) such as inter-rater, test –retest, internal consistency, etc. Finally we can examine various combinations of error sources (e.g. six observers, eight items, three occasions) and see exactly the impact of changing the number of observations on the overall reliability, with a goal to optimally distribute observations over the facets to maximize the overall generalizability.

To begin, it is important to define some terms introduced by Cronbach et al. (1972). First of all, fundamental to the ideas of G theory is the abandonment of any pretense of a 'true' score. After all, the 'true' score for every subject in a study will change with every combination of measures, simply as a consequence of random error. In any case, 'true' confounds issues of reliability and validity. Instead, we begin our G theory analysis by an educated guess of all the likely major sources of error—the rater, the item, the occasion, or whatever. These factors—called *facets* in G theory—define a finite *universe* of observations. In turn, the average score across all of these facets is the *universe score*— the conceptual equivalent of the true score in CTT (or at least the closest equivalent we have to the concept of true score). Note that this is not a true score—there is an explicit acknowledgement that different sets of facets will yield different universe scores, and by implication, the universe score is specific to the defined universe. Such is not the case in CTT, which acts as if there is only one true score (although the substitution of 'universe score' somewhat muddies the water, as no one we have met outside of string theorists and science fiction writers can think about multiple universes).

Before we go further, it is important to try to describe the subtle distinction between a G theory *facet* and a *factor* in ANOVA. Most of the time, they appear to be one and the same; however, they differ in where they enter the process.

Factors are related to the ANOVA which is used to derive variance components from the initial data and are used in the conventional ANOVA sense to conceptualize the design and compute variance components. However, at the point where these are used to calculate G coefficients, Cronbach switches the nomenclature from factor to 'facet'. There are three kinds of facets—the facet of *differentiation*, facets of *generalization*, and facets of *stratification*.

In any measurement situation, there is only one facet of differentiation (also called the object of measurement), usually labelled **p**. This is simply the thing we want to measure, equivalent to 'subjects' in calculating the ICC , as we discussed in Chapter 8. It's a facet of differentiation because, at the end of the day, the G coefficient, like the reliability coefficient, is an index of how well the measure can differentiate among individuals. Realize, though, that 'subjects' can refer to humans (e.g. individuals completing a scale), situations (e.g. OSCE stations), things (e.g. types of Scotch, smart phones), health , or professors , and this is a partial list. The act of measurement, theoretically, can be about differentiating anything; what is critical is that the test designer understands what the object of measurement is, which is not always the case, as we have observed over the years.

Every observation of this object of measurement is subject to error, derived from various sources depending on the 'universe of observation' defined by the researcher. These sources are called *facets of generalization*, or G facets, and address the question: 'To what extent can I generalize from a measurement taken under one situation to another with a different level of the facet (or facets) of generalization?'

Facets of generalization are further subdivided into *fixed* and *random*. In the generalizability analysis, we construct different G coefficients to characterize different kinds of generalizations. For example, if we had 3 raters evaluating a group of students with a 5- item scale, then there are 2 factors / facets in the design. If we are interested in generalizing over raters (inter-rater reliability), then 'rater' is the random facet of generalization and item is fixed; if we want to generalize over items (internal consistency), then 'item' is the random facet of generalization and rater is fixed.

Finally, there is one other kind of facet, called a *stratification facet*. Quite frequently, the facet of differentiation, **p**, can be nested in another facet. For example, if we are studying medical students in the first, second, and third years, we may say that Student is nested in Year, or alternatively, Student is stratified by Year. Another example arises when an examination occurs at different sites, or a study is conducted with patients enrolled from multiple centres. Again, Site or Centre is a stratification facet.

G theory is based on three sequential steps. In the first, having identified the important facets, we create a study design that incorporates all of these facets, and then conduct an ANOVA to compute the variance attributed to each facet and to the interactions among facets.

Next, we use the variances computed by the ANOVA to create families of G coefficients, each an extension of the classical reliability coefficient, looking at the proportion of total variance due to the object of measurement, but differing in what is the facet of generalization—the source of error. In the example above we would compute three coefficients. The first would have 'rater' as the random facet of generalization and 'item' fixed, equivalent to inter-rater reliability; and the second, with 'item' random and 'rater' fixed, equivalent to internal consistency. But in contrast to CTT, both coefficients emerge from the same study and so can be directly compared. Further, the coefficient with both rater and item random (an inter-rater internal consistency reliability) has no classical equivalent.

Finally, we can use the estimates of the variance components to examine the effect of changing the number of levels of each facet to optimize the overall test generalizability. That is, suppose we can have 24 observations. Are we better off to have 6 OSCE stations with 2 raters and 2 items; or 3 stations, 4 raters, and 1 item; etc.? G theory, by estimating the various error variances concurrently, enables us to derive an optimum distribution of observations across the various factors.

Every generalizability coefficient has the same form: an intraclass correlation like we encountered in Chapter 8, the ratio of the variance associated with the facet of differentiation, which Brennan (2001) calls τ (tau), to the sum of this variance and the error variance, called δ (delta) if it is a relative error and Δ (Delta) if it is an absolute error. In other words, the numerator contains the signal, τ, and the denominator contains the sum of signal and noise $(\tau + \delta)$ or $(\tau + \Delta)$, so it looks like:

$$G = \frac{\sigma^2(\tau)}{\sigma^2(\tau) + \sigma^2(\delta)}$$

$$= \frac{\tau}{\tau + \delta}$$

when the coefficient uses the relative error; and

$$G = \frac{\sigma^2(\tau)}{\sigma^2(\tau) + \sigma^2(\Delta)}$$

$$= \frac{\tau}{\tau + \Delta}$$

for the absolute coefficient. For reasons known only to Brennan, the relative coefficient is called $E\rho^2$ (Expected rho squared) and the absolute error coefficient is called Φ (phi).

The formula looks like the standard ICC of CTT. However, it is somewhat misleading, as τ contains the facet of differentiation, but may also contain other terms. The fundamental idea is that all variance components associated with facets of generalization may contribute to τ, δ, or Δ depending on the specific choice of G coefficient. Fixed facets, those that will be held constant, go to τ. Conversely, facets that you want to generalize over contribute to δ or Δ. Whether one uses δ or Δ depends on whether a score is to be interpreted relative to other scores, or in an absolute sense.

An example

To clarify some of the terminology, let us take a relatively straightforward example. Imagine a final examination, consisting of three essay questions, each evaluated by two raters. Assume raters are using 9-point scales. These are the two *facets of generalization* in this design—Rater (2 levels) and Essay (3 levels).

Of course, there is one more facet—the *facet of differentiation*, in this case the student. Presumably the goal of the study is to see how well the ratings can distinguish good from bad students : Student is the *facet of differentiation*. So a design with 2 raters and 3 essay questions (and 1 object of measurement—student) is a three facet design.

There could be many more. For example, if the raters used a number of scale items to judge neatness, logical thought, style, knowledge, and so on, then Item may become another facet.

For simplicity, let us stay with just Essay (3 levels) and Rater (2 levels). With these two facets, we can consider the G theory equivalent of inter-rater reliability ('To what extent can I generalize from a rating made by one rater to a second rater on the same question?'), or of internal consistency ('To what extent can I generalize from one essay to another with the same rater?'), and what might be called inter-rater–inter-essay reliability ('To what extent can I generalize from any rating of any essay to any other rating of any other essay by any other rater?').

We have synthesized a data set for our sample problem, also using G_String_L (the L indicates it's the *Legacy* version). The data base looks like Table 9.1 (for some reason, the program calls the first subject 0, not 1).

Concepts in ANOVA

Just as classical reliability is based on a one-way repeated measures ANOVA, the first step in G theory analysis involves a multifactor repeated measures ANOVA. In the present example, there are six repeated observations on each test—three questions × two raters each—so we have a two-way repeated measures design. However, before we proceed, we must delve deeper into some of the complexities of ANOVA.

Table 9.1 Fictitious data for study of essays measuring student performance for Chapter 9, Example 1

Subject	Essay 1		Essay 2		Essay 3	
	R1	R2	R1	R2	R1	R2
0	2	7	7	6	8	6
1	1	5	2	3	6	1
2	1	3	2	3	6	5
3	4	5	3	7	8	7
4	7	9	6	9	9	9
5	8	9	8	9	9	8
6	1	6	2	6	5	4
7	7	7	6	6	7	6
8	3	9	5	4	9	6
9	6	9	5	5	9	8

Crossed and nested designs

To begin with, there are at least two ways we could conduct the study: we could have two raters rate the first question, a different two raters rate the second, and another pair rate the third. Alternatively, we could have the same two raters rate all three questions. In the language of ANOVA, the first example has raters *nested* in questions (each rater occurs at only one level of question), and the second has raters *crossed* with question (each rater occurs at all levels of question). These issues are covered in most statistics books, for example Norman and Streiner (2014).

Nested designs are quite common in education. One example is teacher ratings, where students in each class rate their teacher. Student is nested in groups (in this case, Teacher), and numbers of students will likely vary. Peer assessments of practicing physicians, called '360-degree evaluation' or 'multisource feedback', is another—different peers with different numbers of observations for each physician. Typically these are not the only two facets, since often ratings are on multi-item questionnaires, so the design would be Peer nested in Doctor crossed with Item. Another common variant is the so-called mini-CEX , where each student is observed on a number of occasions by their supervisor(s), and again, typically each student has different supervisors.

The distinctions matter—if rater is nested in question, we cannot very well ask about the interaction of rater and question ('Do different raters rate different questions differently?') since each rater only rates one question. Furthermore, in nested designs the number of levels may differ in each nest—one teacher may be rated by 5 students and another by 50. This introduces complexities in the analysis, as will emerge later.

Conducting the analysis in G_String

Although the common statistical packages such as SPSS and SAS can deal with fairly complex ANOVA designs, their goal remains to compute Mean Squares so that *F* tests and *p*-values can be determined, and they do not generally compute variance components. There are some exceptions; the 'variance components' subprogram for SPSS, for example, does compute them (naturally); however, it is built on a General Linear Model algorithm that is very demanding. We had the experience of attempting to compute a repeated measures design with nesting, about 50 observations, and 1,000 subjects. A pre-test database of 50 subjects executed in about 20 seconds, 100 subjects took 14 *hours*, and the whole analysis was estimated to need 239 GB of memory (and we had about 64 MB).

The second problem for SPSS is that unless you become very familiar with syntax, it is very limited in the kinds of designs it can handle—nested designs, for example, are not possible.

The solution, to *aficionados*, has always been the family of GENOVA programs written by Brennan and Crick (1999), and available as freeware. These programs were originally written for mainframe computers in the 1970s, and are extremely efficient. The problem described above executed in less than 10 seconds. However, they exist only in a DOS (Disk Operating System, in other words, a very old system!) version, requiring the equivalent of control cards as input, so they are very awkward.

G_String, which we mentioned in the introduction, overcomes these problems. The current version, G_String_L, can compute variance components and G coefficients for a wide variety of complex designs. In particular, it can handle multifaceted unbalanced and nested designs, with correct formulae for dealing with the computed variances of averages. It is written in Java and can execute on both Windows and Mac machines. In addition, it has an extensive manual that describes how to compute a number of common, but complex, designs.

G_String_L is available through GitHub (<https://github.com/G-String-Legacy/GS_MV>). The website contains a number of resources—the program itself, a number of manuals and other print resources, discussion forums, etc. If you are contemplating conducting G theory analysis, we strongly suggest you access the website as a useful resource, both for general approaches to G theory studies and for specific details of the G_String software.

Let us return to the example and proceed with the analysis using G_String. For completeness, let us assume that the exam was administered to 10 students, and let us further assume that we are using a completely crossed design.

Step 1: Analysis of Variance

The first step is to run the ANOVA, yielding the variance components. To do this, G_String first requires that your data are in a '.txt' file, which can be exported from Excel. Further, you cannot have a title line; only numerical data are allowed. Finally, G_String does not recognize subscripts or indices; the design is specified to describe what each cell in the entire data base is. This will (hopefully) become obvious as we proceed.

Step 0 (Fig. 9.1) permits you to identify what you wish to do. You can (1) start a new analysis, (2) reload a set of control instructions from a previous analysis—useful if you are conducting repeated analyses—or (3) create a synthetic data set (as we did to create this example).

Step 1 (Fig. 9.2) allows you to enter a description of the analysis. This can be expanded in Step 2 (Fig. 9.3).

In step 3 (Fig. 9.4) you define the facet of differentiation, give it a one-character label, indicate whether it is nested (within stratification facets), and then indicate how many additional facets there are in the design.

In step 4 (Fig. 9.5) you identify and label the additional facets and indicate whether they are crossed or nested. In the present example, Essay and Rater are both crossed, although we will later recycle the study as a nested design.

In step 5 (Fig. 9.6) you provide more information about the structure of the data. In most designs, there is one record for each subject, so the asterisk is placed on S, and the 3×2 observations appear sequentially on the record. However, if S were nested in a stratification facet, for example a study where there were senior and junior students (stratification facet Level (L)), then S would be dragged below L and the asterisk would follow.

In step 6 (Fig. 9.7) there is a list of all the main effects and interactions. In the case of a completely crossed design like this, nothing more needs to be done at this stage. If there were nested facets, you would drag them from the left box to put them under the facet in which they are nested.

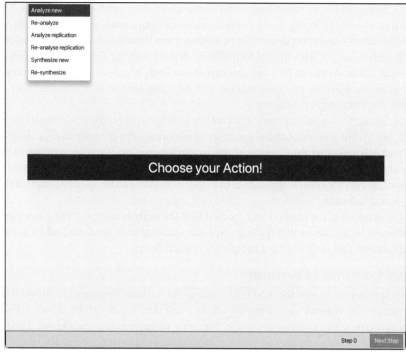

Fig. 9.1 Step 0—Starting the program

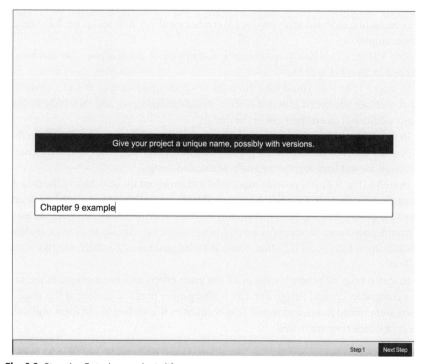

Fig. 9.2 Step 1—Entering project title.

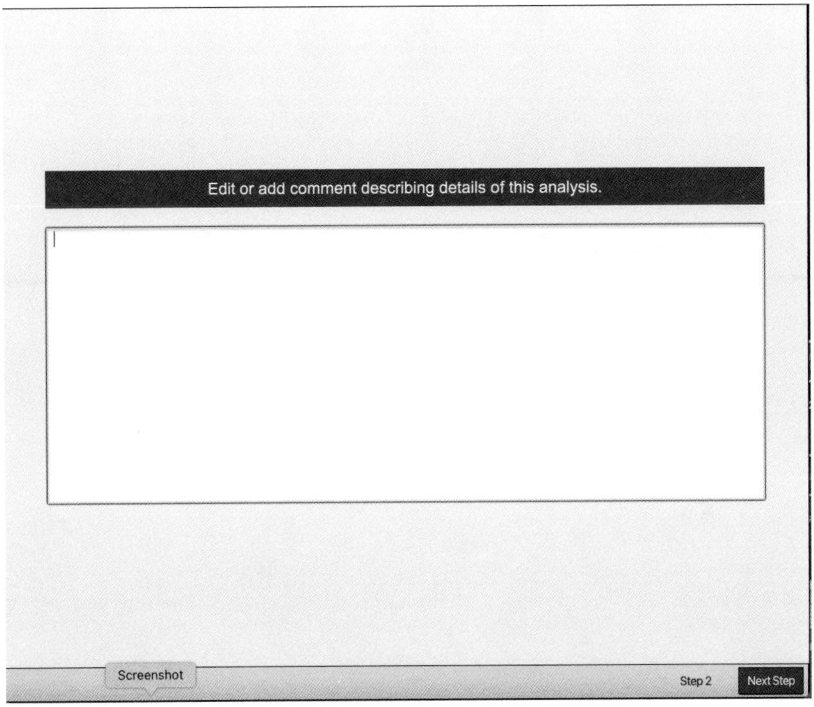

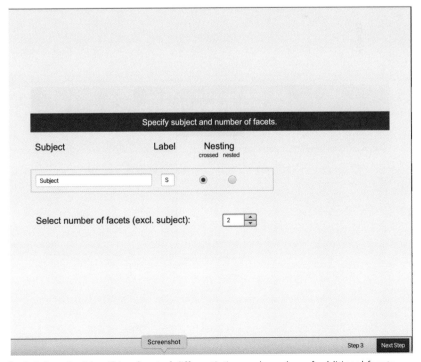

Fig. 9.3 Step 2—Entering optional additional project descriptions.

Fig. 9.4 Step 3—Identifying facet of differentiation and number of additional facets

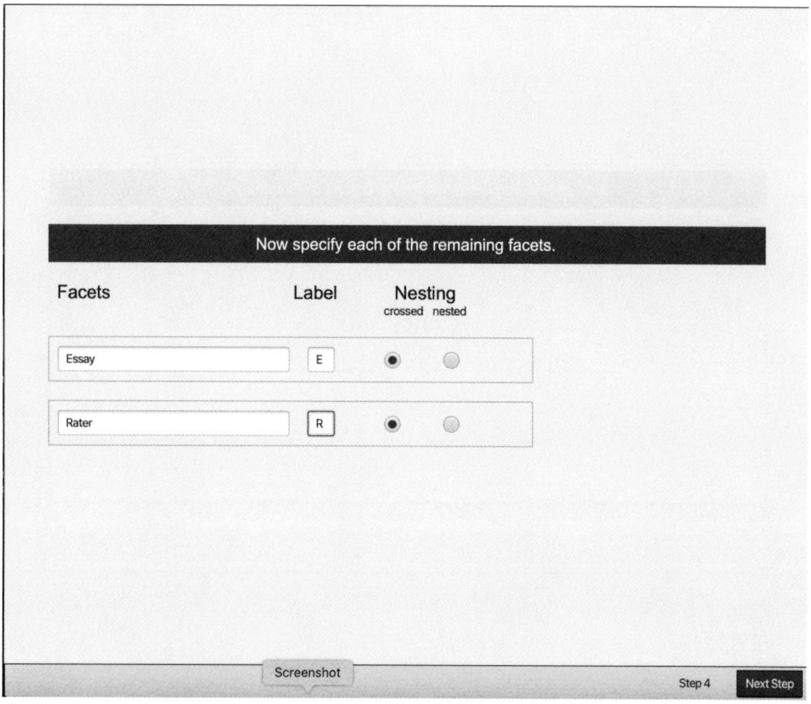

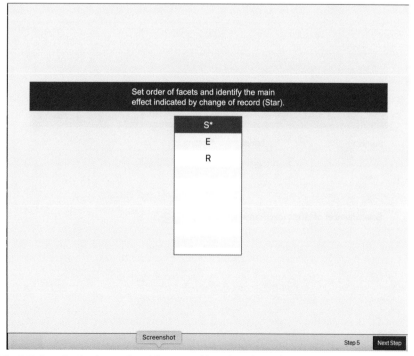

Fig. 9.5 Step 4—Identifying additional facets and characteristics (crossed—nested).

Fig. 9.6 Step 5—Setting order of facets and locating physical record (with asterisk)

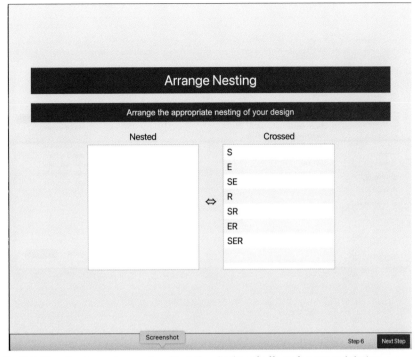

Fig. 9.7 Step 6—Arranging nesting (Part 1) – display of effects for crossed design

In step 7 you specify the location of the data file (Fig. 9.8). The computer retrieves the data file and displays the first 9 records.

You then have the opportunity to skip over leading variables in Step 8. In our example, the first variable (column) is the student ID. By advancing the indicator to '1' you can ignore this (Fig. 9.9).

In step 9 you specify the sample sizes for each facet (10, 3, and 2) (Figs 9.10 –9.12).

In the last screen of Step 9, as shown in Fig 9.13 and 9.14, you can also save the control commands in a retrievable file, so that you can 'Use existing' in Step 0 if you start again.

When the entry of screens 1 –9 complete, G _String prints an output. The first section simply outputs the control language (as used by urGENOVA), then mirrors the data you entered (Table 9.2).

We will now go through the output, one step at a time, beginning with Table 9.2, the first part of the output in Fig. 9.15.

There is then a section that mirrors the input data, except that the grand mean is subtracted from individual values. This is useful to ensure that the data are as you expect them to be.

The next section is the analysis of variance (Table 9.3).

urGENOVA arrives at the variance components by the usual analysis of variance methods, described in statistics books. These include estimates of the three main

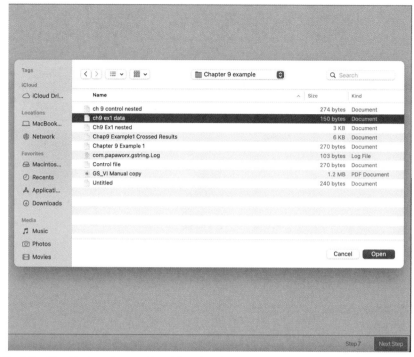

Fig. 9.8 --Step 7—Locating and inputting data base.

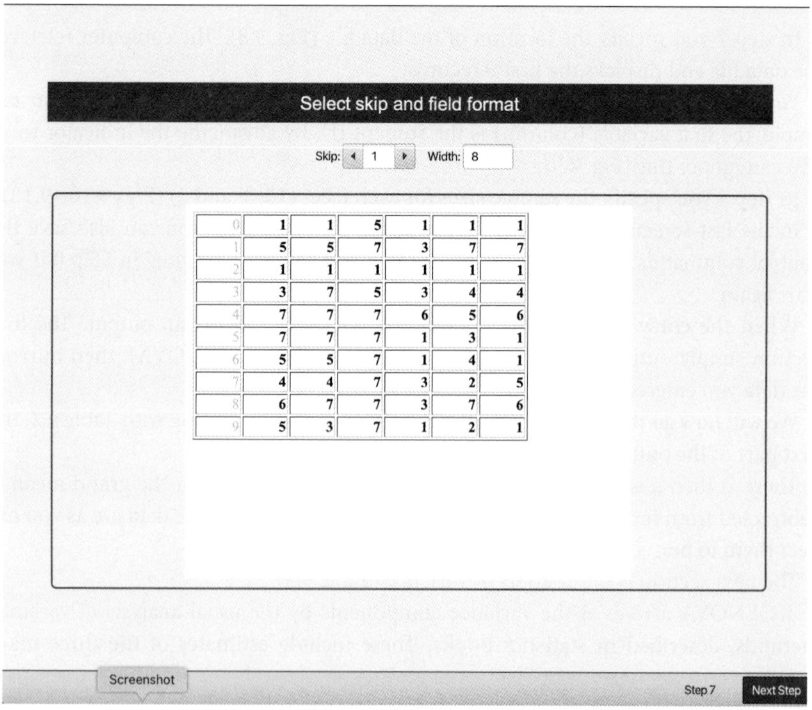

Fig. 9.9 Step 8—Skipping over identifier variables.

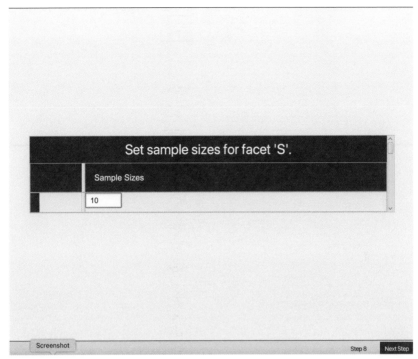

Fig. 9.10 Step 9—Specifying sample sizes for facet.(S)

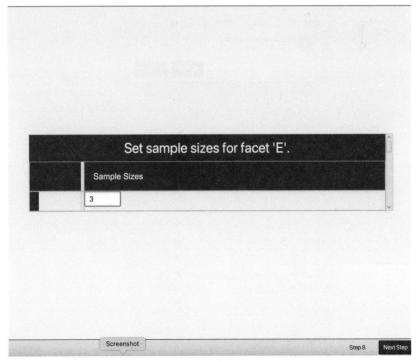

Fig. 9.11 Step 9.—Specifying sample sizes for facet. (E)

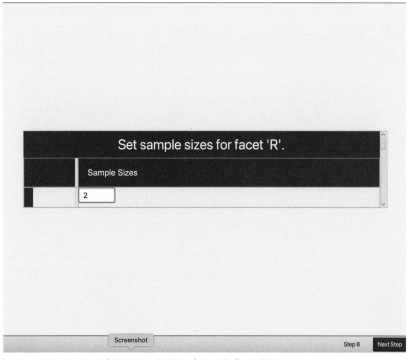

Fig. 9.12 Step 9—Specifying sample sizes for each facet.(R)

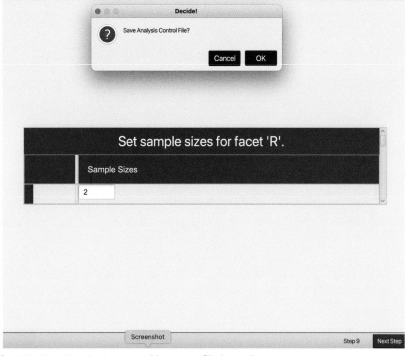

Fig. 9.13 Step 10—Saving control language file (part 1).

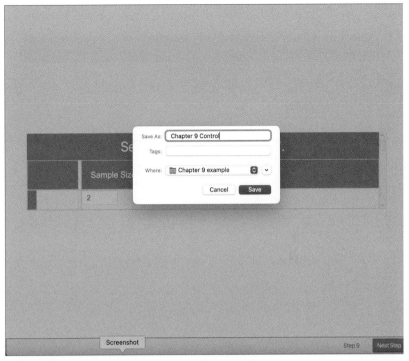

Fig. 9.14 Step 10—Saving control language file (part 2).

Table 9.2 G_String output for Chapter 9, Example 1, Part 1

G study	Chapter 9	Example 1
COMMENT*	Student	(S)
COMMENT*	Essay	(E)
COMMENT*	Rater	(R)
OPTIONS	NREC 5 "*.lis" TIME NOBANNER	
EFFECT	* S	10
EFFECT	E	3
EFFECT	R	2
FORMAT	8 8	
PROCESS	"~data.txt"	

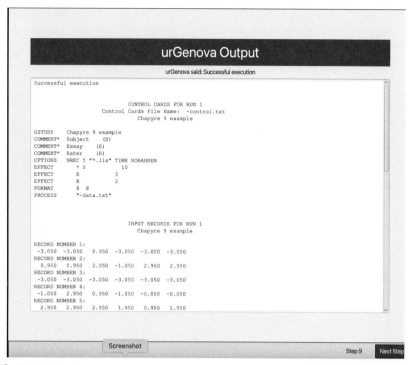

Fig. 9.15 Output.

effects (S, E, and R), three two-way interactions (SE, SR, and ER), and one three-way interaction term, the pure error term, SER.

Note that, in contrast to many statistics programs, this output shows the estimated variance components for each effect and interaction. Note also the omissions; there are no F tests and p-values, nor is there any indication of what lines are effects and what are error terms. There is a good reason for this; G theory is not about testing

Table 9.3 G_String output for Chapter 9, Example 1, Part 2: ANOVA table for RUN 1

Effect	df	T	SS	MS	VC
S	9	165.68333	165.68333	18.40926	2.36296
E	2	12.40000	12.40000	6.20000	−0.93333
R	1	22.81667	22.81667	22.81667	−0.06852
SE	18	225.35000	47.26667	2.62593	0.80000
SR	9	212.18333	23.68333	2.63148	0.53519
ER	2	81.75000	46.53333	23.26667	2.22407
SER	18	336.85000	18.46667	1.02593	1.02593

hypotheses against *Ho*. We use ANOVA to estimate variance components that will then enter into the G coefficients. In fact, in G theory we focus on interactions between facets of generalizability and the facet of differentiation, all of which are viewed as errors in the usual ANOVA, a point we will come back to later.

As you can see, some of the estimated components can come out negative (as in the main effects of E and R above), which is nonsensical for squared quantities. The convention is to set these components to zero for further calculations.

Step 2 : computing overall G coefficient

urGENOVA then goes one step further and uses the variance estimates derived from the G study to determine what the overall generalizability would be, given the number of levels of each facet. That is, it assumes in this case that both Essay and Rater are random facets, and they have 3 and 2 levels respectively. So it asks the question: 'What is the generalizability of a test consisting of 3 essays and 2 raters?'

The relevant output looks like that shown in Box 9.1.

That is to say, for the overall G coefficient, the variances for each main effect and interaction are summed to yield an overall τ, δ, and Δ. For the overall test generalizability, τ contains only the facet of differentiation, S; δ contains all the interactions of other facets with S; and Δ contains these and the main effects of the facets of generalization, E and R.

$$\sigma^2(\tau) = 2.3630$$

$$\sigma^2(\delta) = 0.7052$$

$$\sigma^2(\Delta) = 1.0759$$

Finally, it computes the absolute and relative G coefficients (Box 9.2).

Box 9.1 G_String output for Chapter 9, Example, 1 Part 3

Results G study.

Facet E, random; level = 3.0.

Facet R, random; level = 2.0.

Variance component 'S' (d) is 2.36296; denominator is 1.00; τ only

Variance component 'E' (g) is –0.93333; denominator is 3.00; Δ only

Variance component 'R' (g) is –0.06852; denominator is 2.00; Δ only

Variance component 'SE' (dg) is 0.8; denominator is 1.00 × 3.00; both δ and Δ

Variance component 'SR' (dg) is 0.53519; denominator is 1.00 × 2.00; both δ and Δ

Variance component 'ER' (gg) is 2.22407; denominator is 3.00 × 2.00; Δ only

Variance component 'SER' (dgg) is 1.02593; denominator is 1.00 × 3.00 × 2.00; both δ and Δ

Box 9.2 G_String output for Chapter 9, Example 1, Part 4

GENERALIZABILITY COEFFICIENTS:

Consistency = 0.91

$\qquad E\rho^2 = 0.77$

$\qquad\quad \Phi = 0.69$

Step 3: more G coefficients

However, the analysis does not finish there. G theory can also calculate separate coefficients corresponding to generalizing across Raters and generalizing across Essays—inter-rater reliability, and, if you will, inter-essay reliability (analogous to internal consistency, which generalizes across items on the test).

That is, we can compute coefficients where the error derives from only Raters (inter-rater reliability) or from different Essays (inter-essay reliability). To express these different coefficients, we have to introduce a bit more terminology. If we are examining inter-rater reliability, then we are treating raters as *random* and holding Essays as *fixed*. Conversely, if we want to look at generalization across Essays, then Essay will be random and Rater will be fixed. We deal with this proliferation of possibilities by using the general form of the equation we wrote earlier (see 'Generalizability theory fundamentals'):

$$G = \frac{\sigma^2(\tau)}{\sigma^2(\tau) + \sigma^2(\delta)}$$

when the coefficient uses the relative error; and

$$G = \frac{\sigma^2(\tau)}{\sigma^2(\tau) + \sigma^2(\Delta)}$$

for the absolute coefficient.

However, in contrast to the overall G coefficient computed earlier the τ, δ, and Δ variances change depending on the question. Each is the sum of individual variance components: τ contains the variance due to the facet of differentiation, S, and all variances and interactions associated with only fixed facets; δ contains any variance component with any random facet in it (including interactions between random and fixed facets); and Δ contains all the terms in δ as well as any main effects associated with the random facets.

If we want to look at inter-rater reliability, Rater is a random facet and Essay is a fixed facet. So if we just look at relative error, δ contains variance due to Subject × Rater and the Subject × Rater × Essay interaction (the error term). τ contains the variance due to Subjects and the Subject × Essay term. If we look at the absolute error coefficient, it is the same except that Δ also contains the main effect of Rater.

To accomplish these changes, in Screen 10, we indicate that Essay is fixed, and set sample size for both Essay and Rater to 1. G _String output looks like that shown in Box 9.3.

To arrive at inter-essay generalizability, we set Essay random and Rater fixed and rerun it.

Generalizability of an average

There is one further extension. The coefficients up to now reflect the reliability of a single rating. But we can equally well examine the reliability of the combined score of all three questions with one rater or of both raters on each question. To compute these, we set the sample size of the fixed facet to 3 (for G across Essay) or 2 (for G across Rater). For three essays, the output looks like that shown in Box 9.4.

This then is what G studies look like. The primary goal is to sample across all relevant facets in the measurement situation in order to derive variance estimates. Second, these estimates can be used to determine G coefficients for generalization across the various facets in the design.

Box 9.3 G_String output for Chapter 9, Example 1, Part 5

Facet E, fixed; level = 1.0.

Facet R, random; level = 1.0.

Variance component 'S' (d) is 2.36296; denominator is 1.00; τ only

Variance component 'E' (f) is –0.93333; denominator is 1.00; null

Variance component 'R' (g) is –0.06852; denominator is 1.00; Δ only

Variance component 'SE' (df) is 0.8; denominator is 1.00 × 1.00; τ only

Variance component 'SR' (dg) is 0.53519; denominator is 1.00 × 1.00; both δ and Δ

Variance component 'ER' (fg) is 2.22407; denominator is 1.00 × 1.00; Δ only

Variance component 'SER' (dfg) is 1.02593; denominator is 1.00 × 1.00 × 1.00; both δ and Δ

$\sigma^2(\tau) = 3.163$

$\sigma^2(\delta) = 1.561$

$\sigma^2(\Delta) = 3.785$

GENERALIZABILITY COEFFICIENTS:

Consistency = 0.87

$E\rho^2 = 0.67$

$\Phi = 0.46$

Box 9.4 G_String output for Chapter 9, Example 1, Part 6

Facet E, fixed; level = 1.0.

Facet R, random; level = 1.0.

Variance component 'S' (d) is 2.36296; denominator is 1.00; τ only

Variance component 'E' (f) is –0.93333; denominator is 3.00; null

Variance component 'R' (g) is –0.06852; denominator is 1.00; Δ only

Variance component 'SE' (df) is 0.8; denominator is 1.00 × 3.00; τ only

Variance component 'SR' (dg) is 0.53519; denominator is 1.00 × 1.00; both δ and Δ

Variance component 'ER' (fg) is 2.22407; denominator is 1.00 × 3.00; Δ only

Variance component 'SER' (dfg) is 1.02593; denominator is 1.00 × 3.00 × 1.00; both δ and Δ

$\sigma^2(\tau) = 2.629$

$\sigma^2(\delta) = 0.877$

$\sigma^2(\Delta) = 1.618$

GENERALIZABILITY COEFFICIENTS:

Consistency = 0.92

$E\rho^2 = 0.75$

$\Phi = 0.62$

The power of the G study derives from the ability to estimate concurrently the relative amount of error contributed by various sources so that we can now, by judicious combinations, maximize the reliability for a given number of measurements. That is the purview of the D study.

   NOTE: All of the results shown are accessed by clicking on 'File' 'Save Results' in the top left corner of Screen 9.

Equivalent analysis for a nested design

What if the design were nested? Instead of having every question marked by the same two raters, we use experts in the various knowledge domains, so Essay 1 is marked by Raters 1 and 2, Essay 2 by Raters 3 and 4, and Essay 3 by Raters 5 and 6.

   The way to specify this in G_String_L occurs in Step 6. As we indicated, many of the interactions drop out in nested designs. In this case, to indicate that R is nested in E, we drag R from the left column to directly under E in the right column (R is nested in E) and the screen then changes to indicate the nesting.

   Now, the ANOVA looks a bit different (see Table 9.4), since some of the interactions are missing. When Rater is nested in Essay, we cannot have a Rater × Essay interaction. Instead, the R × E interaction and the R main effect all get absorbed into a single term, the R:E interaction (R nested in E). Similarly the error term, instead of S×R×E, now becomes S×R:E.

Table 9.4 G_String output for Chapter 9, Example 2, Part 1: ANOVA table for RUN 1; Chapter 9, Example 1 nested

Effect	df	T	SS	MS	VC
S	9	165.68333	165.68333	18.40926	2.63056
E	2	12.40000	12.40000	6.20000	–0.89907
R:E	3	81.75000	69.35000	23.11667	2.15556
sE	18	225.35000	47.26667	2.62593	0.53241
sR:E	27	336.85000	42.15000	1.56111	1.56111

Not surprisingly, exactly the same principles for creating G coefficients apply when one or more factors are nested. The generalizability of the total score across all Raters and Essays is shown in Box 9.5.

We could then carry on as before, calculating G coefficient for generalizing across Raters and across Essays. The formulae are completely analogous, except that where before we had *R* and *RS* terms, we now have *R:S*, and where we had *SRE* before, we now have *SR:E*.

Box 9.5 G_String output for Chapter 9, Example 2, Part 2

Results G study

Facet E, random; level = 3.0.

Facet R, random; level = 2.0.

Variance component 'S' (d) is 2.63056; denominator is 1.00; τ only

Variance component 'E' (g) is –0.89907; denominator is 3.00; Δ only

Variance component 'R:E' (g:g) is 2.15556; denominator is 2.00 × 3.00; Δ only

Variance component 'SE' (dg) is 0.53241; denominator is 1.00 × 3.00; both δ and Δ

Variance component 'SR:E' (dg:g) is 1.56111; denominator is 1.00 × 2.00 × 3.00; both δ and Δ

$\sigma^2(\tau) = 2.6306$

$\sigma^2(\delta) = 0.4377$

$\sigma^2(\Delta) = 0.796$

GENERALIZABILITY COEFFICIENTS:

Consistency = 0.92

$E\rho^2 = 0.86$

$\Phi = 0.77$

Generalizability in unbalanced nested designs

The rules for calculating G coefficients for nested designs, when they are unbalanced, are very similar to those for crossed designs, but regrettably, add further complexity to the calculation of G coefficients. Conceptually it is the same as in the section 'Generalizability of an average': simply divide each error variance by the number of observations. The problem arises in determining the number of observations. For some obscure reason, we must use the *harmonic mean*, the inverse of the average of the inverses (yes, you read that correctly). It looks like this:

$$\tilde{n} = \frac{p}{\sum_{p} \dfrac{1}{n_p}}$$

Of course, it is also possible to have unbalanced facets nested in other nested unbalanced facets. For example, we might be attempting to get an overall rating of various graduate programmes, but one programme has 5 courses with varying numbers of students and another has 12 courses. There are equivalent formulae in this circumstance for both facets. However, G_String can handle all these complications, so it is not necessary to know the fine print.

Step 4: from G study to D study

While the section 'Generalizability in unbalanced nested designs' computed the G coefficient for the average of the ratings in the original design, with G theory we have much more flexibility. We can calculate what the G coefficient would be for any combination of different numbers of ratings.

This is the way it works. Since there are different error terms related to different sources of error variance, we can contemplate using different numbers of observations for each; indeed, different numbers is the usual case. Further, it makes good statistical sense to consider different numbers associated with each error term—if we have a finite number of total observations, we would want to average the large sources of error over many observations and the small sources of error over relatively few observations.

A simple extension of these ideas gets us to the D study, where we consider systematically varying the numbers of observations in each facet, using the variance components calculated in the G study, in order to determine what combination of numbers yields the highest generalizability. Herein lies one of the real strengths of G theory : the potential to make significant gains in reliability within a fixed number of total observations, by optimally distributing the numbers of observations over various sources of error.

The difference between G theory and CTT is that in G theory we can simultaneously consider multiple facets with different numbers of levels of each. Therefore, we can work out, more or less by trial and error, what combination of different numbers of each facet optimizes the overall reliability. In the present example, we might begin with the assumption that we can afford a total of 48 observations. That could be 48 essays marked by 1 rater, 24 essays and 2 raters, 16 and 3, 12 and 4, 6 and 8, 4 and 12, 3 and 16, or 1 and 48 . Error due to main effects and interactions will be divided by the number

Table 9.5 G coefficients for various combinations
of sample sizes[a]

Number of raters	Number of essays	Generalizability
48	1	0.913
24	2	0.944
16	3	0.952
12	4	0.954
8	6	0.950
6	8	0.944
4	12	0.929
2	24	0.880
1	48	0.754

[a] This example is not representative and is not based on previous data.
Generally, questions would contribute considerably more error variance
than raters.

of levels of the terms in the variance component. So, for example, if we were considering four raters and three essays, we would divide any term with Rater by 4, any term with Essay by 3, and any term with both by 12. If we distribute the numbers across the error terms in such a way that the larger sources of error are divided by more levels, the end result will be to minimize error and therefore maximize reliability with a given total number of observations.

As we can see in Table 9.5, the overall generalizability peaks at a choice of 12 raters and 4 essays. Reducing the number of essays to 1 (and increasing the number of raters to 48) incurs a relatively small penalty; however, reducing raters to 1 results in a severe loss of generalizability (all with the same total number of observations).

ANOVA for statisticians and ANOVA for psychometricians

As we have seen in the previous simple example, there are three steps in a G study. The first is a repeated measures ANOVA, where every facet in the design is a repeated factor in the ANOVA design. We let the computer do all the work and produce the ANOVA table. This is standard statistical stuff, leading one colleague to dismiss G theory with a haughty hand wave as, 'It's all just applied Analysis of Variance!' Six months later, he was still working out how to apply ANOVA to a G theory problem. The exchange reveals that there are two big differences between the way the G theorist looks at the ANOVA table and how the statistician views it.

First, for the statistician, the goal is to determine what effects (main effects or interactions) are statistically significant. So, the ANOVA proceeds logically from Sums of Squares to Mean Squares to F tests and p-values. G theorists care not at all about the F-ratios or p-values. Instead, we want to use the Mean Squares to estimate variance components. There are some rules to do this, as we've discussed. Second, when statisticians do ANOVA, by and large, they are looking for one or more Treatment effects. Any variation between subjects is viewed as noise, since, if different subjects have different responses, this will make it harder to detect an overall effect of the treatment. As it turns out, corresponding to every effect and interaction in the design, there is a Subject × Effect term listed right underneath it in the ANOVA table. But it is not called that; it is simply labelled Error, and it is up to the researcher to figure out what error belongs to what. Why so sloppy? Because to experimenters, all variation resulting from differences between subjects *is* error. In their ideal world, all subjects in the study would be genetically identical and respond identically to the treatment. But to psychometricians, whose goal is to find measures that differentiate between subjects (i.e. are reliable), variation between subjects is the Holy Grail. The psychometrician's signal is the experimenter's noise—a paradox first noted by Cronbach (1957).

This has practical, as well as conceptual consequences. If you are trying to use a standard statistical package such as SPSS for the analysis, you are going to have a devil of a time figuring out what error is what. The simple rule is that the error term directly underneath any main effect or interaction is the 'Subject X' term. So, the SPSS output for the example in Table 9.3 will list an R × E term, and underneath it, a term labelled 'Error'. This will be the S × R × E term.

Confidence intervals for G coefficients

When we calculated reliability coefficients in Chapter 8, we were able to estimate the confidence interval for the coefficient through application of the Fisher z' transformation. In theory at least, one could do a similar, although even more complex, procedure to calculate confidence intervals (or equivalently, standard errors) for G coefficients. However, such calculations must remain a theoretical possibility for most situations. By the same token, there is no defensible way to estimate required sample sizes. We can only suggest that the sample size estimation procedures used in Chapter 8 be used as a rough rule of thumb for computing sample size in G studies.

Uses and abuses of G theory

While G theory represents a major advance over traditional reliability analyses, there are some situations where it is tempting to conduct a G analysis, and it appears that the data are conducive to G theory, but in fact G theory is not appropriate.

G studies and validity

There are many circumstances where concurrent validation is approached by administering multiple measures to a group of subjects, and then examining correlations among the measures. Often this is done on multiple occasions. As one example, numerous studies of health-related quality of life end up comparing a disease-specific measure like the Asthma Quality of Life Questionnaire (AQLQ) with a general questionnaire such as the Sickness Impact Profile (SIP; Juniper et al. 1993). While it would seem perfectly reasonable to ask a G theory question like 'To what extent can I generalize from scores on the AQLQ to scores on the SIP?', it isn't. The problem is that the two scores have completely different means and standard deviations. Just as the standard ICC is based on the assumption of hypothetically equal means and standard deviations, so is the G coefficient. The correct approach is simply Pearson correlations, or more sophisticated methods like Structural Equation Modelling (again, see Norman and Streiner (2014) for a description).

Information from subanalysis

Occasionally, the ability to average over a number of facets, and, for example, declare that the 'average inter-rater reliability is 0.86', can obscure important information. For example, a study might want to examine the ability of medical students at various levels to read chest X-rays. A study design might include three second-year students, three final-year students, and three radiologists , perhaps with each reading 20 films. An obvious G study is a three-facet design with Film as the facet of differentiation, and Educational Level and Rater within Level as the other two facets. We could compute an inter-rater reliability with Level as a fixed facet, an inter-level reliability with Rater fixed, and an overall reliability. However, this is not really addressing the questions, which are: (1) does inter-rater reliability improve with education, and (2) do raters look more like experts as they get more education? To address these, we really should parse out the analyses and first examine inter-rater reliability separately for each level, to address the first question , and then examine generalizability from Year 2 to expert and separately from Year 4 to expert.

There is one additional observation from this study design. Typically, judgements of radiographs are of the form 'Normal' or 'Abnormal'—0 or 1. It may seem inappropriate to use G theory with a dichotomous outcome, and we should opt for a kappa coefficient. However, as we indicated in Chapter 8, the intraclass correlation yields the same answer as kappa, and is able to deal with multiple raters. Similarly, since all G coefficients are of the form of intraclass correlations, they can be used on dichotomous data and interpreted as if they were kappa coefficients, with much greater flexibility than the kappa. Of course, the strong admonition to avoid dichotomizing continuous data remains true, even though the analysis can handle such data.

Summary

G theory represents a significant advance over traditional approaches to reliability. The strength of the approach lies in its ability to simultaneously consider multiple sources of error variance, which permits rational approaches to optimizing reliability. The major limitation is the difficulty in estimation of confidence intervals for variance components in all but the simplest designs.

Further reading

Brennan, R.L. (2001). *Generalizability theory*. Springer , New York.

Swaminathan, H. (2014). Generalizability theory: A practical guide to study design, implementation, and interpretation. *Journal of School Psychology*, **52**, 13–35.

References

Andersen, S.A.W., Nayahangan, L.J., Park, Y.S., and Konge, L. (2021). Use of generalizability theory for exploring reliability of and sources of variance in assessment of technical skills: A systematic review and meta-analysis. *Academic Medicine*, **96**, 1609–19.

Bloch, R. and Norman, G. (2012). Generalizability theory for the perplexed: A practical introduction and guide: AMEE Guide No. 68. *Medical Teacher*, **34**, 960–92.

Boodoo, G.M. and O'Sullivan, P. (1982). Obtaining generalizability coefficients for clinical evaluations. *Evaluation and the Health Professions*, **5**, 345–58.

Brennan, R.L. (2001). *Generalizability theory*. Springer , New York.

Brennan, R.L. and Crick, J. (1999). *Manual for urGENOVA (Version 1.4)*. Iowa Testing Programs Occasional Paper No. 46. University of Iowa Press, Iowa City, IA.

Cor, M.K. and Peeters, M.J. (2015). Using generalizability theory for reliable learning assessments in pharmacy education. *Currents in Pharmacy Teaching and Learning*, 7, 332–41.

Cronbach, L.J. (1957). The two disciplines of scientific psychology. *American Psychologist*, **12**, 671–84.

Cronbach, L.J., Gleser, G.C., Nanda, H., and Rajaratnam, N. (1972). *The dependability of behavioral measurements: Theory of generalizability for scores and profiles*. Wiley, New York.

Eva, K.W., Neville, A.J., and Norman, G.R. (1998). Exploring the etiology of content specificity: Factors influencing analogic transfer and problem solving. *Academic Medicine*, **73**, S1– 5.

Evans, W.J., Cayten, C.G., and Green, P.A. (1981). Determining the generalizability of rating scales in clinical settings. *Medical Care*, **19**, 1211–19.

Juniper, E.F., Guyatt, G.H., Ferrie, P.J., and Griffith, L.E. (1993). Measuring quality of life in asthma. *American Review of Respiratory Disease*, **147**, 832–8.

Monteiro, S., Sullivan, G.M., and Chan, T.M. (2019). Generalizability theory made simple(r): An introductory primer to G-studies. *Journal of Graduate Medical Education*, **11**, 365–70.

Norman, G. (2010). Likert scales, levels of measurement and the "laws" of statistics. *Advances in Health Sciences Education*, **15**, 625–32.

Norman, G.R. and Streiner, D.L. (2014). *Biostatistics: The bare essentials* (4th edn). PMPH USA, Shelton, CT.

Park, Y.S., Riddle, J., and Tekian, A. (2014). Validity evidence of resident competency ratings and the identification of problem residents. *Medical Education*, **48**, 614–22.

Prion, S.K., Gilbert, G.E., and Haerling, K.A. (2016). Generalizability theory: An introduction with application to simulation evaluation. *Clinical Simulation in Nursing*, **12**, 546–54.

Shavelson, R.J., Webb, N.M., and Rowley, G.L. (1989). Generalizability theory. *American Psychologist*, **44**, 922–32.

Streiner, D.L. (2003). Starting at the beginning: An introduction to coefficient alpha and internal consistency. *Journal of Personality Assessment*, **80**, 99–103.

Torrance, G.W. (1976). Social preferences for health states: An empirical evaluation of three measurement techniques. *Socio-Economic Planning Science*, **10**, 129–36.

Van der Vleuten, C.P.M. and Swanson D.B. (1990). Assessment of clinical skills with standardized patients: The state of the art. *Teaching and Learning in Medicine*, **2**, 58–76.

Vispoel, W.P., Morris, C.A., and Kilinc, M. (2018). Applications of generalizability theory and their relations to classical test theory and structural equation modeling. *Psychological Methods*, **23**, 53–67.

Chapter 10

Validity

Introduction to validity

In Chapters 8 and 9, we examined various aspects of reliability: that is, how reproducible the results of a scale are under different conditions. This is a necessary step in establishing the usefulness of a measure, but it is not sufficient. The next step is to determine if we can draw accurate conclusions about the presence and degree of the attribute for an individual: that is, the scale's *validity*. To illustrate the difference, imagine that we are trying to develop a new index to measure the degree of headache pain. We find that patients get the same score when they are tested on two different occasions, that different interviewers get similar results when assessing the same patient, and so on; in other words, the index is reliable. However, we still have no proof that differences in the total score reflect the degree of headache pain: the scale may be measuring pain from other sources; or it may be tapping factors entirely unrelated to pain, such as depression or the tendency to complain of bodily ailments. In this chapter, we will examine how to determine if we can draw valid conclusions from the scale.

Why assess validity?

The question that immediately arises is why we have to establish validity in the first place. After all, the health care fields are replete with measures that have never been 'validated' through any laborious testing process. Despite this, no one questions the usefulness of taking a patient's temperature to detect the presence of fever, or of keeping track of the height and weight of an infant to check growth, or getting thyroid-stimulating hormone levels on people with suspected thyroid problems. Why, then, is there a multitude of articles addressing the problems of trying to test for validity? There are two answers to this question: the nature of *what* is being measured and the *relationship* of that variable to its purported cause.

Many variables measured in the health sciences are physical quantities, such as height, serum cholesterol level, or bicarbonate. As such, they are readily observable, either directly or with the correct instruments. Irrespective of who manufactured the thermometer, different nurses will get the same reading, within the limits of reliability discussed in Chapters 8 and 9. Moreover, there is little question that what is being measured is temperature; no one would state that the height of the mercury in the tube is really due to something else, like blood pressure or pH level.

The situation is different when we turn to variables like 'range of motion', 'quality of life', or 'responsibility as a physician'. As we discuss later in this chapter when we look at construct validation, the measurements of these factors are dependent upon their definitions, which may vary from one person to another and the way they are measured. For example, some theorists hold that 'social support' can be assessed by counting the number of people a person has contact with during a fixed period of time. Other theories state that the person's perceptions of who is available in times of need are more important; while yet another school of thought is that the reciprocity of the helping relationship is crucial. Since social support is not something which can be observed and measured directly, various questionnaires have been developed to assess it, each reflecting a different underlying theory. Needless to say, each instrument yields a somewhat different result, raising the question of which, if any, gives the 'correct' answer.

The second reason why validity testing is required in some areas but not others depends on the relationship between the observation and what it reflects. Based on years of observation or our knowledge of how the body works, the validity of a test may be self-evident. For instance, since the kidneys regulate the level of creatinine in the body, it makes sense to use serum creatinine to determine the presence of renal disease. On the other hand, we do not know ahead of time whether a physiotherapist's evaluations of patients' level of functioning bear any relationship to their actual performance once they are discharged from hospital. Similarly, we may hypothesize that students who have spent time doing volunteer work for service agencies will make better physicians or nurses. However, since our knowledge of the determinants of human behaviour is far from perfect, this prediction will have to be validated (tested) against actual performance.

Reliability and validity

To begin with, let's consider the relationship between reliability and validity. We already discussed that the two are related, but separate, concepts. But how are they related? Reliability places an upper limit on validity so that the higher the reliability, the higher the maximum possible validity. More formally:

$$Validity_{max} = \sqrt{\left(Reliability_{NewTest}\right)\left(Reliability_{Criterion}\right)},$$

so that if the reliability of the new test is 0.80 and that of the criterion with which we are comparing it is 0.90, the validity of the new test cannot exceed:

$$\sqrt{(0.80)(0.90)} = 0.85.$$

We can also see how the different types of error—random and systematic (bias)—affect both. The traditional way of expressing the variance of observed scores is

$$\sigma^2_{Observerd} = \sigma^2_{True} + \sigma^2_{Error}.$$

That is, as we explained in Chapter 8, the total, or observed, variance of scores is composed of the variance of the true scores (which we never see) plus error variance, which can increase or decrease the true score. Judd et al. (1991) expanded this to read as follows:

$$\sigma^2_{Observed} = \sigma^2_{CI} + \sigma^2_{SE} + \sigma^2_{RE}$$

where *CI* indicates the Construct of Interest, *SE* the Systematic Error, and *RE* the Random Error; and:

$$\sigma^2_{CI} + \sigma^2_{SE} = \sigma^2_{True}.$$

Using this formulation :

$$Reliability = \frac{\sigma^2_{CI} + \sigma^2_{SE}}{\sigma^2_{Observed}}$$

and

$$Validity = \frac{\sigma^2_{CI}}{\sigma^2_{Observed}}.$$

From this, we can see that random error affects both reliability and validity (since the larger the random error is, the smaller the ratio between the numerators and denominators), whereas systematic error affects only the validity of a scale.

Note that in this formulation, systematic error has a somewhat different meaning than we discussed in Chapter 8. There it referred to a bias between raters; whereas here it is a systematic difference between the observation and the construct of interest.

This is why the traditional index of reliability—Pearson's *r*—is 'blind' to systematic differences between raters or time (although, as we discussed in Chapter 8, the intraclass correlation can take this into account).

A history of the 'types' of validity

Prior to the 1950s, the assessment of validity was pretty much restricted to answering the question of how well the scores on a test agree with performance on a task it was meant to predict: what today we would call *criterion validity* (Kane 2001). This was all very well and good in areas where a suitable criterion exists, such as determining whether a university admission test predicts whether or not a person will graduate 4 years hence. However, in many areas, there is no such objective criterion. For example, if one wanted to know a more subtle aspect of a person's behaviour, such as how well a person will do on the job, then the test of validity is how well a placement test predicts the evaluation by a supervisor. But, then the issue arises regarding the validity of the supervisor's ratings, which then must be validated against some other 'soft' criterion, leading to an infinite regress of criterion validational studies (Kane 2001).

It was recognized, though, that some tests were 'intrinsically valid' (Ebel 1961), such as judging how well a person can play a musical instrument or in performance in athletics such as gymnastics (although scandals regarding evaluations of performance during the Olympics can raise legitimate doubts about such an assertion). In the area of achievement testing, this led to examining the content of the items of the test, to ensure that they adequately sampled the subject being evaluated (e.g. knowledge of biochemistry): what we now call *content validity*. The assumption was that if all aspects of the content were included, and there were no items that were irrelevant, then the test would be intrinsically valid, in that it assessed whether or not the person had mastered the course content.

What was missing, though, was a way to assess the usefulness of scales that were more widely used in clinical psychology to evaluate areas such as attitudes, beliefs, and feelings, and pathological states like depression, anxiety, and schizophrenia. In these domains, there is no objective criterion that can be used; and content validity is insufficient, because it does not provide evidence 'in support of inferences to be made from test scores' (Messick 1989, p. 17). To address these concerns, two of the leading theoreticians in measurement theory, Lee J. Cronbach and Paul E. Meehl (1955), introduced what is known as *construct validity*: a framework of hypothesis testing based on the knowledge of the underlying construct (e.g. anxiety or depression). Tests would be validated by devising hypotheses such as 'Because anxious people differ from non-anxious people in carrying out complex tasks, then those who score high on this new test of anxiety should perform differently from those who score low'. If the theory is correct *and if the test is valid*, then the study should come out in the way that was predicted. Because there are an unlimited number of hypotheses that can be derived from the theory, construct validity would be a continual, almost never-ending task of seeing how the scale performs in a variety of situations.

This led to the 'trinitarian' point of view (Landy 1986) adopted by all textbooks on measurement theory and test construction of the time: validity can be divided into the 'three Cs' of *content* validity, *criterion* validity, and *construct* validity. These were seen as three relatively separate attributes of a measure, which had to be independently established. Furthermore, because construct validity can be evaluated in so many different ways, it became subdivided into an ever-increasing number of subtypes, such as convergent validity, discriminant validity, trait validity, and so forth (see, for example, Messick 1980). Much time was spent (or wasted, some would argue) in many classes, debating whether a particular study was an example of criterion validity or convergent validity.

Just when it appeared that there would be as many types of construct validity as construct validators, two trends emerged that reversed the process. The first was a major conceptual shift regarding what was being validated. Until the late 1960s, validity was seen as demonstrating the psychometric properties of the *scale* and was often defined as 'Is the test measuring what I think it is?' (e.g. Cattell 1946; Kelly 1927). Led by Cronbach (1971), though, the focus changed to emphasize the characteristics of the *people* who were being assessed and the scores they achieved. As Landy (1986) put it, 'Validation processes are not so much directed toward the integrity of tests as they are directed toward the inferences that can be made about the attributes of people who have produced those test scores' (p. 1186). In other words, validating a scale is really a process whereby we determine the degree of confidence we can place on the inferences we make about people based on their scores from that scale.

As we shall see later in this chapter, this is more than simply a semantic nicety. Rather, it completely changes the conceptualization of what it is that we do when we run a validation study, and what we can say about the results. In brief, it means that we can never say, 'This scale is valid', because it is not the scale that is being validated. The most that we can conclude regarding the results of any one particular study is, 'We have shown the scale to be valid *with this group of people and in this context*'. It further means that if we use the scale with a different population of people (e.g. those with a different level of education or from a different ethnic background) or in different circumstances (e.g. being evaluated for the courts as opposed to being in a study), the results from the original validational study may not apply, and further validation (more research) is necessary.

It follows from this that any conclusions about validity are not dichotomous (i.e. valid versus invalid) but rather exist on a continuum (Zumbo 2009). It also means that these evaluations involve a synthesis of evidence from many sources, some of which may be conflicting. Thus, judgement is required from the person assessing a scale, involving determining how relevant each study is for the intended inference, how well or poorly the study was done, and how favourable or unfavourable the results were. It is quite possible, then, for two people, looking at the same collection of studies, to arrive at different conclusions, because their values and the intended uses of the scale may vary (Cizek 2012). Cizek summarizes it well when he says that 'validation efforts are integrative, subjective, and can be based on different sources of evidence such as theory, logical argument, and empirical evidence' (p. 36).

The second trend, spearheaded by Messick (1975, 1980) and others, reconceptualized construct validity to encompass all forms of validity testing (and in fact, many aspects of reliability). He wrote that all measurement 'should be construct-referenced because construct interpretation undergirds all score-based inferences—not just those related to interpretive meaningfulness but also the content- and criterion-related inferences specific to applied decisions and actions based on test scores' (Messick 1988, p. 35). That is, correlating a new scale with some criterion in itself is a form of hypothesis testing: 'If my new scale is really measuring a person's adjustment to illness, then it should correlate with tests tapping attributes A and B'. Similarly, an assessment of the individual items is testing a hypothesis: 'I believe that adjustment consists of elements X, Y, and Z'.

This revised conceptualization of validity, which is now enshrined in the latest edition of the *Standards for educational and psychological testing* (American Educational Research Association et al. 2014) means that all validation is a process of hypothesis testing. So, rather than being constrained by the trinitarian Cs mentioned earlier, scale constructors are limited only by their imagination in devising studies to test their hypothesis. Now, rather than arguing which 'type' of validity a study supports, the important questions become 'Does the hypothesis of this validation study make sense in light of what the scale is designed to measure?' and 'Do the results of this study allow us to draw the inferences about the people that we wish to make?'

Unfortunately, this creates difficulties for writers of textbooks, especially those designed for readers in disciplines outside of psychology and education, where these 'new' concepts (now verging on being half a century old) have not yet penetrated. From the new perspective, a chapter on validity would focus primarily on the logic and methodology of hypothesis testing. The reader, though, will continue to encounter terms like and 'criterion validity' in their readings for some time to come. The way we have resolved this conundrum is to speak of 'validity' as a unitary construct, but to refer to different types of *validity testing*. So, for example, the next section will address *content validation*, which is but one way of assessing the validity of an instrument. This is preferable to referring to it as *content validity*, which implies that it is evaluating a different type of validity than, say, criterion validity. Where it may be a bit confusing is that we will use the term *validation* to refer to the process—how we establish the property of the test—and *validity* to refer to the outcome (e.g. 'we have done a study to evaluate the content validity of the scale').

Content validation

We mentioned content validation previously within the context of issues surrounding item construction (see Chapter 3). Here, let us briefly touch on it again from our new vantage point. When we conclude that a student has 'passed' a test in, say, respirology, or that an arthritic patient has a grip strength of only 10 kg, we are making the assumption that the measures comprise representative samples of the disorders, behaviours, attitudes, or knowledge that we want to assess. That is, we do not too much care if the student knows the specific bits of information tapped by the examination, or how much the patient can squeeze a dynamometer. Going back to what validity testing is all about, our aim is *inferential*; a person who does well on the exam can be expected to know more about lungs than a student who does poorly and a patient who has a weaker grip has more severe arthritis than someone who can exert more pressure.

A measure that includes a more representative sample of the target behaviour lends itself to more accurate inferences: that is, inferences which hold true under a wider range of circumstances. If there are important aspects of the outcome that are missed by the scales, then we are likely to make some inferences which will prove to be wrong; our *inferences* (not the instruments) are invalid. For example, if there was nothing on the respirology examination regarding oxygen exchange, then it is quite possible that a high scorer on the test may *not* know more about this topic than a student with a lower score. Similarly, grip strength has relatively poor content validity; as such, it does not allow us to make accurate inferences about other attributes of the rheumatoid patient, such as erythrocyte sedimentation rate, joint count, or morning stiffness, except insofar as these indices are correlated with grip strength.

Thus, the higher the content validity of a measure, the broader are the inferences that we can validly draw about the person under a variety of conditions and in different situations.

We discussed previously that reliability places an upper limit on validity, so that the higher the reliability, the higher the maximum possible validity. There is one notable exception to this general rule: the relationship between internal consistency (an index of reliability) and content validity. If we are tapping a behaviour, disorder, or trait that is relatively heterogeneous, like rheumatoid arthritis, then it is quite conceivable that the scale will have low internal consistency; not all patients with a high joint count have high sedimentation rates or morning stiffness. We could increase the internal consistency of the index by eliminating items which are not highly correlated with each other or the total score. If we did this, though, we would end up with an index tapping only one aspect of arthritis—stiffness, for example—and which therefore has very low content validity. Loevinger (1954) referred to this as the *attenuation paradox*: as internal consistency increases, so does validity, up to a point (also see Chapter 5). After that, increasing homogeneity results in a loss of content coverage and thus results in decreased validity. Under such circumstances, it is better to sacrifice internal consistency for content validity. The ultimate aim of the scale is inferential, which depends more on content validity than internal consistency.

Content validation differs from other forms of validity testing in one important respect: it is not based on the scores from the scale, performance differences between people, or changes based on some intervention; only on the judgement of experts regarding the content of the items. For this reason, some theorists do not consider this to be an aspect of validity at all, although content relevance and representativeness do affect the inferences that can be drawn from a score (Messick 1989).

Criterion validation

The traditional definition of criterion validation is the correlation of a scale with some other measure of the trait, state, or disorder under study, ideally, a 'gold standard' which has been used and accepted in the field. Criterion validation is usually divided into two types: *concurrent* validation and *predictive* validation. With concurrent validation, we correlate the new scale with the criterion measure, both of which are given at the same time. For example, we could administer a new scale for depression and the *Beck Depression Inventory* (an accepted measure of depression) during the same interview, or within a short time of each other. In predictive validation, the criterion will not be available until sometime in the future. Consider college admission tests, where the ultimate outcome is the person's performance on graduation 4 years hence; or diagnostic tests, where we must await the outcome of an autopsy or the further progression of the disease to confirm or disconfirm our predictions.

A major question is why, if a good criterion measure already exists, are we going through the often laborious process of developing a new instrument? Leaving aside the unworthy (if prevalent) reasons of trying to cash in on a lucrative market or having an instrument with one's name as part of the title, there are a number of valid reasons. The existing test can be expensive, invasive, dangerous, or time-consuming; or the outcome may not be known until it is too late. The first four reasons are the usual rationales for scales which require concurrent validation and the last reason for those which need predictive validation. On the basis of these reasons for developing new tests, Messick (1980) has proposed using the terms *diagnostic utility* or *substitutability* for concurrent validation and *predictive utility* for predictive validation; while they are not yet widely used, these are far more descriptive terms for the rationales underlying criterion validation testing.

Let us go through the usual procedures for conducting these two forms of validation and their rationales. As we have mentioned, the most commonly used design for concurrent validation is to administer the new scale and the standard at the same time. As an example, imagine evaluating a new test for TB; in this design, we would give both the Mantoux test (assuming it is the one being validated) and an X-ray (the gold standard) to a large group of people. Since the outcome is dichotomous (the person either has or does not have abnormalities on the X-ray consistent with TB), we would draw up a fourfold table, as in Table 10.1.

We could analyse the results using either the indices of sensitivity and specificity, or some measure of correlation which can be derived from a 2 × 2 table, such as the phi coefficient (φ). This coefficient is related to χ^2 by the following formula:

$$\phi = \frac{\sqrt{\chi^2}}{N}$$

or can be calculated from Table 10.1 using the following equation:

$$\phi = \frac{|BC - AD|}{\sqrt{[(A+B)(C+D)(A+C)(B+D)]}}$$

If our measures were continuous, as would be found if we were validating a new measure of depression against the *Beck Depression Inventory* or *CES-D* (another accepted index of depression), we would use a Pearson correlation coefficient. In either case, we would be looking for a strong association between our new measure and the already existing one. This would indicate that a person who has a high score or comes out 'diseased' on the new test would be expected to have a high score (or have been labelled as diseased) on the more established instrument.

In assessing predictive validity, the person is given the new measure at Time 1 and then the standard some time later at Time 2. Again, we would use a fourfold table to evaluate a scale with a dichotomous outcome and a correlational measure if the outcome were continuous. However, there is one additional point which appears

Table 10.1 Fourfold table to evaluate criterion validity for scales with dichotomous outcomes

		X-ray results	
		TB	No TB
Mantoux test	TB	A	B
	No TB	C	D

obvious, but is often overlooked: *no decision can be made based on the new instrument*. For example, if we were trying to establish the validity of an autobiographical letter as a criterion for admission to medical or nursing school, we would have all applicants write these missives. Then, no matter how good we felt this measure was, we would immediately put the evaluations of the letters in a safe place, without looking at them, and base our decisions on other criteria. Only after the students had or had not graduated would we take out the scores and compare them with actual performance.

What would happen if we violated this proscription and used the letters to help us decide who should be admitted? We would be able to determine what proportion of students who wrote excellent letters graduated 4 years later (cell A in Table 10.1) and what proportion failed (cell B). However, we would *not be able* to state what proportion of those who wrote 'poor' letters would have gone on to pass with flying colours (cell C) nor how well poor letters can detect people who will fail (cell D): they would never be given the chance. In this case, the sample has been *truncated* on the basis of our new test, and as we will describe later in more detail, the correlation between our new test and the standard will be reduced, perhaps significantly.

A somewhat different situation can also occur with diagnostic tests. If the final diagnosis (the gold standard) were predicated in part on the results of our new instrument, then we have artificially built in a high correlation between the two; we are correlating the new measure with an outcome based on it. For example, in the process of validating two-dimensional echocardiography for diagnosing mitral valve prolapse (MVP), we would use the clinician's judgement of the presence or absence of MVP as the criterion. However, the clinician may know the results of the echo tests and temper their diagnosis in light of them. This differs from our previous example in that we have not truncated our sample; rather, we are indirectly using the results of our new scale in both the predictor and the outcome. The technical term for this is *criterion contamination*.

In summary, then, criterion validation assesses how a person who scores at a certain level on our new scale does by comparison against some criterion measure. The usual experimental design is a correlational one; both measures are taken on a series of individuals. In the case of concurrent validation, the two results are gathered close together in time. In predictive validation, the results from the criterion measure are usually not known for some time, which can be between a few days to a few years later.

Construct validation

What is construct validation?

Attributes such as height or weight are readily observable, or can be 'operationally defined': that is, defined by the way they are measured. Systolic blood pressure, for example, is the amount of pressure, measured in millimetres of mercury, at the moment of ventricular systole. Once we move away from the realm of physical attributes into more 'psychological' ones like anxiety, intelligence, or pain, however, we begin dealing with more abstract variables—ones that cannot be directly observed. We cannot 'see' anxiety; all we can observe are behaviours which, according to our theory of anxiety, are the results of it. We would attribute the sweaty palms, tachycardia, pacing back and forth, and difficulty in concentrating experienced by a student just prior to writing an exam to their anxiety. Similarly, we may have two patients who, to all intents and purposes, have the same degree of angina. One patient has quit their job and spends most of the day sitting in a chair; the other continues working and is determined to 'fight it'. We may explain these differences in terms of such attitudes as 'motivation', 'illness behaviour', or the 'sick role model'. Again, these factors are not seen directly, only their hypothesized manifestations in terms of the patients' observable behaviours.

These proposed underlying factors are referred to as *hypothetical constructs*, or more simply as *constructs*. A construct can be thought of as a 'minitheory' to explain the relationships among various behaviours or attitudes. Many constructs arose from larger theories or clinical observations, before there were any ways of objectively measuring their effects. This would include terms like 'anxiety' or 'repression', derived from psychoanalytic theory; or 'sick role behaviour', which was based mainly on sociological theorizing (Parsons 1951). Other concepts, like the difference between 'fluid' and 'crystallized' intelligence (Cattell 1963), were proposed to explain observed correlations among variables which were already measured with a high degree of reliability.

It is fair to say that most psychological instruments and many measures of health are designed to tap some aspect of a hypothetical construct. There are two reasons for wanting to develop such an instrument: the construct is a new one and there is no scale to measure it, or we are dissatisfied with the existing tools and feel that they omit some key aspect of the construct. Note that we are doing more than replacing one tool with a shorter, cheaper, or less invasive one, which is the rationale for criterion validation. Rather, we are using the underlying theory to help us develop a new or better instrument, where 'better' means able to explain a broader range of findings, explain them in a more parsimonious manner, or make more accurate predictions about a person's behaviour.

Construct validational studies

As an example, consider the quest to develop a short checklist or scale to identify patients with irritable bowel syndrome (IBS). First, though, we should address the issue of why we consider IBS to be a construct rather than a disease like ulcers or amoebic dysentery. The central issue is that we cannot (at least not yet) definitively prove that a person has IBS; it is diagnosed by excluding other possible causes of the patient's symptoms. There is no X-ray or laboratory test to which we can point and say, 'Yes, that person has IBS'. Moreover, there is no known pathogen that produces the constellation of symptoms. We tie them together conceptually by postulating an underlying disorder, which cannot be measured directly, in much the same way that we say a large vocabulary, breadth of knowledge, and skill at problem-solving are all outward manifestations of a postulated but unseen concept we label 'intelligence'. Many of what physicians call 'syndromes' would be called 'hypothetical constructs' by psychologists and test developers. Indeed, even some 'diseases' like schizophrenia, Alzheimer's, or systemic lupus erythematosus are closer to constructs than actual entities, since their diagnosis is based on constellations of symptoms, and there are no unequivocal diagnostic tests that can be used with living patients. This is more than just semantics, though. It implies that tests for diagnosing or measuring syndromes should be constructed in an analogous manner to those for more 'psychological' attributes.

The first indices developed for assessing IBS consisted, in the main, of two parts: exclusion of other diseases, and the presence of some physical signs and symptoms like pain in the lower left quadrant and diarrhoea without pain. These scales proved to be inadequate, as many patients 'diagnosed' by them were later discovered to have stomach cancer or other diseases, and patients who were missed were, a few years later, indistinguishable from IBS patients. Thus, new scales were developed which added other—primarily demographic and personality—factors, predicated on a broader view (a revised construct) of IBS, as a disorder marked by specific demography and a unique psychological configuration, in addition to the physical symptoms. The problem the test developers now faced was how to demonstrate that the new index was better than the older ones.

To address this problem, let us go back to what we mean by a 'valid' scale: it is one that allows us to make accurate inferences about a person. These inferences are derived from the construct, and are of the form , 'Based on my theory of construct X, people who score high on a test of X differ from people who score low on it in terms of attributes A, B, and C,' where A, B, and C can be other instruments, behaviours, diagnoses, and so on. In this particular case, we would say, 'Based on my concept of IBS, high scorers on the index should:

1. have symptoms that will not resolve with conventional therapy, and

2. have a lower prevalence of organic bowel disease on autopsy'.

Since we are testing constructs, this form of testing is called *construct validation*. Methodologically, it differs from the types of validity testing we discussed previously in a number of important ways. First, content and criterion validity can often be established with one or two studies. However, we are often able to make many different predictions based on our theory or construct. For example, if we were validating a new scale of anxiety, just a few of the many hypotheses we can derive would be : 'Anxious people would have more rapid heart rates during an exam than low anxious ones'; 'Anxious people should do better on simple tasks than non-anxious subjects, but poorer than them on complex tasks'; or 'If I artificially induce anxiety with some experimental manoeuvre, then the subjects should score higher on my test'.

Thus, there is no one single experiment which can unequivocally 'prove' a construct. Construct validation is an ongoing process of learning more about the construct, making new predictions, and then testing them. Albert Einstein once said that there have been hundreds of experiments supporting his theory of relativity, but it would take only one non-confirmatory study to disprove it. So it is with construct validation; each supportive study serves only to strengthen what Cronbach and Meehl (1955) call the 'nomological network' of the interlocking predictions of a theory, but a single, well-designed experiment with negative findings can call into question the entire construct.

A second major difference between construct validation and the other types is that, with the former, we are assessing both the theory and the measure at the same time.

Returning to our example of a better index for IBS, one prediction was that patients who have a high score would not respond to conventional therapy. Assume that we gave the index to a sample of patients presenting at a gastrointestinal (GI) clinic, and gave them all regular treatment. (Remember, we cannot base any decisions on the results of a scale we are validating; this would lead to criterion contamination.) If it turned out that our prediction was confirmed, then it would lend credence to both our concept of IBS and the index we developed to measure it. However, if high-scoring subjects responded to treatment in about the same proportion as low scorers, then the problem could be that:

1. our instrument is good, but the theory is wrong

2. the theory is fine, but our index cannot discriminate between IBS patients and those with other GI problems, or

3. both the theory is wrong and our scale is useless.

Moreover, we would have no way of knowing which of these situations exists until we do more studies.

A further complication enters the picture when we use an experimental study to validate the scale. Using the example of a new measure of anxiety, one prediction was that if we artificially induce anxiety, as in threatening the subject with an electric shock if they perform poorly on some task, then we should see an increase in scores on the index. If the scores do not go up, then the problem could be in either of the areas already mentioned—the theory and the measure—plus one other; both the theory and the scale are fine, but the experiment did not induce anxiety, as we had hoped it would. Again, any combination of these problems could be working: the measure is valid and the experiment worked, but the theory is wrong; the theory is right and the experiment went the way we planned, but the index is not measuring anxiety; and so forth.

Putting this all together, Cronbach and Meehl's (1955) seminal article on construct validity said that it involves three mandatory steps:

1. Explicitly spelling out a set of theoretical concepts and how they are related to each other.

2. Developing scales to measure these hypothetical constructs.

3. Actually testing the relationships among the constructs and their observable manifestations.

That is, unless there is an articulated theory, there is no construct validity (Clark and Watson 1995). But Clark and Watson go on to state the following (p. 310):

> This emphasis on theory is not meant to be intimidating. That is, we do not mean to imply that one must have a fully articulated set of interrelated theoretical concepts before embarking on scale development. Our point, rather, is that thinking about these theoretical issues prior to the actual process of scale construction increases the likelihood that the resulting scale will make a substantial contribution to the ... literature.

They recommend writing out a brief, formal description of the construct, how it will manifest itself objectively, and how it is related to other constructs and behaviours.

There are a number of implications of this. First, construct validity is not proven just because two groups have different scores on the scale, unless that difference has been postulated a priori and makes sense. If there is no reason that boys and girls should differ on a measure of self-efficacy, then showing that they do proves nothing. Second, exploratory factor analysis is an atheoretical technique, because you cannot postulate beforehand what the factor structure should be. Consequently, its results cannot be taken as demonstrating construct validity. If you can propose what the factor structure should be, you should be using confirmatory factor analysis.

We said that construct validation differs from content and criterion validation methodologically. At the risk of being repetitive, we should emphasize that construct validation does not *conceptually* differ from the other types. To quote Guion (1977), '*All* validity is at its base some form of construct validity ... It is the basic meaning of validity' (p. 410).

It should not be surprising that given the greater complexity and breadth of questions asked with construct validation as compared with the other types of validation, there are many more ways of establishing it. In the next sections, we will discuss only a few of these methods: extreme groups, convergent and discriminant validation, and the multitrait–multimethod matrix. Many other experimental and quasi-experimental approaches exist; the interested reader should consult some of the references listed at the end of this chapter under 'Further reading'.

Extreme groups

Perhaps the easiest experiment to conceive while assessing the validity of a scale is to give it to two groups: one of which has the trait, attribute, or behaviour, and the other which does not. The former group should score significantly higher (or lower, depending on how the items are scored) on the new instrument. This is sometimes called construct validation by *extreme groups* (also referred to as *discriminative valid-ation*, which is not to be confused with *discriminant validation*, discussed in the next section 'Convergent and discriminant validation'). We can use the attempt to develop a better scale for IBS as an example. Using their best tools, experienced clinicians would divide a group of patients presenting to a GI clinic into two subgroups: those whom they believe have IBS and those who have some other bowel disorder. To make the process of scale development easier, all patients with equivocal diagnoses would be eliminated in this type of study.

Although this type of design appears quite straightforward, it has buried within it three methodological problems. The first difficulty with the method is that if we are trying to develop a new or better tool, how can we select the extreme groups? To be able to do so would imply that there is already an instrument in existence which meets our needs. There is no ready solution to this problem. In practice, the groups are selected using the best *available* tool, even if it is the relatively crude criterion of 'expert judgement' or a scale that almost captures what our new scale is designed to tap. We can then use what Cronbach and Meehl (1955) call 'boot-strapping'. If the new scale allows us to make more accurate predictions, or explain more findings, or achieve better inter-observer agreement, then it can replace the original criterion. In turn, then, it can be used as the gold standard against which a newer or revised version can be validated : hence 'pulling ourselves up by the bootstraps'.

The second methodological problem is one that occurs with diagnostic tests and which is often overlooked in the pressure to publish : the extreme group design may be a necessary step, but it is by no means sufficient. That is, it is minimally necessary for our new scale to be able to differentiate between those people who obviously have the disorder or trait in question and those who do not; if the scale cannot do this, it is probably useless in all other regards. However, the question must be asked, 'Is this the way the instrument will be used in practice?' If we are trying to develop a new diagnostic tool, the answer most often is 'no'. We likely would not need a new test to separate out the obvious cases from the obvious non-cases. Especially in a tertiary care setting, the people who are sent are in the middle range; they *may* have the disorder, but then again there are some doubts. If it is with this group that the instrument will be used, then the ultimate test of its usefulness is in making these much finer discriminations. The difficulty is that this middle group, by definition, is more homogeneous than the extreme groups and so, as we have pointed out previously, the reliability of the scale and hence its validity will be lower. In the context of diagnostic tests, therefore, understanding the pathways to diagnosis (pathways through systems of informal and formal care) is critical information for designing validation studies.

For example, many instruments have been designed to detect the presence of organic brain syndrome (OBS). As a first step, we would try out such a tool on one group of patients with confirmed brain damage and on another where there is no evidence of any pathology. These two groups should be clearly distinguishable on the new test. However, such patients are rarely referred for neuropsychological assessment, since their diagnoses (or lack thereof) are readily apparent based on other criteria. The next step, then, would be to try this instrument on the types of patients who *would* be sent for assessment, where the differential diagnosis is between OBS and depression, a difficult discrimination to make. These groups would be formed based on the best guess of a psychiatrist, perhaps augmented by some other tests of OBS—ones we are trying to replace.

The third difficulty is the composition of the control or comparison group. All too often, it is a sample of convenience, and, in university-based studies, undergraduate students. In 1946, Quinn McNemar said that 'The existing science of human behavior is largely the science of sophomores' (p. 333), and the picture has not changed since that was written . Kimmel (1996) estimated that about 70 per cent of studies in personality and social psychology and 90 per cent of those in perception and cognition used students. This raises two issues: to what degree are college students representative of the general population; and is their pattern of responses similar to that of patients? (We will leave aside the broader issue of whether those who volunteer to participate in studies are representative of the general population; see Streiner (2015) to see that the answer is 'no' .)

A number of studies have documented significant differences between college students and the general population. Almost by definition, student groups are more homogeneous, younger, from a higher socioeconomic class, and brighter (although this may be disputed by their professors) than the rest of the population (Foot and

Sanford 2004). Moreover, Peterson and Merunka (2014) have documented differences from one college sample to the next, casting doubts on the replicability of results using these groups.

This latter issue comes to the fore when we use statistical approaches such as factor analysis to look for consistencies among items. Clusters of items may emerge in patient groups but not controls, and vice versa. Delis et al. (2003), for example, found that various tests of cognitive functioning (e.g. long- and short-term memory, immediate and delayed recall) were highly correlated among normals, indicating a global factor of 'memory', but were clearly differentiated when assessed in samples of patients with Alzheimer's disease or Huntington's disease. Thus, be wary of patterns among variables that may appear in special populations (e.g. students) that may not appear in the population of interest (patients) or the reverse.

Convergent and discriminant validation

Assessing the validation by using extreme groups is closely related to *convergent validation*: seeing how closely the new scale is related to other variables and other measures of the same construct to which it should be related. For example, if our theory states that anxious people are supposed to be more aware of autonomic nervous system (ANS) activity than non-anxious people, then scores on the new index of anxiety should correlate with scores on a measure of autonomic awareness. Again, if the scores do *not* correlate, then the problem could be our new scale, the measure of autonomic sensitivity, or our theory. On the other hand, we do not want the scales to be too highly correlated: this would indicate that they are measuring the same thing, and that the new one is nothing more than a different measure of autonomic awareness (what we referred to in Chapter 1 as the 'jangle fallacy'). How high is 'too high'? As usual, it all depends. If ANS sensitivity is, by our theory, a major component of anxiety, then the correlation should be relatively robust; if it is only one of many components of anxiety, then the correlation should be lower.

The other aspect of convergent validation is that the new index of anxiety should correlate with other measures of this construct. Again, while the correlation should be high, it should not be overly high if we believe that our new anxiety scale covers components of this trait not tapped by the existing ones. And of course, once again we must caution that the range of scores in the validation sample should approximate the range in the population to which it is applied; extreme groups lead to high correlations.

Ideally, the new instrument should be tested against existing ones that are maximally different in terms of the nature of the measuring process (Campbell and Fiske 1959). Although it is difficult to define what 'maximally different' means (Foster and Cone 1995), it would imply that a self-report scale should be evaluated against one completed by an observer or a performance task, for example, rather than a different self-report measure. The rationale is that scores on a scale are determined not only by the attribute being measured, but also by aspects of the measuring process itself (this is referred to as *measurement variance*; two or more scales may be correlated simply because the same person is completing the same type of scale, such as self-report). In the next section, on the multitrait–multimethod matrix, we show how correlations between instruments due to similarity of the assessment method can be disentangled from similarity due to tapping the same attribute.

Not only should our construct correlate with related variables, but also it should *not* correlate with dissimilar, unrelated ones: what we refer to as *discriminant validation* (which is also sometimes referred to as *divergent validation*). If our theory states that anxiety is independent of intelligence, then we should not find a strong correlation between the two. Finding one may indicate, for example, that the wording of our instrument is so difficult that intelligence is playing a role in simply understanding the items. Of course, the other reasons may also apply; our scale, the intelligence test, or the construct may be faulty. Further, even though we may have set out to measure construct A, we may be measuring construct B, in whole or in part. As Campbell and Fiske (1959) have said, 'Tests can be invalidated by too high correlations with other tests from which they were intended to differ' (p. 81). One measure commonly used in discriminant validation testing is social desirability bias, for reasons we discussed in Chapter 6 on biases in responding.

Consequential validation

Most of the scales developed for measuring health are used within the context of research. This means that if the scale is invalid in some regard, it may adversely affect the results of the study, but will not have any impact on the individuals who participated. However, if the test is used in a more clinical setting, in which the score dictates whether or not the person will receive some sort of intervention (e.g. physiotherapy if the test indicates restricted use of an upper limb), then the *consequences* of the decisions based on the test should be factored into the evaluation of validity. This aspect of validity, which was introduced by Messick (1989, 1994, 1995), is referred to as *consequential validation*. Messick's concern was 'high-stakes' tests related to education, such as those dictating who will pass or fail a grade in school; who will or will not be admitted to university, professional school, or graduate school; or who will be certified in their professional organization; but his arguments are easily generalized to clinical settings, where the stakes are equally high.

Consequences can be both positive and negative, and deliberate and unintended. For example, a positive, although perhaps unintended, consequence of an assessment of quality of life is to direct the clinician's attention towards this aspect of the patient's response to an illness so that the focus is not exclusively on the biomedical aspect of disorders. This was the motivation to develop such a scale for children with epilepsy, as conventional care focussed solely on seizure control without any regard for quality of life, which is uncorrelated with it (Ronen et al. 2003). Conversely, the requirement in the early 1920s that immigrants to the United States must take an intelligence (IQ) test in English had the negative (albeit likely deliberate) consequence of keeping out those from eastern and southern Europe. In poorly designed achievement tests, such as those used to determine if children in different school districts are meeting certain standards, or if professionals should be certified to practise, the test may drive the curriculum; that is, people will be taught what is assessed, rather than what they need to know. In this regard, the poor content coverage of the test results in poor consequential validity.

A major concern is to differentiate between adverse consequences that are due to various forms of invalidity and those that are valid descriptions of individual or group differences. For example, one impetus for the development of IQ tests in France was that boys were being held back in class to a much larger degree than were girls. The problem was that teachers' recommendations for promotion were based on the ability to sit quietly at the desk, with one's hands folded and ankles crossed. As any parent of children of both genders can tell you, this is a nearly impossible task for young boys; however, it is not related to intellectual ability; that is, it is an instance of construct-irrelevant variance. On the other hand, girls tend to score higher than boys in tests of verbal fluency, which reflects the real phenomenon that females develop language skills earlier than males (e.g. Coates 1993).

It should be noted that this form of validation is not universally accepted. Some people, such as Popham (1997), have argued that validation should be restricted to objective evaluations and that consequential validation involves issues of ethics and social values (Messick 1975). Further, once a test has been published, its developer should not be held responsible for the uses to which others put it (Reckase 1998; see Iliescu and Greiff (2021) for a different view on responsibility). Although this debate is still ongoing, scale designers should at least be aware of possible negative consequences, both intended and unintended.

The multitrait–multimethod matrix

A powerful technique for looking at convergent and discriminant validation simultaneously is called the *multitrait–multimethod matrix*, or MTMM (Campbell and Fiske 1959). Two or more different, usually unrelated, traits are each measured by two or more methods at the same time. The two traits, for instance, can be 'self-directed learning' and 'knowledge' (assuming that they are relatively unrelated), each assessed by a rater and a written exam. This leads to a matrix of 10 correlations, as shown with fictitious data in Table 10.2.

The numbers in parentheses (0.53, 0.79, etc.) along the main diagonal are the reliabilities of the four instruments. The two italicized figures, *0.42* and *0.49*, are the 'homotrait–heteromethod' correlations: the same trait (e.g. knowledge) measured in different ways. Those in curly brackets, {0.18} and {0.23}, are 'heterotrait–homomethod' correlations: different traits assessed by the same method. Finally, the

Table 10.2 A fictitious multitrait–multimethod matrix

		Self-directed learning		Knowledge	
		Rater	Exam	Rater	Exam
Self-directed learning	**Rater**	(0.53)			
	Exam	*0.42*	(0.79)		
Knowledge	**Rater**	{0.18}	[0.17]	(0.58)	
	Exam	[0.15]	{0.23}	*0.49*	(0.88)

heterotrait–heteromethod correlations are in square brackets, [0.17] and [0.15]: different traits measured with different methods.

Ideally, the highest correlations should be the reliabilities of the individual measures; an examination of 'knowledge' given on two occasions should yield higher correlations than examinations of different traits or two different ways of tapping knowledge. Similarly, the lowest correlations should be the heterotrait–heteromethod ones; different traits measured by different methods should not be related.

Convergent validation is reflected in the homotrait–heteromethod correlations; different measures of the same trait should correlate with each other. In this example, the results of the written exam should correlate with scores given by the rater for 'knowledge' and similarly for the two assessments of 'self-directed learning'. Conversely, discriminant validation is shown by low correlations when the same method (e.g. the written exam) is applied to different traits—the heterotrait–homomethod coefficients. If they are as high or higher than the homotrait–heteromethod correlations, this would show that the *method* of measurement was more important than *what was being measured*. This is referred to as *common method variance* (Podsakoff et al. 2003)—that written tests tend to correlate with other written tests and oral exams with oral exams, irrespective of the content. This is obviously an undesirable property, since the manner of assessing various attributes should be secondary to the relationship that should exist between various ways of tapping into the same trait, although the true extent to which this is a serious problem has been questioned by some (Doty and Glick 1998).

It is often difficult to perform studies appropriate for the MTMM approach because of the time required on the subjects' part, as well as the problem of finding different methods of assessing the same trait. When these studies can be done, though, they can address a number of validity issues simultaneously.

Summary—construct validation

Unlike criterion validation, then, there is no one experimental design or statistic which is common to construct validational studies. If one of the hypotheses is that our new measure of a construct is related to other indices of that construct or that the construct should be associated with other constructs, then the study is usually correlational in nature; our new scale and another one (of the same or a related construct) are given to the subjects. If one hypothesis is that some naturally occurring group has 'more' of the construct than another group, then we can simply give our new instrument to both groups and look for differences between the two means. Still another hypothesis may be that if we give some experimental or therapeutic intervention, it will affect the construct and the measure of it: transcutaneous stimulation should reduce pain, while intense radiant heat should increase it. In this instance, our study could be a before/after trial, or more powerfully, a true experiment whereby one group receives the intervention and the other does not. If our construct is correct and the manoeuvre worked and our scale is valid for this population, then we should see differences between the groups.

In summary, it is obviously necessary to conduct validational studies for each new instrument we develop. However, when the scale is one measuring a hypothetical construct, the task is an ongoing one. New hypotheses derived from the construct require new studies. Similarly, if we want to use the measure with groups it was not initially validated on, we must first demonstrate that the inferences we make for them are as valid as for the original population. Finally, modifications of existing scales often require new validity studies. For example, if we wanted to use the D scale of the MMPI as an index of depression, we cannot assume that it is as valid when used in isolation as when the items are imbedded amongst 500 other, unrelated ones. It is possible that the mere fact of presenting them together gives the patient a different orientation and viewpoint.

However, not all changes to a scale necessarily require its revalidation. Some modifications in wording are minor and do not alter the meaning of the stems, such as changing 'his' or 'her ' to 'their ', or perhaps even replacing one disorder with another (e.g. asking how one's migraine headache interfered with work, rather than one's arthritis). On the other hand, changing the period of recall from 'last week' to 'last month' may have a profound change on validity, because of the problems associated with trying to remember past events, which were discussed in Chapter 6; and changing the response options from a Likert scale to a VAS may also affect the responses. Obviously, some degree of judgement is required.

Responsiveness and sensitivity to change

Since the 1980s , two new terms have crept into the psychometric lexicon: *responsiveness* and *sensitivity to change*. While these define useful concepts in evaluating scales, their introduction has also led to two sources of confusion: whether these are synonyms or refer to different attributes of an instrument; and if they refer to a third attribute of a scale (i.e. separate from reliability and validity) or are a component of one or both of them.

Although many authors use the terms interchangeably, Liang (2000) draws a useful distinction between them. He defines sensitivity to change as 'the ability of an instrument to measure change in a state regardless of whether it is relevant or meaningful to the decision maker' (p. 85); and responsiveness as 'the ability of an instrument to measure a meaningful or clinically important change in a clinical state' (p. 85). This, needless to say, leaves open the question of what is meant by a 'clinically important change'. We will discuss this point, as well as the overall issue of how to measure change at all, in Chapter 11.

Accompanying the introduction of these terms has been a tendency for articles to state that their aim is to examine the 'reliability, validity, and sensitivity to change' (or 'responsiveness') of a given instrument. The implication of this statement is that it is not sufficient to establish reliability and validity, and that sensitivity and responsiveness are distinct characteristics. The short response is that this implication is wrong (in addition to erroneously speaking of 'the' reliability and validity of the scale). As a number of theorists have said, responsiveness and sensitivity are part and parcel of validity (e.g. Hays and Hadorn 1992; Patrick and Chiang 2000) and not separate attributes. In Chapter 11, on measuring change, we discuss the mathematical relationship of responsiveness and sensitivity change to reliability. On a conceptual level, they are an aspect of validation, most akin to criterion validation—does the change detected by the new measure correlate with change as measured by some other instrument?

Validity and 'types of indices'

Some authors have proposed that there are different kinds of scales or indices, which vary according to their potential application. For example, Kirshner and Guyatt (1985) state that indices can be *discriminative* (i.e. used to distinguish between individuals or groups when there is no gold standard), *predictive* (used to classify individuals into predefined groups according to an existing gold standard), or *evaluative* (for tracking people or groups over time). Moreover, they state that the purpose of the scale dictates how the items are scaled, which procedures are used to select the items, how reliability and validity are assessed, and how 'responsiveness' is measured. We believe that these are false distinctions that do not reflect the reality of how tests are used in the real world; and more importantly, reflect a misunderstanding of validity testing.

While a scale may have been developed for one purpose, in actual practice it is often used in a variety of different ways. Using their own example of the MMPI, Kirshner and Guyatt state that this is a 'discriminative' tool, 'developed in order to distinguish those with emotional and psychological disorders from the general population' (p. 27). This is undoubtedly true, but it has also been used to diagnose people (what they call the 'predictive' use of a test: e.g. Scheibe et al. 2001), as well as a measure of improvement in therapy, which could also place it within their evaluative category (e.g. Munley 2002). Similarly, they cite the Denver Developmental Screening Test as a 'predictive' tool 'designed to identify children who are likely to have learning problems in the future' (p. 28). Again, though, its use has not been restricted to this; it has also been used as a discriminative tool (Cadman et al. 1988) and to measure change (Mandich et al. 1994).

The bottom line is that scales are used in many ways. Whether or not they can be depends on one, and only one, issue—has it been validated for that purpose? If larger decreases on the Depression scale on the MMPI are seen in a group that receives cognitive behaviour therapy as compared to a control group, for example, then it can be used to measure changes over time, irrespective of the fact that the scale was initially developed to identify patients with depression. It is worth repeating the statement by Nunnally (1970): 'Strictly speaking, one validates not a measurement instrument but rather some use to which the instrument is put' (p. 133).

Biases in validity assessment

Restriction in range

We mentioned in Chapter 8 that an unacceptable way of seeming to increase the reliability of a measure is to give it to a more heterogeneous group than the one it is designed for. In this section, we return to this point from a different perspective: how the range of scores affects the validity of the scale. There are actually three ways this can occur:

1. The predictor variable (usually our new measure) is restricted.

2. The criterion is restricted.

3. A third variable, correlated with both the predictor and criterion variables, is used to select the group which will be given the predictor and criterion variables.

As an example, assume that we have read about a new assay for serum monoamine oxidase (MAO), which is highly correlated with scores on a depression inventory. In the original (fictitious) article, a correlation of 0.80 was found in a large community-based sample. Such an assay would be extremely useful in a hospital setting, where difficulty with the English language and the various biases (e.g. faking good or bad) are often problems with self-administered scales.

We replicate the study on our in-patient psychiatry ward, but find a disappointingly low correlation of only 0.37. Should we be surprised?

Based on our discussion of restriction of range, the answer is 'no'. We can illustrate this effect pictorially by drawing a scatter diagram of the two variables in the original study as in Fig. 10.1.

As a brief reminder, a scatterplot is made by placing a dot at the intersection of a person's scores on the two variables. Alternatively, an ellipse can be drawn so that it includes (usually) 95 per cent of the people. The more elliptical the swarm of points or the ellipse, the stronger the correlation; the more circular the ellipse, the lower the association, with the extreme being a circle reflecting a total lack of any relationship. This scatterplot is fairly thin, as would be expected with a correlation of 0.80.

In our study, all of the subjects were hospitalized depressives, so their scores on the depression inventory are expected to be higher than those in a community

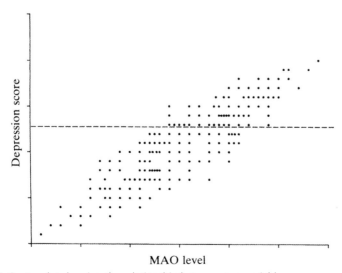

Fig. 10.1 Scatterplot showing the relationship between two variables.

sample, falling above the line in Fig. 10.1. As can be seen, the portion of the ellipse falling above the line is more circular than the whole scatterplot, indicating that for this more restricted sample, the correlation between the two variables is considerably lower.

Using some equations developed by Thorndike (1949), we can predict how much the validity coefficient will be affected by selecting more restricted groups based on the criterion (X), the predictor (Y), or some other variable (Z). The first situation would apply if patients were hospitalized only if their scores on the depression inventory exceeded a certain level. This would be the case if high scores on the scale were one of the criteria for admission and would be analogous to validating a new TB test only on patients who have lesions on an X-ray. In this case, the validity of the predictor would be:

$$r' = \frac{r(s'_X / s_X)}{\sqrt{\left[1 - r^2 + r^2 \left(s'^2_X / s^2_X\right)\right]}}$$

where r' is the restricted validity coefficient, r is the validity coefficient in the unrestricted sample, s'_X is the SD of the criterion for the restricted sample, and s is the SD of the criterion for the unrestricted sample.

If the standard deviation in the unrestricted sample was 10 and it was reduced to 3 in the restricted sample, we would obtain:

$$\frac{0.80 \times (3/10)}{\sqrt{\left[1 - 0.64 + 0.64 \times (9/100)\right]}} = 0.37$$

By the same token, we can work backwards by transforming this formula. If we did a study on a sample that was in some way constrained on the criterion variable, we could figure out what the validity coefficient would be if the full range of the variable were available. In this case, the formula would be:

$$r = \frac{r'\left(s'_X / s_X\right)}{\sqrt{\left[1 - r'^2 + r'^2 \left(s^2_X / s'^2_X\right)\right]}}$$

where the terms have the same meaning as above.

The second case occurs when the group is selected on the basis of the *predictor* variable (Y); using the same example, only patients with increased MAO levels are included. This is the situation that obtains with criterion contamination; students are selected based on their scores on the admission test, which is actually being evaluated to see if it is a valid predictor. The formulae are the same, except that s'_Y is substituted for s'_X, and s_Y for s_X.

The last case is where the subjects are selected on the basis of some other variable (Z), which is correlated with both X and Y. Using our original example, this is the most realistic condition, since patients are admitted because of the severity of their symptomatology, which is related to both MAO level and scores on the depression inventory. The question can again be asked in two ways:

1. If we know the results from an (unrestricted) community-based study, what would the correlation be in our (more restricted) hospital environment?
2. If we correlated X and Y in our restricted sample, what would the correlation be in an unrestricted one?

Since an additional variable is involved (Z, the severity of depression), more information must be known:

1. The correlation of X and Y in the unrestricted sample.
2. The correlations of X with Z and Y with Z in this sample.
3. The standard deviation of Z in the restricted and unrestricted samples.

As these data are rarely known, the equation is mainly of academic interest. For those who are interested, a thorough treatment of this topic can be found in Ghiselli (1964).

Unreliability of the criterion

One pervasive problem in validation occurs when we correlate our new scale with a gold standard. Quite frequently, though, the criterion is not as good as this term suggests (a more accurate term in many instances of clinical medicine would be 'bronze standard'), since it is unreliable in its own right. Thus, the validity coefficient may be attenuated since, even if the predictor (Y) were excellent, it is predicting to an unreliable criterion (X). We can estimate what the validity coefficient would be if the criterion were perfectly reliable by using the following formula:

$$r'_{XY'} = \frac{r_{XY}}{\sqrt{(r_{XX})}}$$

where $r'_{XY'}$ is the estimated correlation with a perfectly reliable criterion, r_{XY} is the actual correlation between tests X and Y, and r_{XX} is the reliability coefficient of the criterion (test X).

If we assume that the criterion is perfectly reliable, and we want to see how much the correlation could improve if the new test were perfectly reliable, we would simply substitute r_{YY} for r_{XX} under the following radical:

$$r'_{XY'} = \frac{r_{XY}}{\sqrt{(r_{YY})}}$$

A more general (and realistic) case assumes that both scales are unreliable, and we want to see what the correlation would be if both were perfectly reliable. The equation now reads:

$$r'_{XY'} = \frac{r_{XY}}{\sqrt{r_{XX}r_{YY}}}$$

Another way this equation can be used is to compare two or more studies that are examining the same construct, but using different tests whose reliabilities vary (Schmidt and Hunter 1999). Let us assume that Study A finds a correlation of 0.42 between a quality of life (QOL) scale and an index of activities of daily living (ADL). Study B, using a different set of scales to measure the same constructs, finds a correlation of 0.22. Why is r nearly twice as high in the first study? Assuming that both studies were sufficiently large enough to rule out sampling error, a possible answer is the differing reliabilities of the measures. If the QOL scale in Study A had a reliability of 0.90 and the ADL scale a reliability of 0.80, then the disattenuated correlation between them is:

$$r'_{XY'} = \frac{0.42}{\sqrt{(0.09)(0.80)}} = 0.49$$

If Study B used shorter scales with lower reliabilities (e.g. 0.50 for QOL and 0.40 for ADL), then its disattenuated correlation is:

$$r'_{XY'} = \frac{0.22}{\sqrt{(0.50)(0.40)}} = 0.49$$

Thus, while the studies report different correlations between the *measures*, the correlations between the *constructs are* the same (Schmidt and Hunter 1999).

The most general (and realistic) case is that perfect reliability never exists, in either the new instrument or in the criterion. However, it may be possible to improve the reliability of one or both, and we would want to know what the correlation between the two indices would be, given these improved (albeit not perfect) reliabilities. In this case, we would use the following equation:

$$r'_{XY'} = \frac{r_{XY}\sqrt{\left(r'_{XY'}r'_{XY'}\right)}}{\sqrt{\left(r_{XX}r_{YY}\right)}}$$

where r'_{XX} and r'_{YY} are the changed reliabilities for the two variables (somewhere between their actual reliabilities and 1.0).

These equations have two possible uses. First, they tell us how much the validity would increase if we were able to increase the reliabilities of the instruments. If the increase is only marginal, then the investment of time and perhaps money needed to improve the psychometric properties may not be worth it, whereas a large potential increase may signal that it could be worthwhile making the investment. The second useful function is in the area of theory development. If our theory tells us that variable *A* should correlate strongly with variable *B*, then correcting for unreliability of the measures gives us an indication of the true validity of the instrument and hence of our construct. A low, uncorrected validity estimate may incorrectly lead us to discard the theory when, in fact, it may be correct and the problem is with the scales.

Whether or not to use any of these formulae depends on the question being asked. If the issue is whether the test, as it currently exists, can predict some other measure as it currently exists, then neither should be corrected for unreliability. Any correction would overestimate how the test performs in the real world, which consists of measures that have some degree of measurement error. Quoting Guion (1965) in this regard, 'The effect of a possible correction for attenuation should never be a consideration when one is deciding how to evaluate a measure as it exists' (p. 32). On the other hand, if we are interested in the degree of improvement that is possible with the new test in predicting an existing criterion, then we should correct only for the predictor variable. However, this corrected coefficient should not be reported as if it were the actual correlation between the two measures, and we cannot perform any tests of significance on it (Magnusson 1967). Finally, if the issue is one of testing a construct—that is, seeing if the construct being measured is related to some other construct—as opposed to establishing the validity of the test itself, then correcting both the predictor and the criterion may make sense (Schmidt and Hunter 1996, 1999).

The final issue is which reliability coefficient to use in the equation—internal consistency, test–retest, or inter-rater. Muchinsky (1996) correctly states that one should 'use the type of reliability estimate that treats as error those factors that one decides should be treated as error' (p. 87). That is, if you feel that the test can be improved by increasing the coverage of the construct (or the criterion is constrained by limited sampling from the domain), then it makes most sense to use Cronbach's α as the estimate of reliability. Conversely, if you feel that error is introduced by unreliability of the raters, then the estimate of inter-rater reliability is the correct one to use, and so on. However, quoting Muchinsky (1996) again, 'There is no acceptable psychometric basis for creating validity coefficients that are the product of correcting for multiple types of unreliability' (p. 87).

Changes in the sample

Life would be simple if we could establish the validity of a measure once by conducting a series of studies and then assume that we could use that instrument under a range of circumstances and with a variety of people. Unfortunately, this is not the case. Estimates of validity, like those of reliability, are dependent upon the nature of the people being measured, and to a greater or lesser degree, the circumstances under which they are being assessed. A tool that can accurately measure the activities of daily living among cancer patients may be quite useless when used with patients who have

COPD; and one that has proven valid in distinguishing OBS from depressed patients may not discriminate between OBS patients and schizophrenics. Every time a scale is used in a new context, or with a different group of people, it is necessary to re-establish its psychometric properties.

Validity generalization

In Chapter 8, we discussed a technique called *reliability generalization*, based on meta-analysis, that allows one to summarize the results from a number of reliability estimates and to determine factors that may affect the magnitude of the reliability coefficients. Needless to say, the same approach can be used with estimates of validity. In fact, validity generalization was developed first (Hunter and Schmidt 2004; Schmidt and Hunter 1977) and only later applied to reliability. Because the methods are the same, we will not discuss them further, and you should read the section in Chapter 8 if you missed it the first time around (readers seeking more might try Murphy 2011).

However, there are some additional issues to keep in mind when doing validity generalization meta-analyses. As we discussed earlier in this chapter, validity coefficients can be attenuated by a variety of factors such as dichotomization of the criterion, unreliability of the measures, and restriction in range in either the new scale, the criterion, or both. In Hunter and Schmidt's excellent book (2004), they discuss how some or all of these factors can be taken into consideration when doing meta-analyses.

Summary

Validation is a process of determining what, if anything, we are measuring with our scale; that is, can we make valid statements about a person based on their score on the index? *Concurrent* validation is most often used when we are trying to replace one tool with a simpler, cheaper, or less invasive one. We generally use another form of criterion validation, called *predictive* validation, in developing instruments that allow us to get answers earlier than current instruments allow. *Construct* validation refers to a wide range of approaches which are used when what we are trying to measure is a 'hypothetical construct', like anxiety or some syndromes, rather than something which can be readily observed.

Further reading

Anastasi, A. and Urbina, S. (1996). *Psychological testing* (7th edn), chapters 5 and 6. Pearson, New York.

Borsboom, D., Mellenbergh, G.J., and van Heerden, J. (2004). The concept of validity. *Psychological Review*, **111**, 1061–71.

Cronbach, L.J. and Meehl, P.E. (1955). Construct validity in psychological tests. *Psychological Bulletin*, **52**, 281–302.

Nunnally, J.C., Jr. (1970). *Introduction to psychological measurement*, chapter 6. McGraw-Hill, New York.

Shadish, W.R., Cook, T.D., and Campbell, T.D. (2002). *Experimental and quasi-experimental designs for generalized causal inference*. Houghton Mifflin, New York.

References

American Educational Research Association, American Psychological Association, and National Council on Measurement in Education (2014). *Standards for educational and psychological testing*. American Educational Research Association, Washington, DC.

Cadman, D., Walter, S.D., Chambers, L.W., Ferguson, R., Szatmari, P., Johnson, N., *et al*. (1988). Predicting problems in school performance from preschool health, developmental and behavioural assessments. *CMAJ*, **139**, 31–6.

Campbell, D.T. and Fiske, D.W. (1959). Convergent and discriminant validation by the multitrait-multimethod matrix. *Psychological Bulletin*, **56**, 81–105.

Cattell, R.B. (1946). *Description and measurement of personality*. World Book Company, New York.

Cattell, R.B. (1963). Theory of fluid and crystallized intelligence: Critical experiment. *British Journal of Educational Psychology*, **54**, 1–22.

Cizek, G.J. (2012). Defining and distinguishing validity: Interpretations of score meaning and justifications of test use. *Psychological Methods*, **17**(1), 31–43.

Clark, L.A. and Watson, D. (1995). Constructing validity: Basic issues in objective scale development. *Psychological Assessment*, **7**, 309–19.

Coates, J. (1993). The acquisition of gender-differentiated language. In *Women, men and language: A sociolinguistic account of gender differences in language* (2nd edn) (ed. J. Coates), pp. 143–67. Longman, London.

Cronbach, L.J. (1971). Test validation. In *Educational measurement* (ed. R.L. Thorndike), pp. 221–37. American Council on Education, Washington, DC.

Cronbach, L.J. and Meehl, P.E. (1955). Construct validity in psychological tests. *Psychological Bulletin*, **52**, 281–302.

Delis, D.C., Jacobson, M., Bondi, M.W., Hamilton, J.M., and Salmon, D.P. (2003). The myth of testing construct validity using factor analysis or correlations with normal or mixed clinical populations: Lessons from memory assessment. *Journal of the International Neuropsychological Society*, **9**, 936–46.

Doty, D.H. and Glick, W.H. (1998). Common method bias: Does common methods variance really bias results? *Organizational Research Methods*, **1**, 374–406.

Ebel, R. (1961). Must all tests be valid? *American Psychologist*, **16**, 640–7.

Foot, H. and Sanford, A. (2004). The use and abuse of student participants. *The Psychologist*, **17**, 256–9.

Foster, S.L. and Cone, J.D. (1995). Validity issues in clinical assessment. *Psychological Assessment*, **7**, 248–60.

Ghiselli, E.E. (1964). *Theory of psychological measurement*. McGraw-Hill, New York.

Guion, R.M. (1965). *Personnel testing*. McGraw-Hill, New York.

Guion, R.M. (1977). Content validity: Three years of talk—what's the action? *Public Personnel Management*, **6**, 407–14.

Hays, R.D. and Hadorn, D. (1992). Responsiveness to change: An aspect of validity, not a separate dimension. *Quality of Life Research*, **1**, 73–5.

Hunter, J.E. and Schmidt, F.L. (2004). *Methods of meta-analysis: Correcting error and bias in research findings* (2nd edn.). Sage, Newbury Park, CA.

Iliescu, D. and Greiff, S. (2021) On consequential validity. *European Journal of Psychological Assessment*, **37**, 163–6.

Judd, C.M., Smith, E.R., and Kidder, L.H. (1991). *Research methods in social relations* (6th edn). Holt, Rinehart, and Winston, New York.

Kane, M.T. (2001). Current concerns in validity theory. *Journal of Educational Measurement*, **38**, 319–42.

Kelly, T.L. (1927). *Interpretation of educational measurements*. Macmillan, New York.

Kimmel, A.J. (1996). *Ethical issues in behavioral research*. Blackwell, Cambridge, MA.

Kirshner, B. and Guyatt, G. (1985). A methodological framework for assessing health indices. *Journal of Chronic Diseases*, **38**, 27–36.

Landy, F.J. (1986). Stamp collecting versus science. *American Psychologist*, **41**, 1183–92.

Liang, M.H. (2000). Longitudinal construct validity: Establishment of clinical meaning in patient evaluation instruments. *Medical Care*, **38**(Suppl. II), S84– 90.

Loevinger, J. (1954). The attenuation paradox in test theory. *Psychological Bulletin*, **51**, 493–504.

Magnusson, D. (1967). *Test theory*. Addison-Wesley, Reading, MA.

Mandich, M., Simons, C.J.R., Ritchie, S., Schmidt, D., and Mullett, M. (1994). Motor development, infantile reactions and postural responses of pre-term, at-risk infants. *Developmental Medicine & Child Neurology*, **36**, 397–405.

McNemar, Q. (1946). Opinion-attitude methodology. *Psychological Bulletin*, **43**, 289–374.

Messick, S. (1975). The standard program: Meaning and values in measurement and evaluation. *American Psychologist*, **30**, 955–66.

Messick, S. (1980). Test validity and the ethics of assessment. *American Psychologist*, **35**, 1012–27.

Messick, S. (1988). The once and future issues of validity. Assessing the meaning and consequences of measurement. In *Test validity* (eds. H. Wainer and H. Braun), pp. 33–45. Lawrence Erlbaum, Mahwah, NJ.

Messick, S. (1989). Validity. In *Educational measurement* (3rd edn) (ed. R.L. Linn), pp. 13–103. Macmillan, New York.

Messick, S. (1994). The interplay of evidence and consequences in the validation of performance assessments. *Educational Researcher*, **23**(2), 13–23.

Messick, S. (1995). Validity of psychological assessment: Validation of inferences from persons' responses and performances as scientific inquiry into score meaning. *American Psychologist*, **50**, 741–9.

Muchinsky, R.M. (1996). The correction for attenuation. *Educational and Psychological Measurement*, **56**, 78–90.

Munley, P.H. (2002). Comparability of MMPI-2 scales and profiles over time. *Journal of Personality Assessment*, **78**, 145–60.

Murphy, K.R. (ed.) (2011). *Validity generalization. A critical review*. Lawrence Erlbaum Associates, Mahwah, NJ.

Nunnally, J.C. (1970). *Introduction to psychological measurement*. McGraw-Hill, New York.

Parsons, T. (1951). *The social system*. The Free Press, New York.

Patrick, D.L. and Chiang, Y.-P. (2000). Measurement of health outcomes in treatment effectiveness evaluations: Conceptual and methodological challenges. *Medical Care*, **38**(Suppl. II), S14– 25.

Peterson, R.A. and Merunka, D.R. (2014). Convenience samples of college students and research reproducibility. *Journal of Business Research*, **67**, 1035–41.

Podsakoff, P.M., MacKenzie, S.B., Lee, J.-Y., and Podsakoff, N.P. (2003). Common method biases in behavioral research: A critical review of the literature and recommended remedies. *Journal of Applied Psychology*, **88**, 879–903.

Popham, W.J. (1997). Consequential validity: Right concern—wrong concept. *Educational Measurement: Issues and Practice*, **16**(2), 9–13.

Reckase, M. (1998). Consequential validity from the test developer's perspective. *Educational Measurement: Issues and Practice*, **17**(2), 13–16.

Ronen, G.M., Streiner, D.L., and Rosenbaum, P. (2003). Health-related quality of life in childhood epilepsy: Moving beyond 'seizure control with minimal adverse effects.' *Health and Quality of Life Outcomes*, **1** , 36.

Scheibe, S., Bagby, R.M., Miller, L.S., and Dorian, B.J. (2001). Assessing posttraumatic stress disorder with the MMPI-2 in a sample of workplace accident victims. *Psychological Assessment*, **13**, 369–74.

Schmidt, F.L. and Hunter, J.E. (1977). Development of a general solution to the problem of validity generalization. *Journal of Applied Psychology*, **62**, 529–40.

Schmidt, F.L. and Hunter, J.E. (1996). Measurement error in psychological research: Lessons from 26 research scenarios. *Psychological Methods*, **1**, 199–223.

Schmidt, F.L. and Hunter, J.E. (1999). Theory testing and measurement error. *Intelligence*, **27**, 183–98.

Streiner, D.L. (2015). Statistical commentary series: Commentary #6 – Are trial participants representative of "real" patients? *Journal of Clinical Psychopharmacology*, **35**, 4–6.

Thorndike, R.L. (1949). *Personnel selection: Test and measurement techniques*. Wiley, New York.

Zumbo, B.D. (2009). Validity as contextualized as pragmatic explanation and its implications for validation practice. In *The concept of validity: Revisions, new directions and applications* (ed. R.W. Lissitz), pp. 65–82. Information Age, Charlotte, NC.

Chapter 11

Measuring change

Introduction to measuring change

The measurement of change has been a topic of considerable confusion in the medical literature. As clinicians and researchers, we view that the ultimate goal of most treatments—medical, surgical, psychosocial, or educational—is to induce change (hopefully positive) in the patient's or student's status. It would appear to follow that the measurement of change in patients' health state or in a student's level of understanding is an appropriate goal of research. A number of articles (Guyatt et al. 1987; MacKenzie et al. 1986) have advocated this position, both on the grounds that the measurement of change in a patient's condition is the goal of clinical care and should be addressed by research methods, and on the methodological basis that instruments which are responsive to changes in health status are more sensitive measures of the effects of clinical interventions than those which simply assess health status after an intervention.

However, this opinion is by no means unanimous. Several authors in education and psychology have taken stands against the use of difference scores (Burckhardt et al. 1982; Cronbach and Furby 1970). In this chapter, we explore the issues surrounding the use of change scores and show that these divergent positions are based on different views of the goals of measurement, and different assumptions regarding the methodological advantages and disadvantages of change measures.

The goal of measurement of change

In order to understand the source of the controversy in the literature, it is necessary to recognize that the measurement of change can be directed at different goals. These have been described by Linn and Slinde (1977):

1. *To measure differences between individuals in the amount of change.* Although apparently similar to the notion of reliability, the intent here is to distinguish between those individuals who *change a lot* and those who *change little*. For example, if we wanted to identify individuals who were responsive to therapy (e.g. in a secondary analysis of a trial of therapy for arthritis), we would proceed by a comparison of individual differences in change scores. Much of the literature in psychology addressing the measurement of change accepts this as the basic goal of change measurement.

2. *To identify correlates of change.* This goal really represents an elaboration of the first. If we were successful at identifying responsive subgroups in a trial of therapy, a logical second step is to attempt to identify those factors which are associated or

correlated with good response. The issues of measurement also follow from the earlier concerns: if we cannot differentiate between those who change a great deal and those who change little, the resulting restriction in range will attenuate any attempt to find correlates.

3. *To infer treatment effects from group differences.* This goal is probably the primary goal of most clinical trials. By randomly assigning individuals to treatment and control groups, measuring the health state before and after treatment, and then comparing the average change in health state in the groups, we can determine a treatment effect—individuals in a treatment group will change, on the average, more than those in a control group.

The first and last goals work against one another. To the extent that there are individual differences in response to treatment, this is an indication that the treatment had different effects on different people, and it will be more difficult to detect an overall treatment effect. However, if there are individual differences in response to treatment, then we will be able to identify responsive subgroups and possible prognostic factors; if there are no individual differences, we will be unsuccessful in this search.

Note, however, that there is no conflict in the goal of discrimination between individuals, as expressed in the reliability coefficient, and the goal of evaluation of change within individuals. It is certainly possible that there may be large and stable differences between individuals on some measure, yet all may change equally in response to treatment, so we can infer an overall treatment effect. If we consider the everyday example of dieting, overweight people may range from 60 to 150 kg; yet a conservative and successful diet would have all losing from 1 to 2 kg per week. As long as there was reasonable consistency in the amount of weight loss experienced by different individuals in the plan, it would not be difficult to demonstrate the efficacy of a treatment programme which showed losses of this order, despite the large differences in individual weights. So the presence of large differences among individuals does not, of itself, preclude the demonstration of small treatment effects.

Why not measure change directly?

The remainder of this chapter will address different ways to combine measures taken at various times (usually two) to best measure the amount of change in individuals or groups. This seems, on the surface, to be a complicated way to go about things. Why not simply ask people how much they have changed, which appears a much more straightforward method? Clinicians do it all the time; for example, the following seem likely ways to ask the question:

'Since I put you on the new drug at your last visit, have you got better or worse? How much?'

'Since your illness began a few months ago, have you been getting better or worse? How much?'

'Thinking back to when you first noticed this symptom, how much worse has it got?'

Although this is a time-honoured approach, there is a very good reason to avoid asking about change directly: people simply do not remember how they were at the beginning.

We have already noted in Chapter 6 that retrospective judgements of change are vulnerable to potential bias. The two biases that are most evident are:

1. *Implicit theory of change.* It is very difficult for people to remember their past state unless there is a salient event associated with it. Ross (1989) showed that, when asked how they felt 'last September', people commonly begin with their present state ('How do I feel today?'), then invoke an implicit theory of change ('How do I think the drug worked?'), and then work backwards to an estimate of what their prior state must have been. As a consequence, the correlation between measures of change and the present state is high, but between the change measure and the prior state is low (Guyatt et al. 2000). So a retrospective assessment of an initial state is not to be trusted.

2. *Response shift.* Conversely, the initial assessment may be wrong. If you are suffering from a chronic illness like an arthritic hip, you may have adjusted to your condition and so rate your health or quality of life fairly high. However, after hip replacement, looking back you realize just how incapacitated you were. This phenomenon is called 'response shift' (Schwarz and Sprangers 1999). In this framework, the subjective estimate of change is based on consistent estimates of initial and current state, and the initial assessment is not to be trusted.

The two theories lead to opposite predictions, and there are many circumstances in assessing health status where the same phenomenon can be interpreted in diametrically opposite ways (Norman 2003). One thing, however, is clear: both theories identify potential for bias in measures based on subjective estimates of change.

Measures of association—reliability and sensitivity to change

The different goals of measurement are reflected in different coefficients, analogous to the reliability coefficient, which express the ability of an instrument to detect change within subjects or the effects of treatment. In order to clarify these distinctions, let us consider a group of six individuals who have entered into a diet plan and are weighed before treatment and again after 2 weeks of dieting. The data might look like Table 11.1.

As we discussed earlier in this chapter, the goal of discriminating among subjects has been incorporated in the notion of *reliability*, which we discussed at length in Chapter 8, and is defined as:

$$Reliability(R) = \frac{\sigma^2_{pat}}{\sigma^2_{pat} + \sigma^2_{err}}$$

In the present example, the reliability focuses on the ability of the measure to distinguish among patients' average weights—for example (from Table 11.1) 106, 128.5, 128.5, and so on. Patient variance, σ^2_{pat}, would be computed from these means, and σ^2_{err} would be calculated as the difference between individual observations and their mean—for example $(110 - 106)^2$, $(125 - 128.5)^2$, $(133 - 128.5)^2$, and so on). Note that

Table 11.1 Weight (in kg) of six patients in a diet clinic

Patient	Before	After 2 weeks	Average	Change
1	110	102	106	−8
2	125	132	128.5	+7
3	133	124	128.5	7
4	98	99	98.5	+1
5	108	98	103	−10
6	86	89	87.5	+3
Mean	110	107.3	108.6	−2.7

this would be a 'pre-test–post-test' reliability, which is not based on repeated observations over a short time.

By analogy, we can also develop a measure to describe the reliability of the change score, that is, an index of the ability of the measure to discriminate between those subjects who *change* a great deal and those who change little. To do so, we need to separately determine the reliability of the pre-test and post-test (e.g. on day 1 and day 2, on day 13 and day 14) in order to distinguish between 'real' change from pre-test to post-test and simple measurement error.

Reliability of the change score

The assessment of the ability of an instrument to detect individual differences in change scores is appropriately labelled as the *reliability of the change score* (Lord and Novick 1968). By analogy to the reliability coefficient, this can be expressed as:

$$Reliability(D) = \frac{\sigma_D^2}{\sigma_D^2 + \sigma_{err(D)}^2}$$

where σ_D^2 expresses the systematic difference between subjects in their *change* score (based on the difference between the initial and final observations 2 weeks later), and $\sigma_{err}^2(D)$ is the error associated with this estimate. In our example, σ_D^2 would be derived from a sum of squares calculated as:

$$SS_D = \left(-8-(-2.7)\right)^2 + \left(7-(-2.7)\right)^2 + \cdots + \left(3-(-2.7)\right)^2.$$

The reliability of the change score can be shown to be related to the variance of pre-test (*x*) and post-test (*y*) scores, their reliability (*R*) (which would come from the observations on days 1 and 2, and days 13 and 14), and the correlation between pre-test and post-test (*r*), in the following manner:

$$Reliability(D) = \frac{\sigma_X^2 R_{XX} + \sigma_Y^2 R_{YY} - 2\sigma_X \sigma_Y r_{XY}}{\sigma_X^2 + \sigma_Y^2 - 2\sigma_X \sigma_Y r_{XY}}$$

If the pre-test and post-test have the same variances, this expression reduces to:

$$Reliability = \frac{R_{XX} + R_{YY} - 2r_{XY}}{2.0 - 2r_{XY}}$$

where R_{xx} and R_{yy} are the reliabilities of the initial and final measurements. In our previous example, assume we measured the reliability as 0.95 for both pre-test and post-test. The calculated correlation between the two measures using the data above is 0.91. Then the reliability of the difference score becomes:

$$Reliability(D) = \frac{0.95 + 0.95 - 2 \times 0.91}{2.0 - 2 \times 0.91} = 0.08 / 0.18 = 0.44$$

This is much smaller than the reliability of the scores themselves. In the limiting case, it can be demonstrated that, under the circumstances where there is a perfect correlation between the pre-test and post-test scores, the reliability of the difference score is zero. Although this appears strange, it actually follows from the basic notion of discriminating between those who change a great deal and those who change little. If an experimental intervention resulted in a uniform response to treatment, all patients would improve an equal amount. As a result, the variance of the change score will be zero, since every patient's post-test score would be equal to their pre-test score, except for a constant; no patients would have changed more or less than any other, and the reliability of the difference score would be zero.

Since a perfectly uniform response to treatment would represent an ideal state of affairs for the use of change scores to measure treatment effects, yet would yield a reliability coefficient for change scores of zero, it should not be used as an index appropriate for assessing the ability of an instrument to measure treatment effects, and some other approach must be used.

Responsiveness—sensitivity to change

In assessing change, it is reasonable to presume that some measures, for whatever reason, may be more sensitive to changes resulting from treatments than others. If so, it is useful to have standard indices, perhaps analogous to the reliability coefficient, to compare one instrument to another.

Although it is possible to create an index of sensitivity to change resulting from treatment effects that is a direct analogy of the reliability coefficient and has the form of an intraclass correlation, this is rarely used in the literature. Instead, there have been a number of indices proposed, most of which are variants on an effect size (average change divided by the standard deviation; Cohen 1988).

First, a word about terminology. As we mentioned in Chapter 10, Liang (2000) differentiates between *sensitivity to change*, which taps an instrument's ability to measure any degree of change, and *responsiveness*, which assesses its ability to measure clinically important change. In this section, we will follow Liang, and deal with sensitivity to change first, then discuss the issue of clinical importance at the end. Further, a number of authors (e.g. Kirshner and Guyatt 1985), primarily in the area of health-related quality of life, have proposed that sensitivity or responsiveness should be considered a third essential measurement property of an instrument, equal with reliability and validity. Not everyone agrees. As we discussed in Chapter 10, we and others (e.g. Hays and Hadorn 1992; Patrick and Chiang 2000) view it as just one form of construct validity, assessing the hypothesis that the instrument is capable of detecting clinically meaningful change. However, if the data are available, it would make sense to report this when discussing validity.

Regardless of its status, the starting point for examining sensitivity to change is a comparison of the mean score (or mean change score) of a group of patients who were given a successful therapy and the mean of a second group who were not. These means, or mean changes, are then used to compute a difference between treatment and control groups. This difference is then compared to some estimate of variability to create a dimensionless ratio.

Regrettably, while there is not universal consensus on the importance of responsiveness as a separate test attribute, there is even less agreement as to how to measure it. As we indicated, most but not all measures are variants on an effect size (ES), but here the similarity ends. Different measures of variability are used, and some numerical multipliers are also used. A brief catalogue of current favourites follows.

Cohen's effect size

The grandfather of all of these measures is Cohen's effect size (Cohen 1988), which is simply the ratio of the mean difference due to treatment to the standard deviation (SD) of baseline scores. Since it is a fairly general construct, initially proposed simply as a basis for sample size calculations, it can be applied to the change observed in a single group from pre-test to post-test, or the difference between the post-test score of a treatment or control group, or, for that matter, the difference between change scores of a treatment and control group. In any case, the denominator would be the SD at baseline of the control group, in which case it is also referred to as *Glass's* Δ (Glass 1976), or the pooled SD at baseline of the treatment and control groups, which is referred to as *Cohen's d* (Rosenthal 1994). The advantage of *d* is that it uses all of the data, and so is a more stable estimate of the SD.

Guyatt's responsiveness

Guyatt's measure (Guyatt et al. 1987) is specific to a pre-test/post-test, two-group design, and is a variant of the ES. In this case, it is the ratio of the mean change *in the treatment group* to the standard deviation of the change scores *in the control group*. It is not at all clear, since there is a control group, why this index would not use a numerator based on the difference between mean change in the treatment group and mean change in the control group. Further, it assumes that there is no change in the control group, although we know that the placebo response in studies of depression ranges between 30 and 50 per cent (Sonawalla and Rosenbaum 2002) , and is almost equal to the effect of analgesics in the treatment of pain (Tuttle et al. 2015). To assume no change in the control group also ignores other phenomena (e.g. regression towards the mean; random fluctuations in symptoms) likely to result in change even in the absence of intervention. For these reasons, Guyatt's measure is likely an overestimate of the effect of the intervention, and we see little use for it.

The standardized response mean

McHorney and Tarlov (1995) have suggested a different effect size, called the standardized response mean, or SRM, which is the ratio of the mean change (in a single group) to the standard deviation of the change scores. This has more of the form of a statistical test of a difference, and is simply the paired t-test multiplied by $\sqrt{n}$, where n is the sample size.

We can actually show a relationship between the SRM and the ES. The standard deviation of the difference score is just $\sqrt{2} \times SEM$ (standard error of measurement), and the SEM, in turn, is equal to:

$$SEM = SD_{Baseline} \times \sqrt{1 - R}$$

so the SRM is just ES divided by $\sqrt{2(1 - R)}$

These indices do not exhaust the possibilities, but are clearly the most common. As we have seen, all are, at their core, variants on the ES, differing only in whether you use the SD of baseline scores of the control group, the pooled SD of both groups, or the SD of difference scores, and whether there is a numerical multiplier. But the differences among them are more ecclesiastical than substantive.

Conceptual problems with sensitivity to change

Aside from the theoretical problems with sensitivity to change and the potpourri of coefficients we just discussed, there are two real problems with trying to calculate it as a property of the instrument.

The first is that, just as reliability is a property of an instrument *as applied to a particular population* and is sensitive to the variance of the sample, sensitivity to change resulting from a treatment is a characteristic of both the treatment and the inherent precision and measurement error of the instrument. Simply put, all instruments are more responsive to large treatment effects than to small ones. But the situation is more tenuous with sensitivity to change than with reliability. It is not all that difficult to select a sample which can be assumed to have, on average, characteristics (mean, standard deviation) of the population to which you ultimately want to apply the measure. But it is a lot more difficult to contemplate selecting a treatment that is representative of the treatments you want to apply the instrument to. That is, presumably you want to show that the sensitivity to change is adequate for the kind of treatments you want to measure. But how can you determine a priori how big those treatment effects are likely to be? And how do you select a single treatment which is right in the middle of them? It clearly matters. Any instrument will be much more sensitive to large treatments than small ones, so it is hard to disentangle characteristics of the instrument from characteristics of the treatment.

One solution is to apply multiple instruments—the new one, and existing validated measures—to the same group of patients who are undergoing a standard and effective treatment, and then look at the relative sensitivity to change of the various measures. But it is very difficult to get funding to examine a group of patients who are given a known efficacious therapy. National agencies most likely will not fund it; drug companies definitely will not.

A second solution that has seen widespread application is to simply follow a group of patients for some period of time and administer the instrument at beginning and end. You then ask the patients at the completion whether they have got better, stayed the same, or got worse and by how much (a little, quite a bit, a lot). Finally you compute the average change on the instrument for those who have got a little better.

However appealing the strategy, it contains a fatal flaw (Norman et al. 1997). The problem is that, in any group of patients followed over time, some will get better, some stay the same, and some will get worse, just through random fluctuation. Even if, on average, there is no overall treatment effect, some people will get better. Indeed, the variability in response is just the statistical fluctuation that makes it difficult to detect treatment effects and ends up in the denominator of statistical tests of treatment effects. In the extreme, you can end up with high responsiveness even in a situation where the average treatment effect is zero or even negative.

Difficulties with change scores in experimental designs

Potential loss of precision

Although it would appear that it is always desirable to measure change, since it removes the effect of variance between patients, this is actually not the case. The calculation of a difference score is based on the difference between two quantities, the pre-test and post-test, and both are measured with some error, σ_{err}^2. If this quantity is sufficiently large relative to the variance between patients, the net result might be to introduce more, rather than less, error into the estimate of treatment effect.

The conditions under which it makes sense to measure change within patients as a measure of treatment effect can be expressed in terms of a reliability coefficient. The use of change scores to estimate treatment main effects is only appropriate when the variance between subjects exceeds the error variance within subjects. This is equivalent to the following expression:

$$\frac{\sigma_{sub}^2}{\sigma_{sub}^2 + \sigma_{err}^2} \geq 0.5$$

Thus, one should only use change scores when the reliability of the measure exceeds 0.5. Reliability is not irrelevant or inversely related to sensitivity—*reliability is a necessary pre-condition for the appropriate application of change scores.* This analysis does not, of course, imply that measures that are reliable are, of necessity, useful for the assessment of change. Even if an instrument is reliable, it remains to be shown that differences in response to treatment can be detected before the instrument can be used for the assessment of change.

Biased measurement of treatment effects

The simple subtraction of post-treatment from pre-treatment scores to create a difference score as a measure of the overall effect of treatment assumes that the effect of treatment will be the same, except for random error, for all patients. This assumption can be shown to be false in many, if not most circumstances. For example, one major cause of an individual having an extreme score on pre-test is simply an accumulation of random processes; that is, the very good scores are to some extent due to good luck, and the very bad scores are due to bad luck. To the extent that chance is operative (and any reliability coefficient less than 1 is an indication of the presence of random variation), then the very good are likely to get worse, and the very bad get better, on retest. This effect is known as 'regression to the mean' (Streiner 2001). In effect, the best line fitting post-test to pre-treatment data in the absence of treatment effects has a slope less than 1 and an intercept greater than 0. The use of change scores assumes a best-fit line with a slope of 1 and intercept of 0. The consequence of regression to the mean is that the use of change or difference scores overestimates the effect of pre-test differences on post-test scores.

The solution to this problem for assessing individual change recommended by Cronbach and Furby (1970) is the use of *residualized gain scores*. Instead of subtracting pre-test from post-test, we first fit the line relating the pre-test and post-test scores using regression analysis. We then estimate the post-test score of each patient from the regression equation. The residualized gain score is the difference between the actual post-test score and the score that was predicted from the regression equation. In other words, the residualized gain score removes from consideration that portion of the gain score which was linearly predictable from the pre-test score. What remains is an indication of those individuals who changed more or less than was expected.

This operation is really designed to identify individual differences in change in an unbiased manner. Cronbach and Furby (1970), among others, have commented on the use of change scores to estimate overall treatment effects, and conclude that analysis of covariance (ANCOVA) methods should be employed when the reliability is sufficiently large, and simple post-test scores otherwise.

The reason for the use of ANCOVA is again related to the phenomenon of regression to the mean. As we discussed, the change score assumes that the line relating pre-test to post-test has a slope of 1 and intercept 0, which is not the optimal line when error of measurement is present. The result is that the denominator of the statistical test of treatment effects includes variance due to lack of fit, resulting in a conservative test. Since ANCOVA fits an optimum line to the data, in general, this will result in a smaller error term and a more sensitive test of treatment effects.

Change scores and quasi-experimental designs

So far, we have addressed the use of change scores in the context of randomized trials, where the primary goal is to increase the sensitivity of statistical tests by reducing the magnitude of the error term. There is another potential application of these methods in situations such as cohort analytical studies, where there are likely to be initial differences between treatment and control groups. In this situation, the change score has an apparent advantage, in that the subtraction of the initial score for each subject will have the effect of eliminating the initial differences between groups.

However, when the change score is used in a situation where there are differences between the two groups on the pre-test measure, as might result if subjects were not allocated at random to the two conditions, additional complications arise. These are directly related to the effect of regression to the mean, discussed in the section 'Biased measurement of treatment effects'. In the absence of treatment effects, individuals measured with some random error will not stay the same on retest. Those who were very good will worsen, on average, and those who were very bad will improve.

Unfortunately this effect also applies to group means, which are simply the average of individual scores. In the absence of any treatment effect, the differences between groups will be reduced at the second testing, confounding any interpretation of differences between groups observed following treatment. One way around this problem is again the use of ANCOVA; however, this method is a refinement to the use of change scores, not a fundamentally different approach.

There are other fundamental reasons to view any attempt at post-hoc adjustment for differences between groups on pre-test, whether by difference scores, repeated measures analysis of variance (ANOVA), or ANCOVA, with considerable suspicion. Implicit in these analytical methods is a specific model of the change process that cannot be assumed to have general applicability. This is illustrated in Fig. 11.1.

Any of the analytical methods assume that, in the absence of any treatment effect, the experimental and control group will grow at the same rate, so that the difference in means at the beginning would equal the difference in means at the end, and any additional difference between the two groups (shown as the difference between the post-test mean of the treated group and the dotted line) is evidence of a treatment effect.

Unfortunately, there are any number of plausible alternative models, which will fit the data equally well. For example, in a rehabilitation setting or in an educational programme for developmentally disabled children, individuals who are less impaired, who thus score higher initially, may have the greatest capacity for change or improvement over time. Under these circumstances, referred to in the literature as a 'fan-spread' model, the observed data would be obtained in the absence of any treatment effect, and ANCOVA or analysis of difference scores would wrongly conclude a benefit from treatment.

Conversely, a situation may arise where a 'ceiling effect' occurs; that is, individuals with high scores initially may already be at the limit of their potential, and thus would be expected to improve relatively less with treatment than those with initially lower scores. In this circumstance, the post-test scores in the absence of an effect of treatment would converge, and the analysis would underestimate the treatment effect.

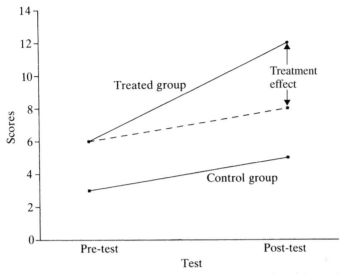

Fig. 11.1 Relation between pre-test and post-test scores in a quasi-experimental design.

It is evident that any analysis based on just one or two means for each group will not permit a choice among these models of growth, and additional points on the individual growth curve would be required (Rogosa et al. 1982). Of course, if such situations were rare, one could argue for the adequacy of change score approaches; however, it is likely that situations of non-constant growth are the rule, not the exception, in health research. As Lord (1967) put it, 'There simply is no logical or statistical procedure that can be counted on to make proper allowances for uncontrolled pre-existing differences between groups' (p. 305). The bottom line is that ANCOVA works well to account for baseline differences *within the context of randomized controlled trials*, when such differences are due to the play of chance. With cohort and case-control studies, its use depends on untestable assumptions and can lead to very different results than simply using difference scores. This situation, referred to as *Lord's paradox*, is discussed by Wainer (1991).

Measuring change using multiple observations: growth curves

In the last section ('Change scores and quasi-experimental designs'), we alluded to the problems associated with inferring change from two observations. In part, these problems result from the very simple model of change that is implied by a simple pre-test/post-test approach. Change looks like a quantum process: first you are in one state, then you are in another state. Individual change obviously does not occur this way. It is a continuous process, whether we are speaking of physical change (e.g. growth or recovery from trauma), intellectual change (learning or development), or emotional change. Moreover, it is probably non-linear. Some individuals may make an initially rapid recovery from an illness and then improve slowly; some may improve gradually at first and then more rapidly; and of course some may deteriorate or fluctuate around a stable state of partial recovery.

It is evident that any reasonable attempt to characterize these individual *growth curves* will require multiple points of observation, so that a statistical curve can be fitted. While this sounds laborious, in many circumstances multiple observations are available, and only await an appropriate method for analysis. For example, many treatment programmes extend across multiple visits, and frequently the clinician makes systematic observations in order to assess response to therapy and possibly adjust treatment. If multiple observations are available, it makes little sense to base an assessment of treatment effect only on assessments at the beginning and end of treatment, which would throw away a great deal of data. Even if the change is uniform and linear, so that there is no apparent advantage of assessment methods based on individual growth, the use of multiple observations amounts to an increase in sample size, with a corresponding reduction of within-subject error and an increase in statistical power.

There is a growing consensus on approaches to the appropriate analysis of data of this form (Bryk and Raudenbush 1987; Francis et al. 1991; Rogosa et al. 1982). The basic idea common to all methods is to develop an analytical model of the relationship between individual growth and time, then estimate the parameters of the model using a variant of regression analysis. In its simplest form, it involves no more than using standard options within some ANOVA packages to break down the variance into linear and higher-order terms. That is, instead of simply estimating the means of all patients at each time point, we first fit a straight line to the means over time, then a quadratic (time^2) term, then a cubic (time^3) term, and so on. If there were repeated observations for a total of k time points, then the data would be fitted with a $(k - 1)$ degree polynomial. Thus, in the simplest case where there are only two time points, the best we can do is fit a $(k - 1) = 1$ degree polynomial : i.e. a straight line. As it turns out, a straight line goes rather well through two points.

To make things more concrete, imagine a series of patients with acute knee injuries enrolled in a physiotherapy programme for treatment. Suppose the therapist aims for biweekly treatments over a total period of 3 weeks. Table 11.2 shows data for eight such patients.

It is always useful to graph the data prior to analysis, and we have done this in Fig. 11.2, which shows the individual data as curves, as well as the mean at each time in the bold line. Examining the overall means first, it is evident that they fall on a nearly straight line as a function of time, with a small amount of curvature. This fact suggests that the data could be modelled quite successfully with a linear function, which has only two parameters, the slope and the intercept, and possibly a small quadratic (time^2) term.

We do not usually approach the analysis this way, however. With ANOVA or ANCOVA , we simply look for differences among means; the data at each time could be interchanged and the results would be the same; and the analysis is completely indifferent to the actual functional relationship between time and the dependent variable. In fact, it does not account for the difference in timing of the follow-up visits, since time is treated as simply a categorical variable. What we really want is an analysis

Table 11.2 Range of motion (in degrees) of knee joints for eight patients enrolled in a treatment programme at baseline and over five follow-up visits

Patient	Baseline	Follow-up visit				
		1	**2**	**3**	**4**	**5**
1	22	23	25	36	42	44
2	30	35	44	51	56	60
3	44	48	50	55	63	66
4	28	32	35	39	42	44
5	40	45	50	57	61	64
6	32	33	35	38	38	37
7	22	27	30	37	42	43
8	40	45	46	55	56	58
Mean	32.25	36.00	39.38	46.00	50.00	52.00

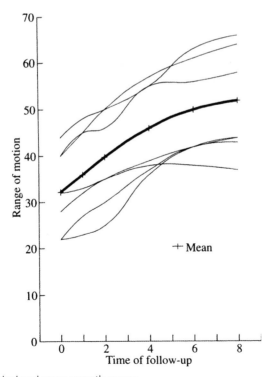

Fig. 11.2 Individual and mean growth curves.

that separately tests the degree of linear change, and any other components. We can show this contrast between the two methods by doing the regular ANCOVA and also conducting a second analysis, called an 'orthogonal decomposition', where the linear, quadratic, and higher order polynomials are modelled. The results are shown in Table 11.3.

The orthogonal analysis confirms our observations from the graph. The linear relationship with time is highly significant ($F = 52.63$, $p = 0.0002$); the quadratic term is also highly significant ($F = 39.42$, $p = 0.0004$); and no other terms are significant. Note that the sums of squares are additive, so that the conventional result can be obtained by simply adding up all the trend sums of squares to get the overall effect of time; and all the patient time sums of squares to get the overall patient × time term. This results in a significant overall effect of time; the F value is slightly lower, but it is more significant (because the degrees of freedom in the numerator are 4 instead of 1).

Why are the results not all that different between the two analyses? In this case, it is because the individual growth curves are quite different. There is a large patient × time interaction, showing that individual patients are changing at quite different rates. This can be tested manually by taking the ratio of the patient time interaction (27.17 in the Mean Square column) to the appropriate error term, which comes from the Sum of Squares column divided by the sum of the corresponding degrees of freedom ([11.64 + 13.85 + 11.38]/21 = 1.75) , resulting in an overall test of the difference in patients in

Table 11.3 Analysis of covariance of range of motion data, compared to conventional analysis

Source	Sum of squares	Degrees of freedom	Mean square	F	Tail probability
Orthogonal decomposition					
Baseline	2509	1	2509	23.40	0.003
Patients	643.5	6	107.2		
Linear trend	1430.1	1	1430.1	52.63	0.0002
Patient × time[1]	190.2	7	27.17		
Quadratic trend	65.5	1	65.5	39.42	0.0004
Patients × time[2]	11.64	7	1.665		
Cubic trend	0.37	1	0.37	0.19	0.67
Patient × time[3]	13.85	7	1.98		
Quadratic trend	0.80	1	0.804	0.50	0.50
Patient × time[4]	11.38	7	1.62		
Conventional analysis					
Time	1496.9	4	374.2	46.14	<0.0001
Patient × time	227.1	28	8.11		

linear trend of $(27.17/1.75) = 15.5$, which is highly significant. As a result, the gain in statistical power is only marginal.

In general, if all the error variance results from systematic differences in the slopes of individual growth curves (i.e. all subjects are changing at different rates), then the overall ANOVA will be more powerful than the trend analysis. Conversely, if all subjects are changing linearly at the same rate, the trend analysis is more powerful.

Modelling individual growth

While the methods outlined in the previous section are a more satisfactory strategy for modelling change when multiple observations are available than the use of standard ANOVA methods, they do have a severe restriction. Ordinary analysis software for repeated measures ANOVA, with or without trend analysis, requires a complete data set; all subjects must be measured at the same times and all subjects must have data at each time point. Any missing data will result in the complete loss of the case. This is an obvious constraint when applied to the real world of scattered follow-up visits or repeated assessments. A more complex analysis to accommodate this involves the idea that each person's data should be fitted separately, since growths are individual (Rogosa et al. 1982). Then each parameter of the overall growth curve (the factor, or *beta weight*, multiplying each term) becomes a random variable with its own mean and standard deviation, rather than a point estimate.

In effect, we reconceptualize the problem as one of modelling individual change, using whatever data are available on each subject, then aggregating these data (that is, the growth parameters) over all subjects. Under this model, it is unnecessarily restrictive to constrain time of assessment to a few standard points. We then analyse the data as two regression problems. The first step is to conduct individual regression analyses for each subject, estimating the intercept plus the linear, quadratic, and other higher-order growth parameters. The second step is to then aggregate the parameters across all subjects, essentially treating the intercept and the growth parameters as random, normally distributed variables. If the goal is to predict individual growth, the parameters are estimated using a second regression equation, where the dependent variable is the growth parameter and the various predictors (e.g. initial severity, age, fitness) are independent variables. The method is called *hierarchical regression modelling* (Bryk and Raudenbush 1987). Over the past few years, a number of software packages, including SPSS, SAS, and others, have implemented routines that are capable of modelling individual growth parameters as random variables. The method uses maximum likelihood estimation procedures, and as a result does not create the usual ANOVA table; instead, the parameters with their standard errors are estimated directly, similar to a regression analysis. A typical computer output, using the same data set, is shown in Table 11.4.

The p-values suggest that the results are similar to those observed previously. This can be confirmed by squaring the Z-scores, which are interpretable as F values. Thus, this analysis results in an F-test for the baseline measurement of 3.86 (1.967^2) vs. 23.40 previously; a linear term of 98.2 (9.911^2) vs. the 52.6 observed previously; and an F-test for the quadratic term of 41.33 vs. 39.42 previously, so we have gained some statistical

Table 11.4 Analysis of individual growth curves using maximum likelihood procedures

Parameter	Estimate	Asymptotic SE	Z-score	Two-sided p-value
1. Baseline	70.9203	36.0466	1.967	0.050
2. Linear	4.63821	0.4680	9.911	<0.001
3. Quadratic	−0.25805	0.0401	-6.429	<0.001

power using this approach. In general, when the data are complete the results will be similar; however, this method accommodates incomplete data sets.

In practice, the analyses are more complex than what is shown here. We begin with a 'null' model (one containing no predictors except group membership). If this explains most of the variance, we can stop. But, if there is unexplained variance, we would add in covariates and see which one(s) can account for the differences in the intercept, the slope, and the interaction between the two (in essence, an index of regression to the mean effects). If the quadratic or cubic effects are significant, we would look for predictors of these, too.

One step up the ladder in sophistication from growth curve analysis is *latent class* growth curve analysis. Rather than assuming the same trajectory for all people, this technique seeks to determine if there may be different classes of trajectories. For example, in a study of the quality of life (QOL) of children with epilepsy, we found that there were six different trajectories, which varied according to the overall level of QOL and whether it increased, decreased, or remained stable over time (Ferro et al. 2017).

How much change is enough?

In this chapter and Chapter 7, we have discussed how to measure change and how to set cut points that differentiate between groups. Astute readers may have noticed that nowhere did we discuss the issue of how much change is 'enough', or whether the groups were 'really' different despite statistically significant differences in scores. In part, this reflects the fact that this is still an open and contentious issue, about which there is little consensus.

In Chapter 7, we discussed one approach to the issue, called the Minimally Important Difference (MID; Jaeschke et al. 1989), and the problems that exist in trying to establish it. In fact, Norman et al. (2003) showed, in a review of 56 MIDs computed in 29 studies, that the mean MID was almost exactly equal to Cohen's 'moderate' effect size of 0.5; and further, that this was equivalent to the detection threshold of humans in a variety of discrimination tasks. In short, it may well be that an ES of 0.5 is a reasonable first approximation to a threshold of important change. Although circumstances will undoubtedly emerge that differ from this approximation, there is remarkable consistency in the empirical estimates of minimal change across a large variety of scaling methods, clinical conditions, and methodologies to estimate minimal change.

In contrast to determining important change for *groups*, techniques have been developed, primarily in the psychotherapy research literature, to evaluate change in *individuals*. Jacobson et al. (1984) outlined three criteria:

1. The patient's score should initially be within the range found for dysfunctional groups.
2. The score at the end of treatment should fall within the 'normal' range.
3. The amount of change is more than would be expected by measurement error.

The first two criteria seemingly raise the issue of cut points again, albeit in a somewhat different context. One solution, proposed by Kendall et al. (1999), is to use data from already existing large 'normative' groups, obviating the circularity of defining change based on the study that is trying to induce it. A different solution, using Bayesian statistics to account for differences in the prevalences of the functional and dysfunctional groups, is to establish a cut point (again from pre-existing data or from the study itself). If the variances of the two groups are similar, Hsu (1996) proposes the formula to derive the cut point (c) as:

$$c = \frac{s^2 \times 2.3026 \times \log_e BR_F / BR_D}{\bar{X}_D - \bar{X}_F} + \frac{\bar{X}_D + \bar{X}_F}{2}$$

where the subscript F refers to the Functional group and the subscript D to the Dysfunctional group; the BRs are the base rates; and s is the pooled standard deviation. (The article also gives the far more complicated formula for the case of unequal variances.)

The third criterion has led to the development of the *reliable change index* (Jacobson and Truax 1991), to take into account the measurement error of the instrument. This was modified by Christensen and Mendoza (1986) to use both the pre- and post-test distributions of scores; and by Hageman and Arrindell (1993) to account for regression to the mean. The RC_{ID} is defined as:

$$RC_{ID} = \frac{\left(x_{post} - x_{pre}\right) r_{DD} + \left(\bar{X}_{Post} + \bar{X}_{Pre}\right)\left(1 - r_{DD}\right)}{\sqrt{SEM_{Pre}^2 + SEM_{Post}^2}}$$

where R_{DD} is the reliability of the change score, as we calculated at the beginning of the chapter. A reliable change has occurred if RC_{ID} is greater than 1.96.

Although this approach was developed to determine if an individual subject has changed, it is possible to calculate the score for each person in various groups and use χ^2 type statistics to see if more people in the experimental group improved compared to the comparison group. A very good summary of the issues involved in the reliable change index is given in Wise (2004).

Summary

This chapter has attempted to resolve some controversies surrounding the measurement of change. There are two distinct purposes for measuring change: examining overall effects of treatments, and distinguishing individual differences in treatment response. Focusing on the former, we demonstrated that reliability and sensitivity to change are different but related concepts. We determined the conditions under which the measurement of change will result in increased and decreased statistical power. We also reviewed the literature on the use of change scores to correct for baseline differences and concluded that this purpose can rarely be justified.

As an extension of the methods to measure change, we have considered in detail the use of growth curves in the circumstances where there are more than two observations per subject. The method is conceptually more satisfactory than the classical approach of considering only a beginning and an end point. In addition, growth curve analyses appropriately use all the data available from individual subjects, even when they are measured at different times after the initial assessment.

Further reading

Collins, L.M. and Horn, J.L. (eds.) (1991). *Best methods for the analysis of change.* American Psychological Association, Washington, DC.

Collins, L.M. and Horn, J.L. (eds.) (2001). *New methods for the analysis of change.* American Psychological Association, Washington, DC.

Nunnally, J.C., Jr. (1975). The study of change in evaluation research: Principles concerning measurement, experimental design, and analysis. In *Handbook of evaluation research* (eds. E.L. Struening and M. Guttentag), pp. 101–37. Sage, Beverly Hills, CA.

References

Bryk, A.S. and Raudenbush, S.W. (1987). Application of hierarchical linear models to assessing change. *Psychological Bulletin*, **101**, 147–58.

Burckhardt, C.S., Goodwin, L.D., and Prescott, P.A. (1982). The measurement of change in nursing schools: Statistical considerations. *Nursing Research*, **31**, 53–5.

Christensen, L. and Mendoza, J.L. (1986). A method of assessing change in a single subject: An alteration of the RC index. *Behavior Therapy*, **17**, 305–8.

Cohen, J. (1988). *Statistical power analysis for the behavioral sciences* (2nd edn). Lawrence Erlbaum, Hillsdale, NJ.

Cronbach, L.J. and Furby, L. (1970). How should we measure 'change'—or should we? *Psychological Bulletin*, **74**, 68–80.

Ferro, M.A., Avery, L., Fayed, N., Streiner, D.L., Cunningham, C.E., Boyle, M.H., et al. (2017). Child- and parent-reported quality of life trajectories in children with epilepsy: A prospective cohort study. *Epilepsia*, **58**, 1277–86.

Francis, D.J., Fletcher, J.M., Stuebing, K.K., Davidson, K.C., and Thompson, N.M. (1991). Analysis of change: Modeling individual growth. *Journal of Consulting and Clinical Psychology*, **59**, 27–37.

Glass, G.V. (1976). Primary, secondary, and meta-analyses of research. *Educational Researcher*, **5**, 3–8.

Guyatt, G., Walter, S.D., and Norman, G.R. (1987). Measuring change over time: Assessing the usefulness of evaluative instruments. *Journal of Chronic Diseases*, **40**, 171–8.

Guyatt, G.H., Norman, G.R., and Juniper, E.F. (2000). A critical look at transition ratings. *Journal of Clinical Epidemiology*, **55**, 900–8.

Hageman, W.J.J.M. and Arrindell, W.A. (1993). A further refinement of the Reliable Change (RC) index by improving the pre –post difference score: Introducing the RCID. *Behaviour Research and Therapy*, **31**, 693–700.

Hays, R.D. and Hadorn, D. (1992). Responsiveness to change: An aspect of validity, not a separate dimension. *Quality of Life Research*, **1**, 73–5.

Hsu, L.M. (1996). On the identification of clinically significant client changes: Reinterpretation of Jacobson's cut scores. *Journal of Psychopathology and Behavioral Assessment*, **18**, 371–85.

Jacobson, N.S. and Truax, R. (1991). Clinical significance: A statistical approach to defining meaningful change in psychotherapy research. *Journal of Consulting and Clinical Psychology*, **59**, 12–19.

Jacobson, N. S., Follette, W. C., and Revenstorf, D. (1984). Psychotherapy outcome research: Methods for reporting variability and evaluating clinical significance. *Behavior Therapy*, **15**, 336–52.

Jaeschke, R., Singer, J., and Guyatt, G.H. (1989). Measurement of health status. Ascertaining the minimally important difference. *Controlled Clinical Trials*, **10**, 407–15.

Kendall, P.C., Marrs-Garcia, A., Nath, S.R., and Sheldrick, R.C. (1999). Normative comparisons for the evaluation of clinical change. *Journal of Consulting and Clinical Psychology*, **67**, 285–99.

Kirshner, B. and Guyatt, G. (1985). A methodological framework for assessing health indices. *Journal of Chronic Diseases*, **38**, 27–36.

Liang, M.H. (2000). Longitudinal construct validity: Establishment of clinical meaning in patient evaluation instruments. *Medical Care*, **38**(Suppl. II), S84– 90.

Linn, P.L. and Slinde, J.A. (1977). Determination of the significance of change between pre- and post testing periods. *Reviews of Educational Research*, **47**, 121–50.

Lord, F.M. (1967). A paradox in the interpretation of group comparisons. *Psychological Bulletin*, **68**, 304–5.

Lord, F.M. and Novick, M.N. (1968). *Statistical theories of mental test development*. Addison-Wesley, Reading, MA.

MacKenzie, C.R., Charlson, M.E., DiGioia, D., and Kelley, K. (1986). Can the Sickness Impact Profile measure change? An example of scale assessment. *Journal of Chronic Diseases*, **39**, 429–38.

McHorney, C.A. and Tarlov, A. (1995). Individual-patient monitoring in clinical practice: Are available health status measures adequate? *Quality of Life Research*, **4**, 293–307.

Norman, G.R. (2003). Hi! How are you? Response shift, implicit theories and differing epistemologies. *Quality of Life Research*, **12**, 239–49.

Norman, G.R., Regehr, G., and Stratford, P.S. (1997). Bias in the retrospective calculation of responsiveness to change: The lesson of Cronbach. *Journal of Clinical Epidemiology*, **8**, 869–79.

Norman, G.R., Sloan, J.A., and Wyrwich, K.W. (2003). Interpretation of changes in health-related quality of life: The remarkable universality of half a standard deviation. *Medical Care*, **41**, 582–92.

Patrick, D.L. and Chiang, Y.-P. (2000). Measurement of health outcomes in treatment effectiveness evaluations: Conceptual and methodological challenges. *Medical Care*, **38**(Suppl. II), S14– 25.

Rogosa, D., Brandt, D., and Zimowski, M. (1982). A growth curve approach to the measurement of change. *Psychological Bulletin*, **92**, 726–48.

Rosenthal, R. (1994). Parametric measures of effect size. In *The handbook of research synthesis* (eds. H. Cooper and L.V. Hedges), pp. 231–44. Russell Sage Foundation, New York.

Ross, M. (1989). Relation of implicit theories to the construction of personal histories. *Psychological Review*, **96**, 341–57.

Schwartz, C.E. and Sprangers, M.A.G. (1999). Methodological approaches for assessing response shift in longitudinal health related quality of life research. *Social Science and Medicine*, **48**, 1531–48.

Sonawalla, S.B. and Rosenbaum, J.F. (2002). Placebo response in depression. *Dialogues in Clinical Neuroscience*, **4**, 105–13.

Streiner, D.L. (2001). Regression toward the mean: Its etiology, diagnosis, and treatment. *Canadian Journal of Psychiatry*, **46**, 72–6.

Tuttle, A.H., Tohyama, S., Ramsay, T., Kimmelman, J., Schweinhardt, P., Bennett, G.J., *et al.* (2015). Increasing placebo responses over time in U.S. clinical trials of neuropathic pain. *Pain*, **156**, 2616–26.

Wainer, H. (1991). Adjusting for differential base rates: Lord's paradox again. *Psychological Bulletin*, **109**, 147–51.

Wise, E.A. (2004). Methods for analyzing psychotherapy outcomes: A review of clinical significance, reliable change, and recommendations for future directions. *Journal of Personality Assessment*, **82**, 50–9.

Chapter 12

Item response theory

Introduction to item response theory

The theory underlying scale construction in the previous chapters is referred to as *classical test theory* (CTT). It has dominated the field for over a century, due primarily to the fact that the assumptions CTT makes about the items and the test are relatively 'weak' ones, meaning that the theory is appropriate in most situations (Hambleton and Swaminathan 1985). The primary assumption is that, for each item, the error score is uncorrelated with the true score: that is, that the variation in error is equal for all values of the true score, and that the average error, summed over all of the items, is zero. If we accept this assumption, then the Spearman–Brown prophesy formula, which we discussed in Chapter 5, tells us that reliability increases as the number of items in the scale increases; and the equation for coefficient alpha, also discussed in Chapter 5, means that reliability also increases as the correlations among the items increase. However, there are a number of problems with the assumptions of CTT, and with the scales constructed using it.

Problems with classical test theory

1. *Sample dependency.* Perhaps the major problem, as we have pointed out in the chapters on reliability and validity, is that the item and scale statistics apply only to the specific group of participants who took the test. This has a number of implications. First, if the scale is to be administered to people who differ in some way, such as being in a special education class, or having a different diagnosis, then it is necessary to re-establish its psychometric properties and perhaps even to develop new norms (e.g. Scott and Pampa 2000). Furthermore, as we have seen when we looked at the formulae for restrictions in the range of scores (Chapter 10), the reliability and validity estimates are dependent on the homogeneity of the sample.

   A second implication is that it is impossible to separate out the properties of the test from the attributes of the people taking it (Hambleton et al. 1991). That is, there is a *circular dependency*, in that the scores on an instrument depend on how much of the trait people in the sample have; while 'how much they have' depends on the norms of the scale. Thus, the instrument's characteristics change as we test different groups, and the groups' characteristics change as we use different tests. For example, the item-total correlations are dependent on the variance of the sample's scores; with a more or less homogeneous sample, these correlations will change. This also means that the test's standard error is sample dependent, and thus the norms are very dependent on the characteristics of the normative sample.

2. *Item dependency.* Just as the properties of the scale are defined by the normative group, it is also dependent on the specific set of items in the scale; the jargon term for this is *test dependency* (Reise and Henson 2003). We would have to go through the same renorming process if any of the items were altered, or if items were deleted in order to develop a shorter version of the scale (e.g. Streiner and Miller 1986), or to extract a subscale from a multifactor inventory (Franke 1997).

3. *Assumption of item equivalence.* In CTT, we assume that each item contributes equally to the final score. That is, unless we attach different weights to each item (and we saw in Chapter 7 why that does not change much in CTT), the total score is most often simply the sum of the scores of the individual items, irrespective of how well each item correlates with the underlying construct. However, both item statistics and clinical (and more broadly, expert) judgement tell us that some items are more important in tapping an attribute than others. For example, responding to an item, 'I am so nervous in social situations that I haven't seen anyone for more than a year' reflects far more anxiety than 'My hands get sweaty when I have to meet people', but there is no way to effectively build this into a scale.

Another way this manifests itself is that there are many ways of achieving the same score on a scale. For example, the Miranda Rights Comprehension Instrument (Grisso 1998) asks prisoners four questions about their Miranda rights: their right to remain silent, the use of their statements as evidence, their right to counsel, and the right to free counsel if they are indigent. Each is scored as 0 (no understanding), 1 (partial understanding), or 2 (full understanding). One person could achieve a score of 4 with a partial understanding of all questions; while another person would get the same score if they had full understanding of two questions and no understanding of the other two. Obviously, the same score reflects very different comprehension of their Miranda rights. (In fact, there are 20 different ways a person could get a score of 4.) This has implications for forming diagnostic groups. There are nine diagnostic criteria for a Major Depressive Disorder, and the person must meet five or more of them to receive a diagnosis. The problem is that there are 126 different ways of receiving five, and at least 227 'subtypes' of five or more (Shader and Streiner 2021).

Summing up the items to create a total score also assumes that all of the items are measured on the same interval scale. This assumption is most often fallacious on two grounds: items are more likely ordinal rather than interval (and therefore should not be added together); and the 'psychological distance' between response options differs from one item to the next (Bond and Fox 2007) and often from one option to another. That is, we are most likely wrong when we assume that the distance between 'agree' and 'strongly agree' is the same for all items, and that it is the same as the distance between 'disagree' and 'strongly disagree'.

4. *Assumptions of the standard error of measurement (SEM).* In CTT, we make the assumption of homoscedasticity: that is, that the error of measurement is the same everywhere along the scale. Again, statistics tells us this is wrong. If the scale is more or less normally distributed, then there will be more people in the middle range. Because the sample size is larger there, the SEM is smallest in the middle,

and increases with higher and lower scores. However, we ignore this assumption because it is too difficult to calculate the actual SEM at each point along the scale, and there is no one summary statistic that captures this. Similarly, once we calculate the SEM, we assume it is the same for every individual. But, by the same logic, and also because of regression towards the mean, it must be higher for people at the extremes of the scale than for those in the middle.

Another consideration to keep in mind is that the SEM for a given individual is dependent on the people with whom they are tested: that is, the distribution of scores for that particular sample. This makes little sense; how much a person's score will change on retesting because of sampling error, which is what the SEM reflects, is a function of the individual, not the other members of the group.

5. *Problems equating tests.* With CTT, it is very difficult to equate scores a person receives on different tests. This poses a particular problem for longitudinal studies for two reasons: (a) over time, scales are revised, with new sets of norms, and (b) as a child matures, they may be given different versions of a test. This makes it difficult to determine growth trajectories over time, as the scores may be influenced by the change in test forms. The usual approach to equating scores is to convert the scores into *T*- or *z*-scores, as we mentioned in Chapter 7, or to use percentile equating. However, this assumes that all of the tests are normally distributed, which is, as Micceri (1989) said, as improbable as unicorns.

6. *Differences between scores are assumed to be equivalent across the entire scale.* In CTT, we interpret a difference of, say, five points as having the same meaning whether it occurs in the middle of the scale or at the tails. We assume that the trait we are measuring has an underlying normal distribution (although the sample data may not be normally distributed). This means, though, that a difference of five points in the middle range reflects less of a difference in ability than the same difference at the extremes.

The introduction of item response theory

In the 1960s, two quite independent groups were modifying CTT in an attempt to overcome these limitations. In North America, Allan Birnbaum (1968) included four previously unpublished papers in what is arguably one of the most seminal books in psychometric theory (Lord and Novick 1968), outlining a new approach to test development; while in Denmark, Georg Rasch (1960) was developing a new mathematical way of separately estimating parameters about the test items and the people taking the test at the same time. These two areas have come together in what is now called *item response theory* or IRT. In fact, though, the foundations had been laid a few decades, earlier, in a paper by D. N. Lawley (1943) at Edinburgh University; and curves showing the proportion of correct responses to items as a function of age on an early IQ test (similar to curves we'll see later in this chapter when we discuss item characteristic curves) were derived by Thurstone even earlier, in 1925. (For a more thorough description of the history of the technique, see Embretson and Reise (2000) or Cai et al. (2016).) IRT does not refer to a specific technique, but rather to a framework that encompasses a group of models, some of which we will discuss in this chapter. A major difference between IRT and CTT is that CTT focuses primarily on test-level information, whereas IRT focuses on item-level information (Fan 1998).

Unlike the 'soft' assumptions of CTT, IRT is based on two 'hard' requirements: that the scale is unidimensional (that is, the items tap only one trait or ability); and that the probability of answering any item in the positive direction (i.e. reflecting more of the trait) is unrelated to the probability of answering any other item positively for people with the same amount of the trait (a property called *local independence*). If these two requirements are met, then two postulates follow. First, the performance of a subject on the test can be predicted by a set of factors, which are variously called 'traits', 'abilities', or 'latent traits' (and the amount of which is referred to in IRT by the Greek letter θ, *theta*). The second postulate is that the relationship between a person's performance on any item and the underlying trait can be described by an *item characteristic curve* or *item response function*.

You may have noticed a slight change in wording in the previous paragraph. In discussing CTT, we used the term 'assumptions', whereas with IRT, we said 'requirements'. This was not done simply to avoid using the same word twice. Unidimensionality and local independence must be assessed before proceeding with IRT. If either requirement is not met, then we cannot pass Go and must either fix the problem or find some other way of analysing the scale. As Reise and Haviland (2005, p. 230) state:

> Any advantage that IRT modeling may have relative to CTT can only be realized in practice when data are judged appropriate for IRT models and the estimated IRT model parameters fit the observed data. If these conditions are not met (they never will be met perfectly, however), researchers should use the more traditional CTT models.

A note about terminology

IRT had its roots in educational testing, and its terminology still reflects that. The probability of endorsing an item is called its *difficulty*, which makes sense if we are trying to measure a person's knowledge of arithmetic or cardiology. An item such as 'What are the factors of $x^2 - y^2$?' is harder to answer than 'What is 2 + 3?', and 'What type of receptors are affected in an AV block?' is more difficult than 'How many chambers does the human heart have?' The terminology seems to make less sense when a scale is tapping pain, or anxiety, or quality of life; it is not any more difficult to respond to the item 'I can run a marathon' than to 'I have difficulty walking up one flight of stairs'. The translation is that when we are measuring these types of constructs, 'difficulty' means how much of the trait or attribute a person must have to endorse the item. A person with only a mild amount of sadness may respond positively to the item 'I sometimes feel dejected', but only a person with a high degree of depression would endorse one that reads, 'I have often thought of killing myself'. Thus, the latter item would be said to be more difficult.

When we are measuring *difficulty*, we count the proportion of people who *failed* or did not endorse that item. Table 12.1 shows how five people did on five items. For Item

Table 12.1 A person-by-item matrix

	Item 1	Item 2	Item 3	Item 4	Item 5	Ability
Person A	1	1	1	1	1	1.0
Person B	0	1	1	1	1	0.8
Person C	0	0	1	1	1	0.6
Person D	0	0	0	1	1	0.4
Person E	0	0	0	0	1	0.2
Difficulty	0.8	0.6	0.4	0.2	0.0	

2, two people endorsed it (or got it correct, if this were an achievement test) and three did not, so it has a *difficulty* level of 3/5 = 0.6.

Similarly, a person's probability of endorsing an item is sometimes referred to as their *ability*. A person with more *ability* is more likely to answer more difficult items correctly. Analogously, then, ability corresponds to how much of the trait or attribute the person has. But, in contradistinction to how we measure difficulty, we assess ability in terms of the proportion of items *passed* (or endorsed), so that Person D, who endorsed two of the five items, has an *ability* level of 0.4.

Item calibration

At this point, we must consider the *difficulties* and *abilities* in Table 12.1 to be tentative, as the responses show a perfect Guttman pattern (discussed in Chapter 4): no person endorses a harder item after failing to endorse an easier one; and no item is passed by a person with less ability and failed by one with more. This is rarely seen in real life. Table 12.2 shows three people who have the same ability score, but the score is based on different items, each with different difficulty levels. In the same way, Table 12.3 shows two items with the same difficulty level (items 1 and 9), but the items are endorsed by people who have varying degrees of ability. These patterns are closer to what usually happens. Consequently, we have to recalibrate our estimates of difficulty and ability, based on these deviations from ideal Guttman scaling.

Table 12.2 Three people with the same ability score but based on items with different difficulty levels

	Item 1	Item 2	Item 3	Item 4	Item 5	Ability
Person C	0	0	1	1	1	0.6
Person F	1	1	0	0	1	0.6
Person H	1	0	1	1	0	0.6

Table 12.3 Two items with the same difficulty level (items 1 and 9) but based on people with different ability scores

	Item 1	Item 2	Item 3	Item 4	Item 9	Ability
Person A	1	1	1	1	0	0.8
Person B	0	1	1	1	0	0.6
Person C	0	0	1	1	0	0.4
Person D	0	0	0	1	0	0.2
Person E	0	0	0	0	1	0.2
Difficulty	0.8	0.6	0.4	0.2	0.8	

The probability of endorsing an item (or getting it correct) is determined by the formula:

$$Pr = \frac{1}{1+e^{-(Ability - Difficulty)}}$$

which is called a *logistic function*. In essence, it means that the probability is the discrepancy between the person's ability and the item's difficulty. In IRT, a person's ability is denoted by the Greek letter theta (θ) and the item's difficulty level by b. When b for a particular item is equal to the person's level of θ, the probability of endorsement is 0.50, or 50 per cent. If θ is greater than b, then the probability is greater than 0.50; and when it is less than b, the probability is less than 0.50. Let's try it out. Person B in Table 12.1 has an ability of 0.8, and item 2 has a difficulty level of 0.6. So, the probability that they will endorse that item is:

$$Pr = \frac{1}{1+e^{-(0.8-0.6)}} = \frac{1}{1+e^{-0.2}} = \frac{1}{1+0.819} = 0.55$$

Since their ability is greater than the item's difficulty, their probability of endorsing the item is greater than 0.5 but less than the 1.0 in the table, which would be the value only if this were a perfect Guttman scale.

Consequently, in calibrating the items' difficulty level and estimating a person's ability, both need to be considered simultaneously. We (or rather the computer program) must go through an iterative process, in which tentative estimates are used to fit a model and then the model is used to predict the data. This iterative procedure continues until there is no discrepancy in the estimates.

As part of the calibration process, both θ and b are transformed, so that, like z-scores, they have a mean of zero and, theoretically, values that can range from $-\infty$ to $+\infty$, but like a bell curve, it's pretty well impossible to get a z-score more than 3 or 4. Over 99.73 per cent of cases fall between zs of -3 and $+3$, and over 99.99 per cent between ± 4, so when plotting them, we usually draw the x-axis to run between ± 3 or ± 4.

In other words, both θ and *b* are measured using the same scale, so that a person with a θ value of 1.0 is one standard deviation (SD) above the mean in terms of ability, and an item with a *b* level of 1.0 is similarly one SD above the mean in terms of difficulty level.

Item characteristic curves

The relationship between difficulty and ability for any given item is shown in an *item characteristic curve* (ICC), also called the *item response function* (IRF), which is the fundamental unit in IRT. ICCs for two items are shown in Fig. 12.1. As we mentioned previously in the section 'Item calibration', the shape of these curves is called a *logistic* function. Why do we use a logistic function rather than some other shape for the function? In Guttman scaling, the shape is a step function—the left tail is a straight, horizontal line along the *x*-axis where the probability is 0.0, then there is a vertical line at a point corresponding to the item's difficulty level, and then the right tail is another horizontal line along the top where the probability is 1.0. However, a Guttman scale is completely deterministic and there is no allowance for any error or deviations from this step function, which is usually unrealistic. From a theoretical perspective, the curve that should have been used is the *cumulative normal distribution*, but in the days before the ready availability of computers, this was too difficult to work with, so the logistic function was used as an approximation. In actual practice, however, there is little difference between them except for a scaling factor.

There are a number of points to note about the ICCs in Fig. 12.1. First, they describe the relationship between a person's ability (θ) and the probability of responding positively to an item (that is, endorsing it or getting the item correct). Second, the curves are *monotonic*; the probability of endorsing the item consistently increases as a person's ability increases.

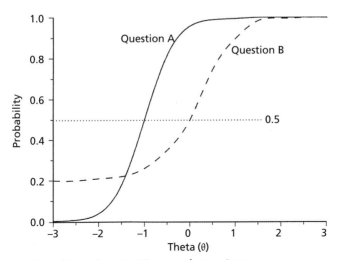

Fig. 12.1 Hypothetical item characteristic curves for two items.

The final point about the ICCs is that each item has its own ICC (as shown in Fig. 12.1 for two Questions, A and B). The curves differ from each other along three dimensions: the steepness of their slopes; their location along the trait continuum; and where they flatten out at the bottom. We shall return to the significance of these differences later in the chapter.

To show some of the attributes of the curves, we have drawn a horizontal line where the probability is 0.5: it intersects the ICC for Question A at a value of the trait (θ) of −1.0, and Question B at a value of 0.0. What this means is that, for a group of people whose value of the trait is −1.0, 50 per cent will answer positively to Question A and 50 per cent will answer negatively; and similarly, 50 per cent of people whose θ level is 0.0 will respond each way to Question B. (Later, in the section on polytomous models, we will discuss items where there are more than two possible responses.)

What can we tell from these two curves? First, Question A is a better discriminator of the trait than Question B. The reason is that the proportion of people responding in the positive direction changes relatively rapidly on Question A as θ increases. The slope for Question B is flatter, indicating that it does not discriminate as well. For example, as we move from $\theta = -2.0$ to $\theta = +1.0$, the proportion of people answering positively to Question A increases from 4 per cent to nearly 100 per cent; while for Question B, a comparable change in the trait is associated with an increase only from 21 per cent to 90 per cent. A highly discriminating item can distinguish between people who have similar (but not identical) levels of the trait; whereas a poorly discriminating item can discriminate only between people with very different levels of it. When the curve has the maximum steepness, it takes the form of a 'step function': no people below the critical point respond positively, and everyone above it responds in the positive direction. The items would then form a perfect Guttman-type of scale (see Chapter 4). Thus, one way of thinking about item characteristic curves is that they are 'imperfect' Guttman scales, where the probability of responding increases gradually with more of the trait, rather than jumping suddenly from a probability of 0 to 100 per cent.

A second observation is that Question B is 'harder' than Question A throughout most of the range of the trait (for values of θ greater than −1.5). That is, the average person needs more of the trait in order to respond in the positive direction. This can also be seen by the fact that the 50 per cent point is further along the trait continuum for Question B than it is for Question A. Finally, the lower asymptote for Question A is 0.0, while it is 0.2 for Question B. When none of the trait is present, nobody responds positively to A, but 20 per cent do to B; later we will discuss possible reasons for this when we look at models with more than one parameter. The various IRT models that we will discuss in this chapter are simply different mathematical functions for describing the item characteristic curves: that is, the relationship between a person's level of the trait (θ) and the probability of a specific response.

So, to summarize, we can think of the item characteristic curve in a number of ways. It shows: (1) the probability of endorsing the item for a given value of θ, (2) the proportion of people who have a given amount of the trait who will endorse the item, or (3) the probability of item endorsement for a specific individual with a given value of θ. Getting information about both the items and the respondents is not possible with CTT.

The one-parameter model

The simplest IRT model is the *one-parameter model*. According to this model, the only factor differentiating the ICCs of the various items is the item difficulty (also called the *threshold parameter*), denoted b_i. That is, it assumes that all of the items have equal discriminating ability (designated as *a*) and reflecting the fact that the slopes of the curves are parallel, but are placed at various points along the trait continuum, as in Fig. 12.2. (Note that when *a* is $+\infty$, the curve becomes a step function, in that the probability jumps suddenly from 0 to 1.0 at some value of θ; this describes a Guttman scale, discussed in Chapter 4.)

Formally, the proportion of people who have θ amount of the trait who answer item *i* correctly is defined by the *item response function*:

$$P_i(\theta) = \frac{e^{a(\theta - b_i)}}{1 + e^{a(\theta - b_i)}}$$

which can also be written as:

$$P_i(\theta) = \frac{1}{e^{-a(\theta - b_i)}}$$

This is the same equation that we used earlier in the section on Item calibration, except that the word 'Ability' has been replaced by the symbol θ, and 'Difficulty' by b_i, where the subscript reflects the fact that each item has a different difficulty level. We've also added the constant parameter *a*, which reflects the relative discrimination of the items; this will become clearer when we discuss more complicated models.

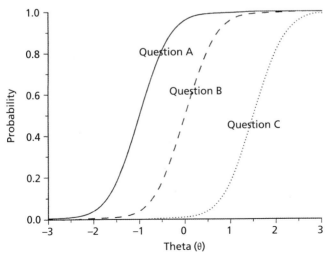

Fig. 12.2 Item characteristic curves for three items with equal discrimination but different levels of difficulty.

Since the form of the equation is called 'logistic', this model and the ones we will discuss in the next section, 'The two- and three-parameter models', are referred to as *logistic models*. (For more detail on logistic models, see Norman and Streiner 2014.)

Because this equation has only one parameter that varies among items (*b*, reflecting item difficulty), it is referred to as the one-parameter logistic model, or 1PLM. When the response option is dichotomous (e.g. True/False, Yes/No), it is also commonly called the *Rasch model*, although Rasch later developed more complicated models (Rasch 1960; Wright 1977).

By definition, half the people have negative values of θ and half have positive ones; this means that Question A in Fig. 12.2 is an easy one that a majority of people will endorse, and Question C a difficult one that most people will not. Note that *b* in the IRT models is related to *p* (the proportion correct score) in CTT, but inversely—the harder the item (that is, the higher the value of *b*), the lower the value of *p*. One important implication of this for the item response function, and one area where IRT differs significantly from CTT, is that the person's true position along the latent trait continuum does not depend upon the specific set of items that comprise the scale (Reise and Henson 2003).

Because of the properties of the logistic function, we can easily convert it to a form that gives us the odds of responding to an item, rather than a probability:

$$Odds = \frac{P_i(\theta)}{1 - P_i(\theta)}$$

If we now take the natural logarithm of the odds, we end up with a function that shows the item response curve as a straight line, as in Fig. 12.3:

$$Log\, Odds = ln\left(\frac{p_i(\theta)}{1 - p_i(\theta)}\right).$$

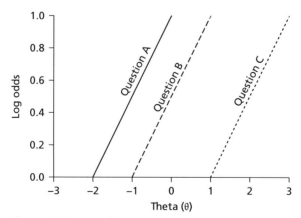

Fig. 12.3 Item characteristic curves from Fig. 12.2, expressed as log odds.

We mentioned earlier in 'The introduction of item response theory' that there are two requirements that must be met in IRT: unidimensionality and local independence. There are two other requirements for the Rasch model: *item difficulty invariance* and *person location invariance*. The first (item invariance) means that the ordering of people is the same for all items; and the second (person invariance) means that the order of difficulty of the items is the same for all people. When these requirements are not met, the ICCs can cross, as in Fig. 12.1, meaning that the item difficulty gradient is not the same for all people. This is permitted in the models discussed below in the section 'The two- and three-parameter models', but not in the 1PLM.

The two- and three-parameter models

The *two-parameter model* (2PLM) allows the ICCs to differ from each other on the basis of both difficulty and discriminating ability; that is, instead of *a* being a constant, there is a different a_i for each item. Consequently, the ICCs are different with respect to their position along the trait line and the slope of the curve, as seen in Fig. 12.4.

The equation for this takes the form:

$$P_i(\theta) = \frac{1}{1 + e^{-a_i(\theta - b_i)}},$$

which differs from the equation presented in the section on Item calibration in that *a* is now a variable, rather than a constant. The discrimination parameter, a_i, is equivalent to the item-total correlation in CTT, which is usually expressed as a Pearson correlation or point-biserial correlation (Fan 1998). It is also similar to a factor loading in exploratory factor analysis, indicating the strength of the association between the item and the latent trait. More formally:

$$a_i \cong \frac{r_i}{\sqrt{1 - r_i^2}}$$

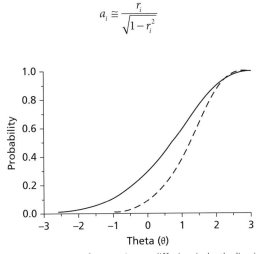

Fig. 12.4 Item characteristic curves for two items differing in both discrimination and difficulty.

where r_i is the biserial correlation for item i. However, a_i is a slope; more specifically, it's the slope of the line at its inflection point, and so, unlike r_p, it can range from 0 (for a totally useless item) to infinity (for a perfect Guttman-type item). Values between 0 and 0.34 are considered very low; 0.35 to 0.64 as low; 0.65 to 1.34 as moderate; 1.35 to 1.69 as high; and 1.70 and above as very high. In practice, we like it to be within the range of 0.75–1.50. If it is much lower, then the item isn't discriminating well. If it is much higher, then the trait may be defined too narrowly, and by the items themselves, rather than by the construct.

Sometimes the equation is written with the constant D just before the $-a_i$ term. D is always equal to 1.701, and is simply a scaling factor so that the logistic function closely approximates the cumulative normal curve, simplifying calculations. Because it is a constant and always there, it is more often left implicit for the sake of simplicity when the equation is written out; don't worry, though, the computer knows it's there.

There is one unfortunate consequence of the two-parameter model. Note than in Fig. 12.4, Question A is easier than Question B. As would be expected, Person 1 has a higher probability of answering Question A than Question B. However, because the ICCs may cross at some point, we have the paradoxical situation where Person 2 has a higher probability of responding positively to the harder question than the easier one. This does not happen in all cases, but should be guarded against in selecting items. This is one reason that adherents of the Rasch model dislike the two- and three-parameter models. Such a situation can never occur in the one-parameter model, because the slope parameter is the same for all items.

Both the one- and two-parameter models assume that at the lowest level of the trait, the probability of responding positively is zero; that is, the left tail of all of the curves is asymptotic to the x-axis. This may be a valid assumption with attitudinal or personality questionnaires, if all of the people are paying attention to the questions at all times and there are no errors in responding. However, it is likely that people will guess on items to which they do not know the answer on multiple-choice achievement tests; and that, on personality tests, some people with very small amounts of the trait may endorse an item because of lapses in attention, bias, or some other factors. The *three-parameter model* (3PLM) takes this into account, and allows the lower end of the curve to asymptote at some probability level greater than zero. This 'pseudo-guessing parameter' is designated as c_i, and the resulting equation is given as:

$$P_i(\theta) = c_i + (1 - c_i)\frac{1}{1 + e^{-a_i(\theta - b_i)}}$$

In Fig. 12.1, Question A has a value of c_i of 0.0 (i.e. the probability of responding positively at the lowest level of the trait is zero), while Question B has a value of 0.2 for c_i. The theoretical limits of c_i are between 0 and 1, although it is rarely above 0.25 (the value for a very difficult multiple-choice item with four alternatives, where nearly everyone is guessing the answer). Although c_i is interpretable in attitudinal and personality measures (it would likely reflect the effects of inattention, difficulty understanding the item, or that people with low levels of the trait interpret the item differently from those with higher levels), the 3PLM is rarely used outside of educational measurement (Panter et al. 1997). (We should note in passing that there is even a 4PLM, in which the right-hand part of the curve asymptotes at a value less than 1.0, but this is even more rarely used than the 3PLM and so deserves even less discussion.)

At one level, the 3PLM can be seen as the general case for IRT: by setting c_i to 0, it is identical to the 2PLM; and when c_i is 0 and a_i is a, then it is the same as the 1PLM and the Rasch model. However, the Rasch model differs from the 2- and 3PLM models in terms of the assumptions of the underlying distributions (which we will not get into here). The result is that only the Rasch model results in a truly interval scale; and only with the Rasch model can the person and item parameters be truly separated. Put somewhat differently, the higher-order models attempt to fit the model to the data; whereas the model is paramount for Rasch, and the data either do or do not fit it. Whether or not this is important depends on the goals of the analyses. If it is to end up with data that conform to an interval scale, then only the Rasch model will do; if it is to describe and model the data, then the Rasch can be seen as a subset of the 2PLM, which in turn is a subset of the 3PLM. For more on the practical and philosophical differences between the Rasch model and the 2- and 3PLM, see Stemler and Naples (2021).

Polytomous models

Up to this point, we have discussed IRT models for scales that have a dichotomous response option: Yes/No, True/False, and so forth. Most instruments, though, consist of items that allow a range of responses, by using Likert scales, visual analogue scales (VASs), adjectival scales, and the like. It is widely accepted that the response options rarely have interval level properties, in that the psychological distance between adjacent points is not constant from one end of the response continuum to the other. However, with CTT, we often close our eyes to this fact, and assume that the actual ordinal data are 'close enough' to interval level for us to ignore the distinction, or that by summing over a number of items, at least the total score will be more or less normally distributed.

Using IRT, we do not have to play 'make believe'. There are many different models for evaluating polytomous response options. When the answers can be considered to be ordered categories, which is most often the case with Likert and adjectival scales, and VAS, the most commonly used models are the *partial credit model* (PCM) and the *graded-response model* (GRM), which are generalizations of the one- and two-parameter logistic models (for a discussion of this and five other models see Embretson and Reise 2000). The difference between the two is that the PCM assumes equal distances between response options, and the GRM does not. Because the GRM is the more general case, and probably a better reflection of reality, we will restrict our discussion to it. The equation is slightly different from the 2PLM:

$$P_i(\theta) = \frac{1}{1 + e^{-a_i(\theta - b_{ik})}}$$

Notice that the difficulty, or threshold, parameter, b, now has two subscripts: i to indicate the item; and k to reflect the different response options for item i. This is called an *unconstrained* model, because the discrimination parameter (a) is free to vary from one response option to the next. Note also that we can use this equation for the one-parameter (Rasch) model, simply by using the same value of a for all items, instead of letting it vary from one item to the next, as reflected by the subscript i. Needless to say, this is referred to as a *constrained* model.

Let us assume that each item is answered on a 5-point Likert scale: Strongly Agree (SA), Agree (A), Neutral (N), Disagree (D), and Strongly Disagree (SD). Conceptually, the GRM would treat each item as if it were a scale with five items, resulting in four dichotomous items, which translates into four thresholds:

For $k = 1$ Test *SA* vs *A, N, D, SD*

$k = 2$ Test *SA, A* vs *N, D, SD*

$k = 3$ Test *SA, A, N* vs *D, SD*

$k = 4$ Test *SA, A, N, D* vs *SD*

These *threshold response curves* can be plotted, as in Fig. 12.5. There are a couple of points to consider. First, there is one value of a_i for the item, meaning that all of the threshold response curves are assumed to have the same slope, or discriminating ability. This slope is actually the average of the slopes for all of the curves for that item. Second, because a has the subscript i, it means that each item can have different discriminating ability (that is, the hallmark of the two-parameter model). Finally, the term b_{ik} is interpreted in the same way as b_i: it reflects the level of θ

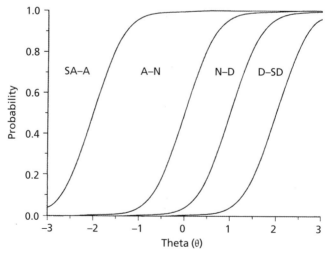

Fig. 12.5 Thresholds for a five-option Likert scale.

where the probability of responding is 50 per cent. Now, though, it's the probability of responding to that threshold between response options, rather than to the (dichotomous) item.

It is obvious that there is a larger threshold between Agree and Neutral (the gap labelled A–N) than between Neutral and Disagree (N–D) and between Disagree and Strongly Disagree (D–SD), and that the latter two thresholds are about the same, reflecting the ordinal nature of the answers; that is, it takes more of the trait to move from Agree to Neutral than it does to move from Neutral to Disagree or from Disagree to Strongly Disagree. The probabilities of giving each response can also be examined, as in Fig. 12.6, where they are plotted for differing levels of θ. The peaks of the curves fall in the middle of the gaps between the thresholds. At any point along the *x*-axis, the sum of the probabilities is 1.0, since there is a 100 per cent probability that one of the options will be chosen.

Now let's look at the response curves for a different item, in Fig. 12.7. What this tells us is that the Agree and Disagree options are not being used by the respondents; most people either strongly agree or strongly disagree with the stem, and a few are neutral, but very few are taking a more tempered position. What this means is that we should either drop the Agree and Disagree options, or, if we prefer to keep the format the same for all items, score them in the respective Strongly category.

Another indication of a problem occurs when the order of the thresholds is disordered: for example, if SA is followed by N, then A, D, and SD. This would indicate that subjects are having difficulty discriminating among the options, because either there are too many of them or the labelling is confusing (e.g. is 'often' more or less than 'frequently'?). Here again, the options would be to rewrite the question or to collapse categories.

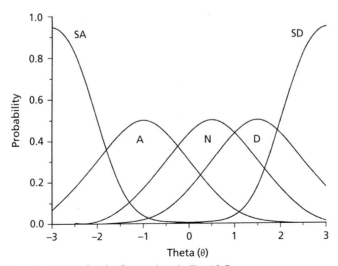

Fig. 12.6 Response curves for the five options in Fig. 12.5.

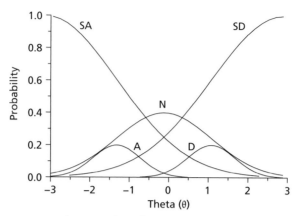

Fig. 12.7 Response curves for a question where Agree and Disagree are not used.

Item information

We would like all of the items in a scale to be equally informative, in that they differentiate among people with varying levels of the trait, but we know that isn't the case. When we discussed the parameter a_i, which reflects the discriminating power of the item in the 2- and 3PLMs, we said that the steeper the slope, the better the discrimination. This is captured in the *item information function* (IIF) for each item:

$$IIF_i \mid \theta = a_i^2 P_i(\theta) Q_i(\theta)$$

where $IIF_i \mid \theta$ means the information for item i at a specific value of θ, and Q_i is $(1 - P_i)$. That means if an item has a slope of 1.0, it has four times the discriminating ability of an item with a slope of 0.5. We can show this in a graph of the IIF, as in Fig. 12.8. The more item information, the taller and narrower is the curve. Good items provide a lot of information, but only around its discriminating function; whereas poorer items provide less information, and it is spread out over a larger range of the trait.

With polytomous items, the IIF depends on two factors: the average slope of the response categories; and the distances among the categories. Consequently, a polytomous item has more information than a dichotomous one, and the information is more spread out along the range of the trait, θ. While the IIF for a dichotomous item resembles a normal curve, that for a polytomous item may be broader, and have a number of peaks.

Item fit

The purpose of IRT is to find a small set of items (usually much smaller than with scales derived using CTT, for reasons we will explain a bit later in this section) that span the range of the construct. Because the item difficulty parameter, b, is standardized on a logit scale to have a mean of 0 and an SD of 1, an ideal situation is to have a

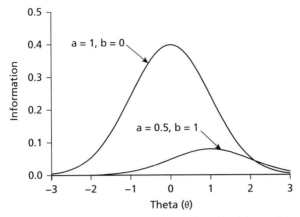

Fig. 12.8 Item information functions for a good ($a = 1$) and bad ($a = 0.5$) item.

set of items where the bs range from about −3 to +3 (that is, 3 SDs above and below the mean). If the bs cluster towards the lower end of this logit scale, with few items near +3, it indicates that the items were too 'easy', with many items measuring small amounts of the trait, and few that are endorsed only by people who have much of it. For example, if we were developing a pain scale, this situation would arise if there were many items about common aches and pains that are experienced by a large number of people, but few items that tap extreme levels of pain, such as endured by patients with bone cancer. Conversely, few items near the −3 end of the scale would reflect the opposite situation—not very many items relating to mild pain, and many at the extreme end. The third situation is where all of the items cluster near the middle, indicating that the scale is restricted at both ends.

Because the logit scale is an interval one, items can be selected from the pool that are relatively evenly spaced along the continuum. How many items to choose depends on how precisely you want to measure the construct. A brief screening test, for example, would need items only near the cut point to define caseness; while many, closely spaced items would be used to make fine distinctions among people, or to measure small amounts of change. The right side of Fig. 12.9 shows the plot of a 10-item scale (for now, we will ignore the left side, where the subjects are plotted). A few points stand out from this. First, the test contains more easy items than hard ones, since seven of the items have logit scores below 0. One consequence is that we jump from a score of just over 1 (item 2) to a score just below 3. This tells us that we may want to write some moderately difficult items in order to discriminate among people within this range. Similarly, it would be helpful to add some moderately easy items, to plug the gap between items 4 and 10. Second, there are a number of items with the same difficulty scores: 3 and 8, and the triplet of 6, 7, and 9. We can eliminate either 3 or 8, and any two of the triplet, and the scale would still have the same discriminating ability.

If a 2PLM was used, then selecting between two items that have similar values of b would depend on the discrimination index for each item, a. Items with higher values have steeper item characteristic curves than those with lower values, and thus

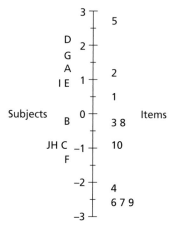

Fig. 12.9 Plot of item difficulty to the right of the axis, and person location to the left.

discriminate better between people whose values of the trait, θ, are similar, but not identical.

We mentioned that one of the strong requirements of IRT is that the scale is unidimensional. This is usually determined by first factor analysing the data; if the scale taps only one attribute, then there should be few significant factors, and the first one should be considerably higher than the others. Even after this has been done, some items may remain that do not fit the requirement of unidimensionality. There are a number of statistics, which vary from one computer program to the next, that indicate the degree to which each item deviates from it. The most common one is a measure of the *residual* of each item, which is evaluated with a likelihood-ratio goodness-of-fit chi-square statistic (χ^2_{GoF}). This assesses the discrepancy between the expected and actual response patterns across respondents, based on their performance on the test as a whole (Fan 1998). Items that meet the requirement of unidimensionality have a low residual value (below 1.96), and a non-significant χ^2_{GoF}, which is conceptually similar to the item having a high item-total correlation. However, χ^2_{GoF} is very sensitive to the sample size, so that if N is large, even slight deviations from unidimensionality may be statistically significant; and conversely, when it is small, large deviations may not be significant.

Because χ^2_{GoF} is difficult to interpret, two other fit statistics are used, called Infit and Outfit. Both are based on discrepancies between actual scores and those predicted by the model, summed over people. Infit focuses on differences near the item's *b*.

Person fit

We mentioned previously when discussing item calibration that both items and people are scored along the same logit scale, which usually ranges from −3 to +3. Consequently, we can determine the degree to which people may be outliers, using a similar type of statistic as was used to see which items fail the criterion of unidimensionality. We can also plot people along the same continuum, which is shown in the left side of Fig. 12.9. In this example, the subjects tend to cluster at the high end of the scale, reflecting the fact that most of them endorsed most of the items. Thus, either this group had a significant degree of pain or, consistent with our evaluation of the items, there are not enough more difficult ones. The ideal situation is one in which the mean location score for all people is around zero.

There are Infit and Outfit statistics for people, too. In this case, they are summed over items, but the meaning and interpretation are similar. Infit looks at discrepancies near people's θ level that are not in line with what is expected; and Outfit at discrepancies far from their θ level, such as easy items failed by people with high values of θ or hard ones passed by people with low values.

Differential item functioning

One of the assumptions of IRT is that the results are independent of the sample. That is, people with the same amount of the latent trait (θ) should have similar IRFs. However, we know that this is not always true. Women with the same amount of depression as men are more likely to endorse items reflecting a tendency to be sad or to cry easily. Whether the assumption is true is examined on a group level through a technique called *differential item functioning* (DIF), where the groups could be males and females, different ethnic groups, patients and non-patients, or people taking the original versus the translated version of a scale. If a scale has a large proportion of items that demonstrate DIF, then this can be a threat to a scale's validity, at least with respect to certain groups of people, as the meaning of the scores would differ from one group to another. As is often the case with advanced statistics that are relatively new, there are literally dozens of methods to evaluate DIF, and no consensus regarding which is the best. One of the more common methods is to run an analysis of variance, with one factor being the group and the other factor being different levels of the trait. Another is to use logistic regression, including an interaction term between ability and the grouping factor (Crane et al. 2004, 2006).

In the Rasch model, because the items are constrained to have a constant slope or discrimination parameter, DIF can occur only when the groups differ in terms of their location along the trait continuum. With the 2PLM and dichotomous items, the groups can differ with regard to discrimination, location, or both. Needless to say, life becomes even more difficult with polytomous items, because now the groups can also differ in terms of the separation among the response alternatives. If the analysis of variance shows a significant effect of group, that would show a uniform DIF; that is, there is a constant difference between the groups across the entire range of the attribute. A group by trait level interaction, on the other hand, points to non-uniform DIF, in which the separation between the item response functions of the two group varies with differing levels of the trait: that is, a difference in discrimination between the groups. Uniform DIF is analogous to confounding, whereas non-uniform DIF would be equivalent to an interaction or effect modification.

What to do when DIF is discovered depends on where you are in the scale development process. If you are developing a scale and hypothesize that there should not be DIF between, say, males and females, then the item can be deleted or rewritten. Similarly, if you are developing a test in two or more languages simultaneously, then DIF may indicate problems with either the concept or the translations. If you are dealing with an existing scale, it may flag why differences between the groups exist.

The problem with all of this, though, is that DIF may occur for reasons having to do with the trait itself. For example, women as a whole are more likely to admit to feeling anxious or depressed than are men, so it would not be surprising that their location parameters for a given item would be different. As we mentioned in the section on translation at the end of Chapter 3, some cultural groups are more likely to use the extremes on adjectival and Likert scales than other groups, so it is to be expected that the threshold values for the response options would differ. We have found subtle but consistent differences between Canadian Anglophones and Francophones on measures of depression and anxiety (Streiner et al. 2005) and DIF on four items. The issue is whether the different prevalences are artefacts due to the DIF, or whether the DIF reflects cultural differences in the expression of affect. Unfortunately, this is a question that can be answered only by anthropology, not statistics, and therefore requires much more effort (and a lot more research).

Unidimensionality and local independence

In the introduction to this topic, it was mentioned that IRT has two 'hard' requirements: those of unidimensionality and of local independence. As we will see, both requirements are highly related to each other. Unidimensionality means that the scale is measuring only one attribute, and the amount of that attribute is the only factor influencing the probability of endorsing an item.

Unidimensionality

The most common way of testing for unidimensionality is to use a technique called factor analysis; a very brief introduction to factor analysis is given in Appendix B, and a more complete description can be found in Norman and Streiner (2014). If the scale is unidimensional, then all of the items should be highly correlated with (the technical term is 'load on') the first factor; and the amount of variance accounted for by the first factor (called the factor's 'eigenvalue') should be considerably higher than the eigenvalues of succeeding factors. The problem is defining 'considerably higher'. Some people (e.g. Reckase 1979) have said that it should account for at least 20 per cent of the variance, while others (Carmines and Zeller 1979) have said 40 per cent, but no rationale has been given for either criterion. Others (Lumsden 1957, 1961) use a ratio of the variances between the first two factors (e.g. the first eigenvalue should be about ten times higher than the eigenvalue for the second factor), but again, there was no justification for this amount. Unfortunately, as Hattie (1985) has concluded, 'Yet, there are still no satisfactory indices' (p. 158). Even though this was written years ago, the conclusion still stands. An extension of using factor analysis is to run it twice: once on the raw data and again on the *residuals*. If there is only one dominant factor, then once its effect on the variables is taken into account, what's left over (the residuals) should just be noise, and the correlations among the variables should be close to zero. If the factor analysis of the residuals does show a pattern, then there is another construct at play, and the scale is not unidimensional (Linacre 1998).

Compounding the difficulty, 'unidimensionality' is itself a slippery concept. Anxiety, for example, can be seen as a single attribute. But we can also divide anxiety into a number of subcomponents, such as physiological (e.g. tachycardia, dry mouth, and sweatiness), behavioural (avoidance of certain situations, anticipation of being fearful), and cognitive (fearfulness, rumination), each of which can be tapped by its own subscale. However, as long as these subcomponents are correlated with each other, the scale as a whole may still be unidimensional. That is, unidimensionality is not an all-or-nothing phenomenon; judgement is required, as well as knowledge of the underlying construct, in order to determine if a scale is 'unidimensional enough'. Pure unidimensionality is impossible; what we are interested in is 'sufficient' unidimensionality. Bear in mind the sage advice of Hill et al. (2007): 'It is less important for the model to be perfect than it is for it to be useful' (p. S41).

A note of caution is in order, though. Most of the more common computer packages that can do factor analysis (e.g. SAS, SPSS, or Stata) begin with a correlation matrix based on the Pearson correlations among the items. This should not be done if the response options are dichotomous or polytomous, as with a Likert scale, for reasons outlined in Appendix B. There are specialized programs that first calculate the correlation matrix based on tetrachoric or polychoric correlations before running the factor analysis, and it is these programs that should be used.

Local independence

Local independence means that, once we remove the influence of the trait being measured (i.e. the first factor in the factor analysis), then the probability of endorsing a specific item is unrelated to the probability of answering any other item. In other words, it is the latent trait (or 'construct' in measurement terminology, or 'factor' in factor analysis terminology) and only the latent trait that influences the answer. The reason that the items are correlated is that they are all affected, albeit to different degrees, by the trait; once the effect of the trait is removed, the items are uncorrelated. This is simply another way of defining a strong first factor, so that local independence and unidimensionality can be seen as saying the same thing in different ways.

The reason it is called 'local independence' is based on what we just discussed. Among people who span the entire range of the trait, there will be strong correlations among the items. But for any subsample of people who are at the same level of θ (which is one way to remove the effect of the trait), there will be no correlation among the items.

Violation of local independence (called, for obvious reasons, 'local dependence') can be due to a number of factors. The first is that the scale isn't unidimensional, but rather is tapping two or more attributes. This is often revealed in a strong second or even third factor in the factor analysis. Something else that can lead to local dependence is the presence of redundant items: those that ask the same question in two different ways, so that if one is endorsed, the other one will be, too. There can be local dependence even if the two items aren't totally redundant. For example, if a person endorses an item stating, 'I can walk for 10 blocks without any difficulty', they will al-most certainly endorse the item 'I can walk one block without any difficulty'. Looking at the correlations among the items may point to problems in this area; you shouldn't include items that correlate above, say, 0.80. A third source of problems in this area oc-curs when two or more answers are linked. For example, the respondent may be asked to read a paragraph and then answer a number of questions based on it. If the person did not understand the paragraph, then all of the items will be answered incorrectly. Finally, local dependence can be caused by the context or content of the preceding items, so that there is 'carryover' in answers from one item to the next. If local de-pendence is present, it can cause the slope parameters to be misleadingly high, and the reliability of the scale to be exaggerated.

However, local independence is similar to unidimensionality in that it is not an all-or-nothing phenomenon. If, as mentioned earlier, the underlying construct is a com-plex one, then different items tapping various facets of it may be redundant. Again, judgement comes into play. If the first factor is much stronger than the others, then it is possible to live with the redundancy; otherwise, one of the two similar items should be eliminated. (For a somewhat sophisticated approach to this problem, see Reise and Haviland 2005.)

Monotonicity

Based on the requirements we have already mentioned—that the scale is unidimen-sional and that the probability of responding to an item increases at higher levels of θ—the items should satisfy one further condition: *monotonicity*. This means that the probability of responding to a given item should increase monotonically with higher scores on the scale (Reise and Haviland 2005).

To test a specific item, we calculate the total score, omitting that item (i.e. the partial-total score) for each person. Then for all of the people with a given score, we determine the proportion who have endorsed the target item. A good item, such as Question 1 in Fig. 12.10, has a probability close to 0 per cent at the lowest score and increases to nearly

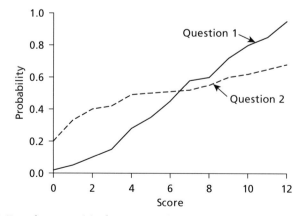

Fig. 12.10 Test of monotonicity for two questions.

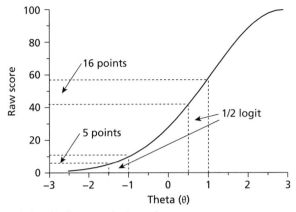

Fig. 12.11 The relationship between logits and raw scores.

100 per cent at the highest. A poorly performing item, such as Question 2 in the same figure, has a much flatter line, starting well above 0 per cent and ending well below 100 per cent. Such items are poor discriminators and probably should be dropped from the final scale. We can also calculate the point-biserial correlation between the item score and the test score, which should be high (Nandakumar and Kumar 2004).

Logits and raw scores

As has been mentioned in various sections in this book, scores resulting from scales developed by CTT do not have interval level properties and, unless they have been normalized using the procedures outlined in Chapter 7, they are rarely normally distributed. This means that a 5-point difference in the mid-range of the scale cannot be presumed to be equivalent to a 5-point difference at the lower or upper extreme. Logits, on the other hand, especially those resulting from the Rasch model, are interval. The relationship between logit scores and raw scores is shown in Fig. 12.11. In the middle of the range of scores, where the item characteristic curve is straight, there is a one-to-one relationship between changes in logits and changes in the raw score. But, as the figure shows, this breaks down at the ends. Equal changes in logits translate into proportionately smaller raw score changes. This means that, at the two extremes, differences in the trait are underestimated using raw scores, making it more difficult to discriminate among people with high or low levels of θ, or to determine the meaningfulness of changes within an individual (Cella and Chang 2000).

Test information and the standard error of measurement

In CTT, there is one SEM for the test, defined as:

$$SEM = \sigma\sqrt{1 - r_{XX}}$$

where r_{xx} is the estimated reliability of the scale and σ its estimated standard deviation. As we mentioned in the introduction to this chapter, this is an unrealistic simplification, because the error is actually smaller in the middle of the scale, and larger at the extremes where there are usually far fewer items and people. Further, the SEM varies from one population to another, because each has a different reliability and variance. In IRT, the concept of reliability is replaced by one of item or test *information*, which is a function of the model parameters. In the dichotomous Rasch model, item information (I) is the probability of a correct or positive response, $p_i(\theta)$, times the probability of an incorrect or negative one, $q_i(\theta)$:

$$I(\theta) = p_i(\theta)q_i(\theta)$$

that is, it is the IIF we discussed earlier (in the section 'Item information'), but without the slope parameter, because that is constant for all items. For the 2- and 3PLM, the discrimination parameter, a_i, also plays a role:

$$I(\theta) = a_i^2 p_i(\theta)q_i(\theta)$$

Test information is additive across items and is simply the sum of all of the item information curves, and the SEM at any given trait level is:

$$SEM(\theta) = 1/\sqrt{I(\theta)} = 1/\sqrt{\sum a_i^2 p_i(\theta)q_i(\theta)}$$

These formulae tell us two things. First, the more information there is (items where p_i is around 50 per cent, and with good discrimination), the smaller the error of measurement. Second, the SEM is a U-shaped function, smallest when θ is zero (and roughly equal to the SEM estimated from CTT) and increasing as we move towards the extremes (Embretson 1996). Thus, the level of SEM for a given individual depends only on their trait level and the levels of $I(\theta)$ to which they responded (Reise and Haviland 2005). Third, if items are added to or eliminated from a scale, the new value of SEM can be easily calculated by simply adding the item information values of the resulting scale. Finally, this information can be used to design tests for different purposes. For example, in qualification exams, where a person either surpasses the cut point and passes, or falls below it and fails, the actual score is of little importance. Thus, items can be chosen that have high information values near the cut point, resulting in very efficient tests.

Having said that, it is often useful to have an index that is applicable for the scale as a whole. This is given by the *Person Separation Index*, R_θ, which is analogous to Cronbach's alpha. It is defined as:

$$R_\theta = \frac{var\left(\hat{\theta}\right) - var(\varepsilon)}{var\left(\hat{\theta}\right)}$$

where the error term, ε, is the mean squared error of the person estimate, summed across people.

Equating tests

It is possible to equate instruments in CTT, and it is common practice with aptitude, achievement, admission, licensing, and other high-stake tests (see, for example, Kolen 1988; Kolen and Brennan 1995). This is done so that people taking one version of a scale are not disadvantaged if a parallel version is slightly less difficult; in essence, a linear transformation is found so that scores on one version can be equated with scores on the other version. It is also extremely useful in health measurement when different scales are used to measure the same attribute, such as quality of life or depression. In Chapter 7, we outline some simple techniques that can be used, such as transforming raw scores into deviation scores (z- or T-scores). However, this approach is based on a number of assumptions, such as the normality of the distributions and interval level properties of the scores—assumptions that are rarely met.

IRT provides another method for equating tests. However, a few caveats are necessary before discussing some of the details. Strictly speaking, test equating in IRT (as in CTT) is designed for parallel forms of the same test. It should *not* be used if the scales differ markedly with respect to their content, difficulty, or reliability; no equating method works well if the scales do differ in any of these aspects (Cook and Eignor 1991). Two tests are considered to be equated if: (1) they both measure the same attribute, (2) the conversion from one to the other is independent of the groups used to derive the raw scores, (3) the tests are interchangeable after the conversion, and (4) either scale can be used as the comparator (Angoff 1984).

Another use of this technique in IRT is to create an *item bank*, in which items from a number of scales are equated and calibrated so that they can be placed on one continuum. For example, McHorney and Cohen (2000) used functional status items from 75 different activities of daily living instruments. As a result of this exercise, they were able to identify items that were redundant, in that they had equivalent item difficulty and discrimination parameters, and to determine that there were very few items across all of the scales that would be considered very difficult. Furthermore, it is now possible for others to tailor scales for specific groups, by selecting items that are germane to the disorder and span the activities of daily living continuum.

However, there is a heavy cost associated with this procedure. McHorney and Cohen bemoaned the fact that they were able to get 'only' 2,306 usable questionnaires, a 'smaller analytic sample than desired' (p. S44), and their concern was not unfounded. Kolen and Brennan (1995) recommend a minimum of 400 subjects for a 1PLM and about 1,500 for a 3PLM, but these are the sample sizes for each form; as we shall see, these recommended numbers often have to be doubled.

Because we imagine that relatively few readers of this book will have either the need or the resources to do equating themselves, we will describe the technique only briefly. Those who need more information are directed to Cook and Eignor (1991) and Kolen and Brennan (1995).

The simplest method for equating is the *single group design*: all subjects are given all of the items. This may be infeasible, though, if the total number of items becomes onerous, or if the individual scales are intended to be used with different groups. The first problem can be solved with the *random groups design*, in which two or more equivalent groups are given different forms of the test. The second problem (as well as the first) can be dealt with using the *anchor test design*. Here, the groups, which need not be equivalent, are given the separate forms, but there is a block of items which they both receive—the anchor test. This smaller pool of items is then used to derive the equations that equate the items. With these last two designs, though, we pay the price of needing twice the sample size.

Sample size

Although we have been discussing both the 'simple' Rasch model and the more complex 2- and 3PLMs in the same chapter, they differ greatly with respect to sample-size requirements. For the Rasch model with dichotomous variables, Linacre (1994) and Wright and Tennant (1996) state that, to be 95 per cent confident that no item calibration score (b) is more than 1 logit from its stable value, 30 subjects are required; and about 100 subjects are needed for 1/2 logit. However, as the number of parameters increases, and when we move from dichotomous to polytomous items, the sample size requirements increase rapidly. If the Rasch model is used with a Likert-type scale, for example, Linacre (1999) recommends at least 10 subjects for each category. If the responses are not equally divided among the response options, this may mean that there would have to be 100 or more subjects in the more commonly endorsed ones. Thus, paradoxically, we often need a larger sample size to evaluate a more informative polytomous scale than a less informative dichotomous one. Embretson and Reise (2000) state that 'some of the category threshold parameters were not well estimated in the GRM with 350 examinees' (p. 123); and Reise and Yu (1990) recommend 500 responders for the GRM with a 25-item test; longer questionnaires may require even larger sample sizes. As with CTT, all we have are recommendations based on experience and simulations. Our (tentative) suggestions at this point are:

1. For a 1PLM with a dichotomous response option, the minimum requirement is 30 subjects.
2. The more parameters that are estimated, the larger the sample size that is needed.
3. With the GRM and the 2- and 3PLMs, aim for a minimum of 500 people.
4. The finer the discriminations among people you want to make, the more subjects are needed to derive the scale.

The other consideration is how many items there needs to be in a scale. Especially with respect to the GRM, Dai et al. (2021) recommend an absolute minimum of five, with parameter estimates improving as the number of items increase.

Mokken scaling

Falling somewhere between Guttman scaling, which was discussed in Chapter 4, and IRT is a technique called *Mokken scale analysis* (MSA). A perfect Guttman scale imposes a fairly strict criterion on the pattern of answers, in that a person who responds positively to a given item *must* also respond positively to less difficult items; and if an item is scored negatively, then all more difficult items *must* be answered negatively, too. That is, Guttman scaling is *deterministic*; the response to one item predicts the response to all less difficult items. MSA (Mokken 1971; Mokken and Lewis 1982) relaxes this criterion, so that answering positively to one item increases the *probability* of answering less difficult items the same way, without regarding reversals as errors in scaling, as is the case with Guttman scales. Both types of scales assume that the underlying trait is measured with a set of hierarchical items that can be ordered by item difficulty. Thus, the person's score is simply the total number of positive responses, or the rank of the highest item on the hierarchy.

MSA also shares assumptions with the Rasch model: in particular, unidimensionality, local independence, and monotonically non-decreasing IRFs. Where they part company is that all of the IRT models are parametric, in that they assume that the IRFs follow a logistic function, whereas MSA is a non-parametric technique (or, more accurately, a set of techniques).

There are two versions of MSA: the Monotone Homogeneity (MH) and the Double Monotone (DM) models. The MH model assumes that the IRFs are monotonically decreasing, but the shapes of the response curves can differ from one item to the next. Thus, the MH model is the non-parametric equivalent of the 2PLM in IRT. The DM model makes the additional assumption that the IRFs do not intersect. This implies that the curves all have the same slope, and so it is the non-parametric counterpart of the 1PLM (van Schuur 2003).

Mokken scaling is much less commonly used than IRT. One reason is that, because the IRF is not defined parametrically, the person parameters that come out of IRT cannot be estimated in MSA (Sijtsma and Verweij 1992). Also, some have questioned whether the scaling procedures that are used result in unambiguous results (e.g. Roskam et al. 1986). However, it remains a viable alternative to IRT, especially when the number of items in the scale is low. If you want to learn more, you should read Sijtsma and Molenaar (2002).

Advantages

IRT has many advantages over CTT, which are both theoretical and practical. On the theoretical side, the primary one is that there is no need to play 'let's pretend' that what is really an ordinal scale can be treated as if it were interval; the scale that emerges from an IRT analysis truly has interval level properties. Consequently, moving from a score of $+2$ to $+1$ logits on a pain scale would represent the same distance as changing from 0 to -1. Because many of the mathematical models of change described in Chapter 11 assume that the scale is interval (that is, difference scores are constant across the range of possible answers), the results are more likely to be valid. It should be noted, though, that some authors, such as Bond and Fox (2007), maintain that interval level scales arise only from the one-parameter Rasch model, and that adding the other two parameters eliminates this property.

A second theoretical advantage is that IRT provides a more precise estimate of measurement error. In CTT, as we discussed, there is one value for the reliability and the SEM, which then pertains to all respondents, irrespective of where they fall on the scale. IRT is more realistic, in that these values vary, depending on what the respondent's score is. Because most people fall in the middle range, scores with intermediate values of θ are estimated more accurately than those at the two extremes.

On the practical side, a major advantage is that IRT allows *test-free measurement*; that is, people can be compared on a trait or attribute even if they took completely different items! Assume that we have developed a test of physical mobility using IRT, and have derived a 30-item scale that spans the range from complete immobility at the low end to unrestricted, pain-free movement at the top. These items can be thought of as comprising a Guttman-ordered scale; responding positively to the eighth item, for example, means that the person must have responded positively to the previous seven. Conversely, if a person answers in the negative direction to item 15, then they would not answer positively to any item above number 15. Knowing this, we do not need to give all the items to all people—only those items that straddle the point where the person switches from answering in one direction to answering in the other. That point places the person at a specific point on the mobility continuum; and that point can be compared directly to one from another person, who was given a different subset of items. In actuality, because the slopes of the item characteristic curves are never perfectly vertical, a number of items spanning the critical point must be used.

This form of administration has received its widest application in achievement testing. Many tests developed over the past four decades, such as the revised version of the *Wide Range Achievement Test* (Wilkinson 1993), the *Keymath Diagnostic Arithmetic Test* (Connolly et al. 1976), and the *Woodcock Reading Mastery Tests* (Woodcock 1987), have used it, so that people at different levels can be given different items, yet be placed on the same scale at the end. This means that people with less of the trait (e.g. spelling ability) are not frustrated by being given a large number of items that are beyond their ability; nor are people with more of the trait bored by having to spell very easy words like 'cat' or 'run'. In addition to reducing frustration, it lessens testing time, since candidates do not spend large amounts of time on items that are trivial or beyond their capacity. This 'adaptive' or 'tailored' testing is not dependent on IRT (e.g. the Wechsler intelligence tests were not developed using IRT, but use a degree of adaptive testing), but it is greatly facilitated by it.

Combining IRT with computers leads to the next logical step, which is *computerized adaptive testing* (CAT). The examinee is presented with a few items near the mid-point of the difficulty range (i.e. $\theta = 0$). If most of them are answered in the keyed direction (correct for ability tests; endorsing the item for personality scales), then items with a higher value of θ are given; if not, then less difficult items are presented. This continues until some criterion is reached, usually that the person's ability is estimated with a sufficient degree of accuracy (that is, the standard error falls below some established value). Waller and Reise (1989) determined that there is no loss of precision when fewer than 50 per cent of the items were administered. This is one reason that companies administering high-stakes exams have widely adopted CAT. However, it is rarely used for most scales of attitudes and beliefs, primarily because large sample sizes are needed in order to derive accurate parameter estimates for each of the items.

One concern that may be raised is that a shortened subtest would have a much larger SEM and lower reliability than the whole test, and this would be true in CTT. However, in IRT, the SEM is dependent solely on the probability of endorsing an item at a given value of θ, so that short tests can be as reliable, or even more reliable, than long ones (Embretson 1996; Embretson and Reise 2000). Another reason is that, in CTT, the assumption is that all items come from a common pool, so that the Spearman–Brown prophecy formula, discussed in Chapter 5, applies—increasing the number of items increases the test's reliability. However, in adaptive testing, the items that are presented are tailored to the person's ability level, and those that are too extreme for that person are not given (Embretson 1996).

A second practical advantage of IRT is that, in CTT, it is usually undesirable to have items with different response options in the same scale (e.g. mixing True/False items with 5- and 7-level Likert scales) because this leads to the items contributing differentially to the total score, simply because of the answering scheme. This is not a problem using IRT, since the weight assigned to each item is a function of its difficulty level, not the raw answer. This gives the test designer much greater flexibility in phrasing the questions, rather than the usual Procrustean solution of forcing all items into the same format.

Disadvantages

Given the many practical and theoretical advantages of IRT, the question can be raised why it is used so widely in aptitude and achievement testing, but is rarely used for measuring attitudes, traits, quality of life, and other areas tapped by this book. In fact, Reise (2003) found that over 57 per cent of articles in two leading journals that focus on innovations in psychometrics (the *Journal of Educational Measurement* and *Applied Psychological Measurement*) involved IRT, but fewer than 4 per cent of articles in two equally prestigious scale-oriented journals (the *Journal of Personality Assessment* and *Psychological Assessment*) did.

One reason is that, with the large sample sizes generally found in developing educational tests, the differences between scales constructed with IRT and CTT are trivial. Fan (1998), for example, found that the correlations between the parameters a, b, and θ derived from IRT, and the equivalent values of r_{pb}, p, and the T-score derived from CTT were in the high 0.80s and 0.90s. Further, as mentioned previously in 'Advantages', none of the versions of the widely used intelligence tests developed by Wechsler was developed using IRT, yet no one within the psychometric community challenges their validity, and the IQ scale that results from them is most often considered an interval one.

Second, one purported advantage of IRT is its *invariance* property: that is, that item characteristics are independent of the sample from which they were derived. This has been shown on a theoretical level (e.g. Hambleton and Swaminathan 1985), but Fan (1998) states that 'the superiority of IRT over CTT in this regard has been taken for granted by the measurement community, and no empirical scrutiny has been deemed necessary' (p. 361). In fact, a number of studies have found relatively large differences from one population or test condition to another, suggesting that invariance does not hold (e.g. Cook et al. 1988; Miller and Linn 1988). One possible reason for the disagreement regarding the invariance of item characteristics may have to do with the populations studied. IRT was developed within the context of educational tests, where the population being assessed is relatively homogeneous. Cella and Chang (2000) suggest that clinical populations are more heterogeneous, so that issues such as context, the sequence of questions, and the nature of the specific sample may affect the item parameters. This is still an open question.

A third reason that IRT is not as widely used is its 'hard' assumption of unidimensionality. One implication of this is that IRT cannot be used to construct indices, where the items are causal rather than effect indicators (this was discussed in Chapter 5: 'When homogeneity does not matter'). Thus, it would be wrong to use IRT to construct indices of quality of life, symptom checklists, and other tools where the items themselves define the construct, rather than being manifestations of an underlying latent trait. A second implication is that IRT cannot be used when the underlying construct is itself multifaceted and complex, as are many in the health field. For example, Koksal and Power (1990) postulate that anxiety consists of four components—affective, behavioural, cognitive, and somatic—which Antony (2001) states can operate independently from one another. Although IRT can be used to create four subscales, it cannot be used in this case to make a 'global' anxiety scale.

Fourth, adaptive testing makes sense when, as with aptitude, achievement, and admissions tests, there is a very large pool of items, and it is impractical to administer them all to each person. However, most scales used in personality and health-related areas are relatively short, consisting of 20 or 30 items at most, so that there is little advantage in using adaptive or tailored tests. Finally, as Reise and Henson (2003) point out, testing in these fields has not come under the close public and legal scrutiny about fairness and validity that exists (at least in the United States) in the realms of achievement and aptitude testing, so there is less pressure to develop scales that meet the more stringent psychometric demands of IRT.

Reporting results of a Rasch analysis

Very recently, a comprehensive set of guidelines has been published regarding how to report the results of a Rasch analysis. The two papers can be found in Mallinson et al. (2022) and Van de Winckel et al. (2022). To the best of our knowledge, there are no equivalent guidelines for the two- and three-parameter models.

Computer programs

When this chapter was first written, there were relatively few computer programs that could handle IRT models. Now, there is a proliferation of them, especially for the 1PLM. Perhaps the most popular are RUMM for the polytomous Rasch model (Sheridan et al. 1996); BILOG (Mislevy and Bock 1990), which can handle up to a three-parameter model for dichotomous data; an extension of it, called PARSCALE (Muraki and Bock 1993), for polytomous items; and MULTILOG (Thissen 1991), for up to three parameters and dichotomous or polytomous data. Guides to these and other of the more popular programs can be found in Bond and Fox (2007), Embretson and Reise (2000), and Thorpe and Favia (2012). Since version 14, Stata can run different IRT models; and macros have also been developed for widely used statistical software packages such as SAS (<http://www2.sas.com/proceedings/sugi30/204-30.pdf>) and SPSS (<https://www.ibm.com/support/pages/item-response-theoryrasch-models-spss-statistics>). For those who use *R*, there are a number of packages to run IRT, such as *cran* and *irtplay*. A good resource for *R* is Rizopoulos (2006).

Further reading

Allen, M.J. and Yen, W.M. (1979). *Introduction to measurement theory*. Wadsworth, Belmont, CA.

Bejar, I.I. (1983). *Achievement testing*. Sage, Beverly Hills, CA.

Bond, T.G. and Fox, C.M. (2007). *Applying the Rasch model: Fundamental measurement in the human sciences* (2nd edn). Routledge, New York.

Crocker, L. and Algina, J. (2006). *Introduction to classical and modern test theory*. Wadsworth, Belmont, CA.

Embretson, S.E. and Reise, S.P. (2000). *Item response theory for psychologists*. Lawrence Erlbaum Associates, Mahwah, NJ.

Hambleton, R.K. (ed.) (1983). *Applications of item response theory*. Educational Research Institute of British Columbia, Vancouver.

Lord, F.M. (1980). *Application of item response theory to practical testing problems*. Erlbaum, Hillsdale, NJ.

Reise, S.P. and Henson, J.M. (2003). A discussion of modern versus traditional psychometrics as applied to personality assessment scales. *Journal of Personality Assessment*, **81**, 93–103.

Stemler, S.E. and Naples, A. (2021). Rasch measurement v. item response theory: Knowing when to cross the line. *Practical Assessment, Research, and Evaluation*, **26**, Article 11 .

Traub, R.E. and Wolfe, R.G. (1981). Latent trait theories and assessment of educational achievement. In *Review of research in education 9* (ed. D.C. Berliner), pp. 377–435. American Educational Research Association, Washington, DC.

References

Angoff, W.H. (1984). *Scales, norms, and equivalent scores*. Educational Testing Service, Princeton, NJ.

Antony, M.M. (2001). Assessment of anxiety and the anxiety disorders: An overview. In *Practitioner's guide to empirically based measures of anxiety* (eds. M.M. Antony, S.M. Orsillo, and L. Roemer), pp. 7–17. Kluwer Academic/Plenum, New York.

Birnbaum, A. (1968). Some latent trait models and their use in inferring an examinee's ability. In *Statistical theories of mental test scores* (eds. F.M. Lord and M.R. Novick), pp. 397–479. Addison-Wesley, Reading, MA.

Bond, T.G. and Fox, C.M. (2007). *Applying the Rasch model: Fundamental measurement in the human sciences* (2nd edn). Routledge, New York.

Cai, L., Choi, K., Hansen, M., and Harrell, L. (2016). Item response theory. *Annual Review of Statistics and Its Application*, **3**, 297–321.

Carmines, E.G. and Zeller, R.A. (1979). *Reliability and validity assessment.* Sage, Beverly Hills, CA.

Cella, D. and Chang, C.-H. (2000). A discussion of item response theory and its applications in health status assessments. *Medical Care*, **38**(Suppl. II), S66–72.

Connolly, A.J., Nachtman, W., and Pritchett, E.M. (1976). *Keymath Diagnostic Arithmetic Test.* American Guidance Service, Circle Pines, MN.

Cook, L.L. and Eignor, D.R. (1991). *IRT equating methods. Instructional Topics in Educational Measurement, Module 10.* National Council on Measurement in Education, Mount Royal, NJ.

Cook, L.L., Eignor, D.R., and Taft, H.L. (1988). A comparative study of the effects of recency of instruction on the stability of IRT and conventional item parameter estimates. *Journal of Educational Measurement*, **25**, 31–45.

Crane, P.K., van Belle, G., and Larson, E.B. (2004). Test bias in a cognitive test: Differential item functioning in the CASI. *Statistics in Medicine*, **23**, 241–56.

Crane, P.K., Gibbons, L.E., Jolley, L., and van Belle, G. (2006). Differential item functioning analysis with ordinal logistic regression techniques: DIFdetect and difwithpar. *Medical Care*, **44**, S115–23.

Dai, S., Vo, T.T., Kehinde, O.J., He, H., Xue, Y., Demir, C., *et al.* (2021). Performance of polytomous IRT models with rating scale data: An investigation over sample size, instrument length, and missing data. *Frontiers in Education*, **6**, Article 721963 .

Embretson, S.E. (1996). The new rules of measurement. *Psychological Assessment*, **8**, 341–9.

Embretson, S.E. and Reise, S.P. (2000). *Item response theory for psychologists.* Lawrence Erlbaum Associates, Mahwah, NJ.

Fan, X. (1998). Item response theory and classical test theory: An empirical comparison of their item/person statistics. *Educational and Psychological Measurement*, **58**, 357–81.

Franke, G.H. (1997). 'The whole is more than the sum of its parts': The effects of grouping and randomizing items on the reliability and validity of questionnaires. *European Journal of Psychological Assessment*, **13**, 67–74.

Grisso, T. (1998). *Instruments for assessing understanding and appreciation of Miranda rights.* Professional Resources, Sarasota, FL.

Hambleton, R.K. and Swaminathan, H. (1985). *Item response theory: Principles and applications.* Kluwer Nijhoff, Boston, MA.

Hambleton, R.K., Swaminathan, H., and Rogers, H.J. (1991). *Fundamentals of item response theory.* Sage, Newbury Park, NJ.

Hattie, J. (1985). Assessing unidimensionality of tests and items. *Applied Psychological Measurement*, **9**, 139–64.

Hill, C.D., Edwards, M.C., Thissen, D., Langer, M.M., Wirth, R.J., Burwinkle, T.M., *et al.* (2007). Practical issues in the application of item response theory: A demonstration using items from the Pediatric Quality of Life Inventory (PedsQL) 4.0 Generic Core scale. *Medical Care*, **45**(Suppl. 1), S39–47.

Koksal, F. and Power, K.G. (1990). Four systems anxiety questionnaire (FSAQ): A self-report measure of somatic, cognitive, behavioral, and feeling components. *Journal of Personality Assessment*, **54**, 534–45.

Kolen, M.J. (1988). Traditional equating methodology. *Educational Measurement: Issues and Practice*, **7**, 29–36.

Kolen, M.J. and Brennan, R.L. (1995). *Test equating: Methods and practices*. Springer, New York.

Lawley, D.N. (1943). XXIII.—On problems connected with item selection and test construction. *Proceedings of the Royal Society of Edinburgh Section A: Mathematics*, **61**, 273–87.

Linacre, J.M. (1994). Sample size and item calibration stability. *Rasch Measurement Transactions*, **7**, 328.

Linacre, J.M. (1998). Why principal components analysis (PCA)? *Rasch Measurement Transactions*, **12**, 636.

Linacre, J.M. (1999). Investigating rating scale category utility. *Journal of Outcome Measurement*, **3**, 103–22.

Lord, F.M. and Novick, M.N. (1968). *Statistical theories of mental test development*. Addison-Wesley, Reading, MA.

Lumsden, J. (1957). A factorial approach to unidimensionality. *Australian Journal of Psychology*, **9**, 105–11.

Lumsden, J. (1961). The construction of unidimensional tests. *Psychological Bulletin*, **58**, 122–31.

Mallinson, T., Kozlowski, A.J., Johnson, M.V., Weaver, J., Terhorst, L., Grampurohit, N., et al. (2022). Rasch reporting guideline for rehabilitation research (RULER): The RULER statement. *Archives of Physical Medicine and Rehabilitation*, **103**, 1477–86.

McHorney, C.A. and Cohen, A.S. (2000). Equating health status measures with item response theory. *Medical Care*, **38**(Suppl. II), S43–59.

Micceri, T. (1989). The unicorn, the normal curve, and other improbable creatures. *Psychological Bulletin*, **105**, 156–66.

Miller, M.D. and Linn, R.L. (1988). Invariance of item characteristic functions with variations in instructional coverage. *Journal of Educational Measurement*, **25**, 205–19.

Mislevy, R.J. and Bock, R.D. (1990). *BILOG3: Item analysis and test scoring with binary logistic models*. Scientific Software, Mooresville, IN.

Mokken, R.J. (1971). *Theory and procedure of scale analysis*. Mouton, The Hague.

Mokken, R.J. and Lewis, C. (1982). A nonparametric approach to the analysis of dichotomous item responses. *Applied Psychological Measurement*, **6**, 417–30.

Muraki, E. and Bock, R.D. (1993). *PARSCALE: IRT based test scoring and item analysis for graded open-ended exercises and performance tasks*. Scientific Software International, Chicago, IL.

Nandakumar, R. and Ackerman, T. (2004). Test modeling. In *The Sage handbook of quantitative methodology in the social sciences* (ed. D. Kaplan), pp. 93–105. Sage, Thousand Oaks, CA.

Norman, G.R. and Streiner, D.L. (2014). *Biostatistics: The bare essentials* (4th edn). PMPH USA, Shelton, CT.

Panter, A.T., Swygert, K.A., Dahlstrom, W.G., and Tanaka, J.S. (1997). Factor analytic approaches to personality item-level data. *Journal of Personality Assessment*, **68**, 561–89.

Rasch, G. (1960). *Probabilistic models for some intelligence and attainment tests.* Nielson and Lydiche, Copenhagen.

Reckase, M.D. (1979). Unifactor latent trait models applied to multifactor tests: Results and implications. *Journal of Educational Statistics*, **4**, 207–30.

Reise, S.P. and Haviland, M.G. (2005). Item response theory and the measurement of clinical change. *Journal of Personality Assessment*, **84**, 228–38.

Reise, S.P. and Henson, J.M. (2003). A discussion of modern versus traditional psychometrics as applied to personality assessment scales. *Journal of Personality Assessment*, **81**, 93–103.

Reise, S.P. and Yu, J. (1990). Parameter recovery in the graded response model using MULTILOG. *Journal of Educational Measurement*, **27**, 133–44.

Rizopoulos, D. (2006). ltm: An R package for latent variable modeling and item response theory analyses. *Journal of Statistical Software*, **17**(5).

Roskam, E.E., van den Wollenberg, A.L., and Jansen, P.G.W. (1986). The Mokken scale: A critical discussion. *Applied Psychological Measurement*, **10**, 265–77.

Scott, R.L. and Pampa, W.M. (2000). The MMPI-2 in Peru: A normative study. *Journal of Personality Assessment*, **74**, 95–105.

Shader, R.I. and Streiner, D.L. (2021). How homogeneous are diagnostic groups? *Journal of Clinical Psychopharmacology*, **41**, 620–1.

Sheridan, B., Andrich, D., and Luo, G. (1996). *Welcome to RUMM: a Windows-based item analysis program employing Rasch unidimensional measurement models. User's guide.* RUMM Laboratory, Perth.

Sijtsma, K. and Molenaar, W. (2002). *Introduction to nonparametric item response theory.* Sage, Thousand Oaks, CA.

Sijtsma, K. and Verweij, A.C. (1992). Mokken scale analysis: Theoretical considerations and an application to transitivity tasks. *Applied Measurement in Education*, **5**, 355–73.

Stemler, S.E. and Naples, A. (2021). Rasch measurement v. item response theory: Knowing when to cross the line. *Practical Assessment, Research, and Evaluation*, **26**, Article 11 .

Streiner, D.L. and Miller, H.R. (1986). Can a good short form of the MMPI ever be developed? *Journal of Clinical Psychology*, **42**, 109–13.

Streiner, D.L., Corna, L., Veldhuizen, S., and Cairney, J. (2005). *Anglophone and Francophone rates of depression: Cultural or language differences?* Paper presented at the Canadian Academy of Psychiatric Epidemiology, Vancouver.

Thissen, D. (1991). *MULTILOG user's guide: Multiple category item analysis and test scoring using item response theory.* Scientific Software International, Chicago, IL.

Thorpe, G.L. and Favia, A. (2012). Data analysis using item response theory methodology: An introduction to selected programs and applications. *Psychology Faculty Scholarship*, Paper 20. DigitalCommons@UMaine.

Thurstone, L.L. (1925). A method of scaling psychological and educational tests. *Journal of Educational Psychology*, **16**, 433–51.

Van de Winckel, A., Kozlowski, A.J., Johnson, M.V., Weaver, J., Grampurohit, N., Terhorst, L., *et al.* (2022). Reporting guideline for RULER: Rasch reporting guideline for rehabilitation research—Explanation and elaboration manuscript. *Archives of Physical Medicine and Rehabilitation*, **103**, 1487–98.

Van Schuur, W.H. (2003). Mokken scale analysis: Between the Guttman scale and parametric item response theory. *Political Analysis*, **11**, 139–63.

Waller, N.G. and Reise, S.P. (1989). Computer adaptive personality assessment: An illustration with the Absorption Scale. *Journal of Personality and Social Psychology*, 57, 1051–8.

Wilkinson, G.S. (1993). *Wide Range Achievement Test 3 manual.* Jastak Associates, Wilmington, DE.

Woodcock, R.W. (1987). *Woodcock Reading Mastery Tests—Revised.* American Guidance Service, Circle Pines, MN.

Wright, B.D. (1977). Solving measurement problems with the Rasch model. *Journal of Educational Measurement*, 14, 97–116.

Wright, B.D. and Tennant, A. (1996). Sample size again. *Rasch Measurement Transactions*, **9**, 468.

Chapter 13

Methods of administration

Introduction to methods of administration

Having developed the questionnaire, the next problem is how to administer it. This is an issue which not only affects costs and response rates but also, as we shall see, may influence which questions can be asked and in what format. Traditionally, the most commonly used methods involved participants completing questionnaires by themselves, often by mail, or in groups at the same time such as in a classroom setting. For many years, questionnaires were also completed using the telephone, where an interviewer asked structured questions and then recorded the responses of the participant. In some cases, particularly in clinical settings, face-to-face interviews are used to collect responses to questionnaire items, especially if the participant (or patient) has difficulty understanding the wording or requires assistance in answering. For much of the twentieth century, responses from questionnaires were collected with all these methods using pen and paper. The responses were then entered into a database for analysis. Today, responses are digitally converted to data at the point of collection, via survey assistive software on computers, tablets, and mobile devices. As we'll see, this opens up new opportunities as well as new issues that must be faced. Social media, for example, is now commonly used to recruit participants.

In the first five editions of the book, we retained all the methods including those that were outdated, because it provided an opportunity to discuss some methodological issues that even with the advancement of online technologies, we believed were still worth considering. In this edition, we have rewritten the chapter, focusing primarily on contemporary methods, and devoting less space to those methods which are almost never used, except in specific contexts, such as where access to online methods and mobile technologies are limited.

Face-to-face interviews

As the name implies, this method involves a trained interviewer administering the scale or questionnaire on a one-on-one basis, either in an office or, more usually, in the participant's home. The latter setting serves to put the respondents at ease, since they are in familiar surroundings, and may also increase compliance, because the subjects do not have to travel. However, home interviewing involves greater cost to the investigator and the possibility of interruptions, for instance, by telephones or family members. For this reason, it is typically not used except in situations where the respondents might need assistance, either with interpretation of the items, or in answering the questions. For example, a large multisite intervention study targeting homeless individuals with mental illness (the At Home/Chez Soi project) used face-to-face interviews for follow-up because of the precarious circumstances of the participants and the need to ensure comprehension of items (Goering et al. 2011). Some methods, such as structured clinical interviews used in assessing mental illness (Kessler and Ustun 2004), also continue to rely on interviewee -based protocols.

Advantages

The advantages of face-to-face interviewing begin even before the first question is asked—the interviewer is sure who is responding. This is not the case with telephone or mail administration, since anyone in the household can answer or provide a second opinion for the respondent. In addition, having to respond verbally to another person reduces the number of items omitted by the respondent: it is more difficult to refuse to answer than to simply omit an item on a form (Quine 1985). Face-to-face interviews allow non-verbal communication between the two parties, which can motivate the respondent to reply (Holbrook et al. 2003). The interviewer can also determine if the subject is having any difficulty understanding the items, whether due to a poor grasp of the language, limited intelligence, problems in concentration, or boredom. Further, since many immigrants and people with limited education understand the spoken language better than they can read it, and read it better than they can write it, fewer people will be eliminated because of these problems. This method of administration also allows the interviewer to rephrase the question in terms the person may better understand, or to probe for a more complete response. Although it is now possible to interview people using Voice-over-Internet Protocols (VoIP), richer information is gathered with in-person rather than remote interviews (Johnson et al. 2019).

Another advantage is the flexibility afforded in presenting the items, since questions in an interview can range from 'closed' to 'open'. Closed questions, which require only a number as a response, such as the person's age, number of children, or years of residence, can be read to the subject. If it is necessary for the respondent to choose among three or more alternatives, or to give a Likert-type response, a card with the possible answers could (and most likely *should*) be given to the person so that memory will not be a factor. Open questions can be used to gather additional information, since respondents will generally give longer answers to open-ended questions verbally rather than in writing. This can sometimes be a disadvantage with verbose respondents.

Complicated questionnaires may contain items that are not appropriate for all respondents: men should not be asked how many pregnancies they have had; native-born people when they immigrated; or people who have never been hospitalized when they were last discharged. These questions are avoided with what are called 'skip patterns': instructions or arrows indicating that the section should be omitted by skipping to a later portion of the questionnaire. Unless they are very carefully constructed and worded, skip patterns can be confusing to some respondents—and therefore likely to induce errors—if they have to follow these themselves. In contrast, interviewers, because of their training and experience in giving the questionnaire many times, can wend their way through these skip patterns much more readily, and are less likely to make mistakes. Moreover, with the advent of laptop computers, the order of questions and the skip patterns can be programmed to be presented to the interviewer, so that the potential for asking the wrong questions or omitting items is minimized.

Disadvantages

Naturally, there is a cost associated with all of these advantages, in terms of both time and money. Face-to-face interviews are significantly more expensive to administer than any other method. Interviewers must be trained, so that they ask the same questions in the same way, and to handle unusual circumstances similarly. As noted in the 'Advantages' section, one advantage of the face-to-face interview is that the interviewers can rephrase a question, if they feel that the respondent does not understand what is being asked. The converse of this, though, is that without sufficient training, the interviewer may distort the meaning of questions. In many studies, random interviews are recorded, to ensure that the interviewers' styles have not changed over time, that they have not become lazy or slipshod, or do not sound bored. This entails further expense, for the recording equipment itself, and for the supervisor's time to review the session and go over it with the interviewer.

If the interview is relatively short, the interviewer can arrive unannounced. This, though, takes the chance that the respondent is at home and is willing to be disturbed. The longer the session, the greater the danger that it will be seen as an imposition. Further, there is an increasing trend for people to live in settings that restrict unwanted or uninvited visitors, such as gated communities, locked apartment buildings, and retirement homes (Tourangeau 2004).

For these reasons, especially when an hour or more of the person's time is needed, it is better to announce the visit beforehand, checking the respondent's willingness to participate and arranging a convenient time to come. This requirement imposes the added costs of telephoning, often repeatedly, until an answer is obtained. Further, since many people work during the day, and only evening interviews are convenient, the number of possible interviews that can be done in one day may be limited.

The opposite side of the difficulty of gaining access to homes or apartments with security procedures is having to meet respondents in unsafe or unsanitary settings, or being alone with people who may be dangerous. For example, the At Home/Chez Soi project mentioned earlier (Goering et al. 2011) involved interviewing homeless, mentally ill individuals, some of whom had been given apartments. In some instances, the research assistants were threatened, and in other cases there was the possibility of contact with bed bugs, cockroaches, and other unpleasant creatures. The solutions included having two interviewers present if there was fear of physical harm (which increases the cost) or meeting in a public place that still afforded some degree of privacy. In these instances, safety and comfort concerns for the interviewer end up trumping the potential advantages of having the respondent feel at ease about participating in the interview.

Another potential cost arises if, for instance, English is not the native language for a sizable proportion of the respondents (especially in North America, the United Kingdom, and Australia). Not only must the scales and questions be translated into one or more foreign languages (as would be the case, regardless of the format), but bilingual (or in some cases multilingual) interviewers must be found. This may not be unduly difficult if there are only a few major linguistic cultures (e.g. English and French in Quebec, Spanish in the southwestern United States, Flemish and French in Belgium), but can be more of a problem in cities that attract many immigrants from different countries. In Toronto, Canada, for example, there are over 140 languages and dialects spoken, and 30 per cent of the people speak a language other than English or French at home. There are more languages to take into account and, if immigration has been recent, there may be few people sufficiently bi- or multi lingual who can be trained as interviewers.

Finally, attributes of the interviewer may affect the responses given. This can be caused by two factors: biases of the interviewer, and their social or ethnic character-istics (Weiss 1975). It has been known for a long time that interviewers can subtly communicate what answers they want to hear, often without being aware that they are doing so (e.g. Rice 1929). This is the easier of the two factors to deal with, since it can be overcome with adequate training (Hyman et al. 1954). The more difficult problem is that differences between the interviewer and respondent, especially race, also have an effect (Pettigrew 1964; Saltier 1970). During a gubernatorial campaign in the United States, for example, white telephone interviewers found that 43.8 per cent of those polled preferred the black Democratic candidate, while black interviewers found that his level of support was 52.2 per cent, a difference of 8.4 per centage points (Finkel et al. 1991). The interaction between the perceived race of the interviewer and the background characteristics of the interviewees was even more striking: among Republicans, there was only a 0.5 per centage point difference, while Democrats' re-ported level of support increased by 24.2 per centage points with black interviewers. Among those who reported themselves to be 'apolitical', support increased from 16.7 per cent to 63.6 per cent, although the sample size for this group was small. The reasons usually given for this phenomenon include social desirability, deferring to the perceived preferences of the interviewer because of 'interpersonal deference', or 'cour-tesy to a polite stranger' (Finkel et al. 1991). As is obvious from the results of this and other studies (e.g. Meislin 1987), the race of the interviewer can be detected relatively accurately over the telephone, although it is not known whether the subjects respond to the interviewer's accent, speech patterns, inflections, or other verbal cues.

The effect of sex differences is less clear. Female interviewers usually have fewer refusers and higher completion rates than males (Backstrom and Hursh-Cesar 1981; Hornik 1982), which in part may explain why the majority of interviewers are women (Colombotos et al. 1968). The responses women elicit may be different from those given to male interviewers, especially when sexual material is being discussed (Hyman et al. 1954), but also when the topic of the interview is politics (Hutchinson and Wegge 1991). Pollner (1998) found that both men and women reported more symptoms of depression, substance abuse, and conduct disorder to female interviewers than to males, and suggested that 'female interviewers may create conditions more conducive to disclosure and be perceived as more sympathetic than male interviewers' (p. 369). Furthermore, the differences in response rates seem to occur more with male inter-viewees than with females. Although both men and women prefer female interviewers, it is quite conceivable that there are some survey topics for which it is better to use same-sex interviewers, such as studies of sexual inadequacy or attitudes towards the opposite sex.

Age differences between the interviewer and interviewee have not been extensively studied. The general conclusion, though, is that to the degree that it is possible, the two should be as similar as possible, since perceived similarity generally leads to improved communication (Hutchinson and Wegge 1991; Rogers and Bhowmik 1970).

Before concluding this section, we would be remiss if we did not highlight that the very notion of face-to-face, which implies spatial proximity, is itself evolving. With the ability to FaceTime using mobile devices, and the rise in popularity of platforms such as Zoom and Microsoft Teams, it is no longer necessary to be in the same place as the participant to conduct an interview. With the requirements of physical distancing during the COVID19 pandemic, we increasingly saw interviews, including qualitative interviews, being conducted online (Lobe et al. 2020). While many of the same advantages and disadvantages apply to so-called web conferencing approaches to interviews (Glassmeyer and Dibbs 2012), the technology might offer some interesting possibilities. For example, both the image and voice of the interviewer could be changed, if the attributes of the interviewer were thought to be of concern. Of course, this raises potentially ethical concerns, as concealing or altering the identity of the interviewer is a form of deception. Perhaps the most obvious advantage of this approach is the cost savings. Whereas in the past, a researcher might have had to travel to another part of the country or even another country to do interviews, web conferencing allows the researchers to do their work from anywhere, at any time. This may also address some of the safety concerns noted above under 'Disadvantages'. At the same time, the obvious limitation is the availability of the technology. For vulnerable or marginalized populations, access to these platforms may be limited or non-existent. Privacy may also be a concern. For individuals living in small dwellings with large families or groups, finding a place to do the interview in private may be a challenge. Finally, the technology is dependent on Internet access; if connectivity is poor, the quality of the experience can be significantly compromised. Nevertheless, the technology is likely to continue to grow in use, making face-to-face interviews likely less common over time.

Self-administered

Arguably the easiest way to administer a scale is to simply hand it to people and have them complete the questionnaire themselves. The instructions can be written out on the top, or they can be read to the respondents, or both.

Advantages

The advantages of self-administered scales are obvious. They can be 'delivered' to the respondents in a variety of ways: handed out in class, mailed to them, or sent and responded to over a smartphone or the Internet. This means that no trained interviewers are required, and many people can complete the inventories simultaneously. If sent out electronically, the responses can often be scored and stored automatically, obviating the need to later enter the responses into a computer, with all of the time and probable entry errors this entails. Especially when paper forms are handed out and collected, it is easier to guarantee anonymity. This can be promised when the scales or questionnaires are sent out electronically, but some people may believe that their names can somehow be linked to their responses (and indeed they can be). However, it raises a problem if it's necessary to readminister the scale to test for reliability, or to link it to other sources of information.

Disadvantages

Counterbalancing the many advantages are a number of disadvantages. First, the researcher has lost control over how the questions are answered, or if they are even answered at all. The person may not answer the questions sequentially, but may rather skip around and even change early answers in light of later questions. This may not be an issue in most cases, but may be if the order of questions is important or first associations to them are important. As we discussed in Chapter 6 on biases in responding, poorly motivated respondents can resort to satisficing, by giving the same response to all items, choosing the 'neutral' option with Likert scales, or just not answering some or all of the questions.

However, most if not all of these disadvantages are now limited to self-administered questionnaires completed using pen and paper; surveys administered digitally can be set up to ensure questions are answered in the order intended by the designer, and that each item or question has a response logged before the respondent is allowed to proceed. There is no digital solution for poor motivation, however; moreover, problems of interpretation of items remains a possibility.

Telephone questionnaires

For most of the latter part of the twentieth century, telephone surveys were a popular method for administering surveys, largely because of the ubiquity of the technology. For example, in the United States in 2000, the proportion of households with a telephone was over 95 per cent by 2000 (Keeter 1995; Tourangeau 2004), with comparable figures for the United Kingdom (Nicolaas and Lynn 2002). However, the picture of telephone use has changed dramatically in the twenty-first century with the near universal adoption of mobile phones. A survey by Statistics Canada (2006) found that between mid -2003 and December 2005, the number of homes having only a mobile phone increased from 1.9 to 4.8 per cent. By 2019, this had jumped to 45 per cent (Statistics Canada 2019). In the United States, the numbers are even more dramatic. A 2021 survey by the National Center for Health Statistics reported that two-thirds of American homes had only mobile telephones (Blumberg and Luke 2021), up from one-third only a decade earlier. Moreover, the distribution was not uniform across the country or in different demographic characteristics. Among low-income households, 74 per cent had only a mobile phone, higher than the rate in higher-income groups (67 per cent), although the gap was much less than it had been 10 years previously. Those who rented apartments were more likely to have only mobile service (82 per cent) than those who owned their own home (61 per cent), and again, the gap had narrowed significantly. As would be expected, age was also a factor; 85 per cent of adults aged

25–29 did not have landlines, compared to only 41 per cent for those 65 and older. At this rate, there will be very few people using landlines in the foreseeable future. On the positive side, a recent review of over 250 surveys found that excluding people who had only landlines resulted in very little change in the results (Kennedy et al. 2018).

This decline in landline use has implications for surveys. First, the fact that many mobile phone companies charge the recipient of a call for the time used cannot auger well for response rates, especially for long surveys. Second, until recently, random digit dialling samples (described in the next section) excluded households that have only mobile phones, and even now, methodological, operational, and legal challenges exist which make including them difficult. In the United States, for example, automatic telephone dialling systems are specifically barred from calling mobile phones without the user's expressed consent. While the absolute number of people missed in surveys is small (although likely to grow), the results from the Statistics Canada (2006) and Tucker et al. (2007) national surveys show that it is a biased sample, with those not called being younger, more likely to be single, less well educated, and living in rented apartments. Other implications for random sampling are more subtle. Landline numbers are geographically based, allowing researchers to make their sample representative of the population. Mobile phone numbers, though, are not, meaning that a random selection of mobile phone numbers reflects the geographic distribution of mobile phone users, which is not uniform in the general population. Furthermore, a landline most often represents a household (except, perhaps, if teenagers have their own numbers), whereas mobile phones represent an individual, and some individuals may have multiple phones. Finally, there are unresolved issues of liability: if a driver answers their mobile phone to respond to a survey and is involved in a car accident, who is at fault?

Two other common advances in technology that have affected use of both landlines and mobile devices are call display and voicemail. In the latter case, the surveyor may be frustrated when their attempts to reach persons continually results in being pushed to a voicemail box. Sometimes, this is directly the result of the would-be participant not recognizing the number on call display and letting the call go to voicemail directly. There have been a few studies conducted to assess the effect of call display. In 2006, the National Immunization Survey (NIS), through the Centers for Disease Control at the University of Chicago, conducted an experiment to see if response rates were affected by the use of caller ID (Barron and Khare 2008). Respondents were randomly assigned to one of three groups: no-ID, ID on ('Norc U Chicago'), and a toll free number displayed. The results showed that blocking ID led to a lower response rate by almost 2 per centage points. Mostly this has to do with who answered the phone; respondents were less likely to pick up if the caller ID was blocked. A similar experiment was conducted by the Gallup Organization (Callegaro et al. 2010). The results showed that knowing a survey company was calling (via Caller ID) tended to act similarly to a 'business card', adding credibility and reducing fears that the person on the other end might be a telemarketer or collection agent.

One effect of all of these new telephone-related technologies, as Dillman (2002) has pointed out, is to alter our relationship to the telephone. Before voicemail and call display, it would have been unthinkable to ignore a ringing telephone. It would be interpreted as rude, and there was the concern that the caller would not be able to make contact. Now, rather than our behaviour being controlled by the telephone, we control it and use it at our convenience. One manifestation of this is that response rates that approached 80 per cent in the 1970s have been cut to 8 per cent by 2014 (Zukin 2015).

Random digit dialling

A technique called *random digit dialling* (RDD) was designed to bypass the problem of unlisted numbers. A computer-driven device dials telephone numbers at random, using either all seven (in some places, ten) digits of the number or the last four once the area code and the three-digit exchange has been chosen by the researcher. (This applies in the U.S. and Canada; other countries use a different number of digits for the area code and number.) Because there are a number of disadvantages to RDD, and as more and more households have abandoned landlines in favour of mobile devices, it is mostly obsolete today. Moreover, technologies such as call display and voicemail, which also are used on landlines, mean would -be respondents can still be difficult to reach if their landline number is not publicly available.

Advantages of telephone surveys

Many of the advantages of face-to-face interviewing also pertain to telephone surveys. These include:

1. A reduction in the number of omitted items.
2. Skip patterns are followed by the trained interviewer or a computer rather than the respondent.
3. Open-ended questions can be asked.
4. A broad, representative sample can be obtained.
5. The interviewer can be prompted by a computer (a technique often referred to as CATI, or computer-assisted telephone interviewing).
6. The interviewer can determine if the person is having problems understanding the language in general or a specific question in particular.

Another advantage of telephone interviewing is that, even when the person is not willing to participate, they may give some basic demographic information, such as age, marital status, or education. This allows the researcher to determine if there is any systematic bias among those who decline to participate in the study.

Moreover, there are at least three areas in which the telephone may be superior to face-to-face interviews. First, any bias that may be caused by the appearance of the interviewer, due to factors such as skin colour or physical deformity, is eliminated. However, one interviewer characteristic that cannot be masked by a telephone is gender. There is some evidence that male interviewers elicit more feminist responses from women and more conservative answers from men than do female interviewers , and more optimistic reports from both sexes regarding the economic outlook (Groves and Fultz 1985). These authors also report higher refusal rates for male interviewers, which is consistent with other studies.

A second advantage is that nationwide surveys can be conducted out of one office, which lowers administrative costs and facilitates supervision of the interviewers to ensure uniformity of style. Last, there is some evidence that people may report more health-related events in a telephone interview than in a face-to-face one (Thornberry 1987), although it is not clear that the higher figure is necessarily more accurate.

Disadvantages

A potential problem with telephone interviewing is that another person in the household may be prompting the respondent. However, this risk is fairly small, since the person on the phone would have to repeat each question aloud. A more difficult issue is that there is no assurance who the person is at the other end of the line. If the sampling scheme calls for interviewing the husband, for instance, the masculine voice can be that of the chosen respondent's son or father. This may be a problem if the designated person is an immigrant unsure of their grasp of the language and asks a more fluent member of the household to substitute.

Another difficulty with telephone interviews, as with face-to-face ones, is that unless a specific respondent is chosen beforehand, the sample may be biased by *when* the call is made. During the day, there is a higher probability that parents with young children, those who work at home, shift-workers, the ill, or the unemployed will be reached. Evening calls may similarly bias the sample by excluding shift-workers. Traugott (1987) found that people reached during the day did not differ significantly from those who could be contacted only in the evening with respect to age, race, or sex, but the latter group were more likely to be college graduates, since they tended to be employed and not work shifts.

A major problem with telephone interviewing, as opposed to face-to-face interviewing, is the difficulty with questions that require the person to choose among various options. With the interviewer present, they can hand the respondent a card listing the response alternatives—an option not available over the telephone. A few suggestions have been offered to overcome this problem. The easiest to implement is to have the respondent write the alternatives on a piece of paper and then to refer to them when answering. This is feasible when one response set is used with a number of items, such as a Likert scale, which will be referred to in responding to a set of questions. However, if each item requires a different list, the method can become quite tedious and demanding, and the respondent may either hang up or not write the alternatives down, relying on their (fallible) memory. In the latter situation, a 'primacy effect' is likely to occur, with subjects tending to endorse categories that are read towards the beginning rather than towards the end of the list (Locander and Burton 1976; Monsees and Massey 1979).

A second method is to divide the question into parts, with each section probing for a more refined answer. For example, the person can be asked if they agree or disagree with the statement. Then the next question would tap the strength of the endorsement: mild or strong. It also helps if the response format is given to the person as an introduction to the question: for example, 'In the following question, there will be four possible answers: strongly agree, mildly agree, mildly disagree, and strongly disagree. The question is …'.

A third method involves a pre-interview mailing to the subjects. This can consist of the entire questionnaire itself, or a card with the response alternatives. With the former, the interviewer then reads each question, with the respondent following in their version. The telephone call allows for probing and recording answers to open-ended questions. If a card with the alternatives is mailed, it is often combined with features like emergency telephone numbers or other items which encourage the person to keep it near the telephone, readily available when the call comes (Aneshensel et al. 1982).

These various techniques make it more feasible to ask complicated questions over the telephone. However, the major consideration with this form of interviewing remains to reduce complexity as much as possible. If detailed explanations are necessary, as may be the case if the person's attitudes towards public policy issues are being evaluated, face-to-face or mailed questionnaires may be preferable.

Whatever technique is used, it is highly likely that repeated calls may be necessary to reach a desired household: people may be working, out for the evening, in hospital, or on holiday. It has been recommended that three to six attempts may be required; after this, the law of diminishing returns begins to play an increasingly large role. Research Ethics Boards may also place a limit on the number of callbacks, based on the concern that overzealous recruitment can easily become harassment. Moreover, the call should not be made at times such that the respondents feel it would be an intrusion: on holidays, Sundays, or during major sports events.

Computerized administration

Scales and surveys can be completed digitally on a number of different devices (desktops, laptops, mobile devices) which are collectively referred to as *computerized administration*. This can be as simple as presenting the form on the screen as opposed to on paper; through incorporating skip patterns, as we discussed previously under the advantages of face-to-face interviews; to having the computer select which questions to present based on previous responses. Over the past decade or so, a number of free or inexpensive programs have appeared that allow researchers to construct computer-based questionnaires with these advanced features; some of these are discussed later in this chapter under Implementation. As with any method, there are benefits and drawbacks.

Advantages

There are at least five major advantages to computerized administration. First, it can free the interviewer to do other things, or to administer the scale to a number of people simultaneously. Second, every time data are transferred from one medium to another, there is the potential for transcription and entry errors. When the subject is interviewed in person, there are many steps where these errors can creep in: the participant means to say one answer but gives another; or the interviewer mishears the response; intends to write one thing but puts down something else; errs in transcribing a check mark in one box to a number; or finally keys the wrong number into the computer. Having the person enter their responses directly into the machine eliminates all sources of error but one—unknowingly hitting the wrong key (or touching the wrong response option on a screen). With so many steps eliminated, there is also a commensurate saving of time and money to the researcher.

A third advantage is that neither the subject nor the interviewer can inadvertently omit items or questions. As we have already discussed under the advantages of face-to-face interviews, a related advantage is that the skip patterns can be automated, eliminating another source of error.

Fourth, people may be more honest in reporting unacceptable or undesirable behaviours to an impersonal machine than to a human. A number of studies have shown that people admit to more drinking when seated in front of a computer than an interviewer (e.g. Lucas et al. 1977; Skinner and Allen 1983).

Fifth, online questionnaires and surveys are returned much faster than other forms of administration (Lazar and Preece 1999; Raziano et al. 2001). For example, Farmer (cited in Granello and Wheaton 2004) found an average turnaround time for online surveys of 2–3 days, compared with 2–3 weeks for telephone interviews and 4–6 weeks with mailed surveys. Moreover, the cost is lower than mailed surveys. McMorris et al. (2009) found that the cost of online surveys was half that of in-person ones, due primarily to the number of calls necessary to arrange a time for face-to-face interviews plus travel time.

Finally, it is sometimes possible to administer only part of a long questionnaire: what is referred to as *variable-length testing*. This is based on *countdown* procedures, in which items are presented until one of two outcomes are reached: (1) the person meets the criteria for the condition being studied; or (2) it would be impossible for the person to meet the criteria (Finkelman et al. 2018). Two countdown methods have been developed: the *classification* method and the *full scores on elevated scales* (FSES) method (Forbey and Ben-Porath 2007). The classification method is predicated on the assumption that what is of interest is not the total score, but whether or not the person has reached some minimum, criterion score. For example, many diagnoses in the *Diagnostic and Statistical Manual of Mental Disorders* (American Psychiatric Association 2013) are based on the patient having at least a given number of symptoms; anything beyond that number doesn't affect either the diagnosis or a severity score. Using the classification method, items are administered until (1) the person reaches the criterion, or (2) it is impossible for the person to reach the criterion even if all of the remaining items are endorsed.

In the FSES method, testing is again discontinued if it is impossible to reach some criterion score, as with option (2) of the classification method. However, if the person does reach the criterion, then all of the remaining items are presented, thus generating a continuous, full-scale score (Ben-Porath et al. 1989). Using long, multiscale inventories such as the *MMPI*, it is possible to save about 30 per cent in administration time (Roper et al. 1995).

Disadvantages

One potential disadvantage of computerizing scales stems from the direct transfer of existing instruments to a computerized format. In most cases, it has not been established whether or not the translation has adversely affected their reliability and validity. Paper-and-pencil questionnaires allow subjects to see how many items there are and to pace themselves accordingly; to skip around, rather than answering the questions in sequence; and to go back easily to earlier questions, in order to change them or to check for their own consistency. While scale developers may deplore these deviations from the way the instrument was intended to be taken, the results of the original reliability and validity studies were conducted with these factors possibly playing a role. Modifying these factors *may* affect the psychometric properties of the scale. However, the evidence to date suggests that if there are any differences between the paper-and-pencil and the computerized versions, they are very small (e.g. Merten and Ruch 1996; Pinsoneault 1996; Watson et al. 1990).

A second, again potential, disadvantage is the belief, especially among healthcare workers, that some subjects or patients may be apprehensive about computers. These machines still retain the mystique of 'giant brains', which can, nevertheless, be brought to their knees by the press of a wrong key. However, their apprehension about subjects' reactions to these machines is probably not well founded. Most studies have found that far more people are comfortable in front of a terminal or computer than are uncomfortable. Indeed, in many studies, a majority of responders preferred the machine to a human (for a review of this see Stein 1987). Moreover, this may be a concern for specific age cohorts, particularly those born before the Second World War, but may be less of a concern for younger age cohorts. A related problem is that attitudes towards computerized interviewing may be sex related: men tend to be more comfortable 'talking' to machines about sensitive material than to a human interviewer, while the reverse is true for women (e.g. Skinner and Allen 1983). At present, there is insufficient information to indicate whether this is due to the greater use of computers by men, or whether this attitude transcends familiarity with the machines. In either case, though, the sex difference tends to be small and disappearing, as computers have become just another ubiquitous electronic gadget.

Implementation

In implementing a computerized scale or questionnaire, some considerations should be kept in mind. First, there should be an ability for the subject to interrupt the testing and return later to the place where they stopped, without either losing the original data or having to go through questions already answered. This is particularly true for long scales, when it is one of many scales, or when the person may become tired or distracted easily. Second, there must be a provision for the subjects to modify their answers, both to the item they are completing at the time and to previous ones. Respondents should be able to review their earlier answers, modify them if desired, and return to the same place in the instrument. Last, there must be a way for the subject to indicate that they cannot or do not want to answer a question. This option is often missing on paper-and-pencil questionnaires, since the person can simply leave the offending item out. If the subject cannot proceed to the next question without entering some response into the machine, the option must be explicit. When he was in the university town of Madison, Wisconsin, one of the pioneers in computerized interviewing, Warner Slack (cited in Fishman 1981), used the phrase 'None of your damn business' as the option the person could use to avoid a question. This was changed to 'Skip that one' when Slack moved to Boston, emphasizing the importance of cultural factors.

The questionnaire can be designed to have 'drop-down windows' for each question, giving it a less cluttered look, and reducing the possibility of erroneous responses. It is also possible to track how long it took the respondents to complete the questionnaire. A very short time may be a flag that the respondent used satisficing or did not bother to read the questions carefully (King et al. 2014). The responses themselves are entered into a database automatically, eliminating another source of error. However, this requires that there is someone with computer knowledge who can design the questionnaire and the database. There are other problems with this approach. First, various browsers have different capabilities; a scale that looks well-formatted on one browser may have items wrapped around onto a second line, or elements that are no longer aligned, with a different browser (Weinman 1996). Similarly, computer screens themselves vary in size and resolution, so that even with the same browser, a questionnaire that looks good on one computer may not on another. Second, more 'fancy' questionnaires can use advanced features of high-level programming languages. Unfortunately, these take longer to load and require more computer memory, overwhelming the capabilities of some older home machines, and may actually decrease the response rate. Third, people have to know that the questionnaire exists. This could involve sending e-mails to people, with links to the online questionnaire; posting links on existing sites that are likely to be read by the intended audience; or simply hoping that people will stumble on the site. Fourth, because the site is available for anyone to see, more control must be exercised if it is to be completed only by specific people. Fifth, the rule of thumb is that if more than three mouse clicks are needed to get to the questionnaire, people will become frustrated and leave.

Just as there are guidelines for reporting how a randomized controlled trial was conducted (CONSORT) or a meta-analysis was carried out (PRISMA), there is one for reporting how online surveys were done. It is called the Checklist for Reporting Results of Internet E-Surveys (CHERRIES; Eysenbach 2004), and contains items such as how contact was made, whether adaptive questions were used (those that are displayed conditioned on responses to previous questions), whether there were checks for completeness, various response rate indices (discussed later in this chapter under Reporting response rates), and so forth. It also serves as a very useful guide for planning such surveys.

A questionnaire sent directly by e-mail is a 'low tech' method that avoids some of these problems, but may introduce others. Web browsers are not required, eliminating the issue of incompatibility. However, without careful design, entering the responses into the questionnaire may in itself alter the format of the page and result in lines being split. Because drop-down menus cannot be used, the questionnaire may appear more cluttered, and there is more chance for entering erroneous answers. Finally, the answers have to be entered manually into the database.

A compromise between e-mailed questionnaires and posting them on a website is to develop a new questionnaire or to 'translate' existing ones using Web-based survey construction tools. These often allow branching logic: formats that force the respondent to choose one option, allow for multiple responses, or rank order responses; room for open-ended answers; and so forth. The researcher can then send an e-mail message to selected people, with a link to the Web-based questionnaire.

Over time , it has become easier to construct questionnaires and scales for online distribution. Two of the most popular platforms are HubSpot (<https://hubspot.com>) and SurveyMonkey (<https://surveymonkey.com>). Both are 'freemium' services, meaning that there is a free version, with limits on the number of items and responses; and more extensive and expensive versions. While the upgrades can be quite costly, the free versions should meet the needs of most researchers. For those based at non-profit organizations, REDCap (Research Electronic Data Capture; <https://www.project-red cap.org>) is a free and secure platform. It is very popular in university and healthcare settings, because it can be used to build scales and create databases, and is compliant with legislation governing the privacy of medical information.

Another consideration for both ways of using the Internet is that many people pay for the time they are connected. This imposes yet another burden on them, which must be overcome in order to ensure compliance. Also, with the exponential increase in the number of 'junk' and 'spammed' messages, there is growing resentment over unsolicited and unannounced e-mail. One study, cited by Kaye and Johnson (1999), drew so many hostile messages from their mailing that it had to be aborted. It is estimated that the average academic professional receives about 50 e-mails a day and responds to about 30 of them (Pignata et al. 2015). The other side of the coin is that institutions are increasingly installing spam detectors and firewalls to prevent unsolicited e-mails and those with attachments from getting through. The results of one international study (Hartford et al. 2007) were jeopardized because all e-mails to the National Health Service in the United Kingdom were rejected by filters that blocked mass mailings. Even if the message does get through, the fear of computer viruses, worms, and other forms of malware may inhibit people from clicking on a link from an unknown source.

Some suggestions for improving the quality of online questionnaires are given by Kaye and Johnson (1999) and Dillman et al. (2014). Whereas personalization has a positive effect in influencing the return rate of mailed questionnaires, its effects on online questionnaires are more mixed. On the one hand, it does improve response rates (e.g. Heerwegh 2005; Heerwegh and Loosveldt 2006; Heerwegh et al. 2005). But, in mailed questionnaires with personalized envelopes, the respondent can return the form without any identifying information; the answers themselves remain anonymous. This is not the case with questionnaires posted online, where the respondent's name can be (or, more importantly, is *perceived* to be) linked to the answers, thus jeopardizing anonymity. There is some indication that this results in a greater tendency for people to respond with, 'I prefer not to answer' (Joinson et al. 2007), and to give socially desirable answers to personal questions (Heerwegh and Loosveldt 2006; Heerwegh et al. 2005). Thus, personalization of online surveys should be considered carefully; when sensitive information is involved, the increase in response rate may be offset by the decrease in usable answers. There are two other aspects of the e-mail header: the address of the sender and the subject line. Data are sparse, but one study found that academics are more likely to open and respond to surveys if the address is from another academic institution (e.g. ending with '.edu' in the United States or containing a university's name in other parts of the world) rather than an address from an Internet service provider (e.g. 'gmail' or 'hotmail'). Paradoxically, an unclear subject line leads to better compliance, possibly due to curiosity or a feeling of being deprived of information (DeAngelo and Feng 2019). It's also a good idea to avoid using the terms 'lottery' or 'free gift' (which, by the way, is a redundancy) in the subject line, because some spam filters may either delete the message or relegate it to the garbage folder.

To date, there are limited and conflicting data comparing questionnaires completed by e-mail or online to more traditional methods of administration. On the one side, Pettit (2002) did not find that completing scales digitally introduces any additional biases. However, Heerwegh and Loosveldt (2008) found greater tendencies towards satisficing—either omitting a question or responding with 'don't know'—with Web-based questionnaires, possibly because respondents were 'multitasking' (Holbrook et al. 2003). Further, response rates appear to be lower to e-mail than to postal mail (Eley 1999; Jones and Pitt 1999; Raziano et al. 2001). However, comparing online to mailed questionnaires amongst 5,600 healthcare professionals, Lusk et al. (2007) found that being younger and male was associated with a greater probability of responding online. This, though, may change over time, as those brought up online enter the work force. The other issue is whether the mode of administration affects people's responses. Again, the data are still limited, but the answer seems to be 'Yes'. Dillman et al. (2014) report more positive answers being given on telephone surveys as opposed to online and conclude that 'obtaining the same results on scalar questions across survey modes remains an unresolved challenge' (p. 457).

Finding the sample

If the computer is used to present (and possibly score) scales to people who are already enrolled in a study, then there are no concerns regarding locating the sample; it already exists. However, there are times when the aim of the study includes locating people via the Internet, either because they share some attribute or to generate a random sample. The issue then becomes locating the sample. On the positive side, there are thousands of list servers and 'chat rooms' composed of people with similar interests, concerns, or disorders; and there is even a website that indexes them (<http://www.tile.net/tile/listserv/index.html>): for example, Cinà and Clase (1999) administered the Illness Intrusiveness Rating Scale (Devins et al. 1983–1984) online to 68 patients with a relatively rare disorder, hyperhidrosis. Without the Internet, it would have been almost impossible to locate such a group of people who are scattered around the world. Another advantage of using social networks to recruit subjects is that it reduces the number of fraudulent participants. Especially if the site offers clinical or social support, it is unlikely that people without the disorder being studied will stumble across it (Quagan et al. 2021). (Various ways to find samples online and to administer scales and surveys are discussed by Bradley (1999).) However, if the object of a survey is to gather a representative sample of the population, using opt-in samples online is less accurate than probability samples using the Web or telephone (MacInnis et al. 2018).

In 2005, Amazon introduced a service called Mechanical Turk (MTurk; <www.mturk.com>), named after an automaton built in 1770 by Wolfgang von Kempelen that purportedly played chess and beat Napoleon Bonaparte and Benjamin Franklin (in fact, a man was hidden inside). For a relatively low price, researchers can post questionnaires and surveys that can be completed by people around the world—an approach called 'crowdsourcing'. Mortensen and Hughes (2018) estimated that there were over 17,000 studies published by 2017 that used this service. The allure is obvious: a large sample can be gathered quickly and cheaply, from people all over the world. However, the validity of this research has been called into question. First, 'world-wide' means people primarily in the United States (60 per cent) and India (30 per cent) who do not mind working for less than $1 per hour (if they are very fast). It has also been found that 30 per cent of surveys are completed by very active participants, who constitute just 0.25 per cent of the population, and who complete on average one survey a day (Miller 2006). There are a number of studies showing that MTurk responders are not representative of the general population (e.g. Huff and Tingley 2015; Mullinix et al. 2015), although others have argued that, by controlling for easily measurable sample features, most differences can be reduced (Levay et al. 2016). Further, responders who complete a large number of surveys tend to provide better quality responses than those who complete fewer surveys (Zhang et al. 2019). Other platforms for recruiting participants are discussed later in this chapter under the heading 'Social media'.

The opposite side of the coin, though, is that it is often difficult to determine how many people received the questionnaire, so it is difficult to establish the response rate or the sampling error because the probability of a person being selected is unknown. There is no list of e-mail addresses, equivalent to a telephone directory, so that a computer-based version of random digit dialling is not possible . This then makes it impossible to generalize the results to the entire population, since the latter is undefined. By the same token, care must be taken to ensure that people do not respond a number of times, especially if the questionnaire taps an area about which the respondents feel very strongly. An online survey about events in the Middle East, for example, had to be cancelled when it was found that some groups were flooding the website with thousands of copies of their answers. Both of these problems can be obviated if the researcher has the names of all eligible respondents. For example, Dhalla et al. (2002) and Kwong et al. (2002) were able to obtain the e-mail addresses for over 95 per cent of Canadian medical students, and assigned each one a unique code number, which was needed to open up the questionnaire. This meant that each person could respond only once.

Social media

The rapid adoption of smart phones has been paralleled by an equal growth in social media. It has been estimated that, by the end of 2021, there were nearly 3 billion users of Facebook worldwide, of whom about 180 million were in the United States and 35 million in the United Kingdom. These numbers increase when other platforms, such as Twitter (now called X), Google Plus, LinkedIn, Reddit, Pinterest, and TikTok, are added to the mix (Backlinko n.d.). Many of these sites allow researchers to solicit participants through advertisements, which charge the advertiser either for each time the link is clicked, or by the number of times the ads are shown to viewers. On Facebook, for example, the advertisers are given a range of suggested prices, and those willing to pay more are more likely to have their ads viewed. Researchers can also specify the sociodemographic characteristics of those who should see their ads, such as location, age, sex, gender, occupation, and so forth (King et al. 2014). There are many advantages to this, in addition to finding the appropriate participants. It is not necessary to then ask questions about sociodemographics, making the survey shorter. In fact, it is possible to reach a larger audience than just those who see the ads through 'snowball sampling'. That is, people who find the site through the ad could forward the link to their friends, allowing the sample to grow like a snowball rolling down the hill. This has been used very successfully to recruit many participants for a study (Kosinski et al. 2015). The downside is that this sample tends to be more homogeneous than the general population, because friends tend to share common interests and demographic characteristics. For the most part, the other platforms offer few options to target the audience.

Soliciting participants through social media presents the same problems in estimating the response rate as does recruitment using the Web or newspaper advertisements: we don't know the size of the readership, so we cannot determine the proportion of people who responded. There are, however, some other metrics that can be used. One is the *click-through rate* (CTR), which is the ratio of the number of times the link to the ad was clicked divided by the number of times it was presented. So, a CTR of 5 per cent means that for every 20 times the ad was seen, one person clicked on it. However, one person may see the ad numerous times, and even click on it many times. The *unique* CTR counts each person only once (King et al. 2014).

Another widely used platform for recruiting participants is Reddit, and specifically its 'subreddit' called r/ SampleSize (<https://www.reddit.com/r/samplesize/>). As of the middle of 2023, there were nearly 210,000 users. It does not have the range of options that MTurk offers but does have the distinct advantage that it is free and respondents are not paid. One study, which compared Reddit responders to university students (the most commonly used participants in psychological studies) found that both groups gave reliable results, but there were significant demographic differences between the groups, with the Internet sample having a higher proportion of males, being more educated, and ethnically diverse (Jamnik and Lane 2017).

Based in Germany, SurveyCircle (<https://www.surveycircle.com/en/>) bills itself as 'the largest community for online research'. Like SampleSize (whatever happened to spaces between words?), it is free. Respondents earn points, which they can transfer to the researcher, raising that survey's ranking. It divides the world into regions (e.g. German -speaking countries are in Region 1; North America, much of Europe, South Africa, and India are in Region 2), and researchers' surveys are made available with their home region.

In summary, the use of social media to recruit participants for surveys has some problems regarding the representativeness of the samples, but these likely can be overcome to some degree through the use of selection criteria and post hoc stratified sampling of the results. It can easily reach a large and diverse group of people, often at little expense, and will most likely grow in popularity.

Increasing response rate and the quality of responses

Dillman et al. (2014) have a number of suggestions for increasing the response rate for e-mailed and online surveys, similar to those he proposed for mailed surveys (Dillman

1978). Other suggestions can be found in King et al. (2014) and Edwards et al. (2009). For e-mailed ones, these include:

1. *Use multiple contacts.* Even more so than with mailed surveys, letting people know that a questionnaire will be coming is an essential first step. Especially with the plethora of spam, it is too easy to hit the Delete key, so that notification that a legitimate message (at least to the sender) will be coming is vital. There should be no more than 2 or 3 days between the initial mailing and the survey itself.

2. *Personalize the address.* Do not list all of the people who are receiving the message or indicate that it comes from a list server. If this is not possible, then use bcc (blind carbon copy) and use a generic greeting.

3. *Keep the message in the initial contact e-mail brief.* Many e-mail systems preview the contents of the message below the list of messages, and it is often on this basis that the respondent decides whether or not to hit the Delete key. The information needed to entice the person to open the message and read further should appear in these first few lines.

4. *Allow alternative ways of responding.* Some people prefer to print the questionnaire and mail it back. This is especially true if it is long, or if the respondent is concerned about confidentiality. This means that a mailing address must be part of the message. Also, the researcher should ensure that the downloadable file is in a format compatible with multiple systems (Mac, PC), and that it will not be filtered out by spam detection software, if at all possible.

5. *Send a replacement questionnaire with the reminder.* This parallels the procedure used with mailed questionnaires; the reminder message to those who have not responded should include the survey itself, under the assumption that the recipient has cleared out their mailbox (or can't find the original message because it is lost amidst all of the other messages).

6. *Limit the length of the questions.* As we mentioned, the number of characters that can be displayed in one line differs depending on the person's e-mail system, size of screen, and other factors. If a sentence has to wrap around to the next line, it is unpredictable how this will look from one computer to the next. Limiting the length of each question to about 70 characters (including spaces) will minimize this problem. And, as we discussed in Chapter 3 on Devising the items, shorter questions tend to be more reliable than longer ones.

7. *Start with an interesting question that is easy to answer.* With paper-and-pencil questionnaires, it is easy to thumb through the pages to see if it is interesting, relevant, and easy to answer. This is much more difficult to do with e-mailed ones. An initial question that is seen as irrelevant or hard to answer will lead people to hit the dreaded Delete button, so entice them in gently.

8. *Limit the length of the questionnaire.* As with paper-and-pencil questionnaires, the length affects both the overall response rate and the quality of the answers. Deutskens et al. (2004) found a response rate of about 25 per cent when the length was 15 to 30 minutes, but only 17 per cent when the length was 30 to 45 minutes. In addition, the longer questionnaires had more 'don't know' responses. Respondents in another study were told beforehand how long it will take to complete the

questionnaire. For the group told it would take 10 minutes, 75 per cent began the survey and 59 per cent completed it; for the 20 -minute group, the numbers were 65 per cent and 55 per cent; and for those told it would take 30 minutes, the figures were 62 per cent and 53 per cent. Moreover, the quality of the responses declined as the time increased (Galesic and Bosnjak 2009).

9. *Use progress bars.* Progress bars allow the respondents to see what proportion of the questionnaire they have completed and how much remains. This tends to reduce the discontinuation rate, because if they see that they have already completed 80 per cent of it, they may be less likely to stop answering. On the flip side, if they have been working away for 15 minutes and see that they are only one-quarter of the way through, a progress bar may result in them discontinuing. But, as we said in the previous point, such long questionnaires are unlikely to be completed in any case.

10. *Recognize the limitations of the medium.* Some response formats, such as 7-point, horizontally arranged Likert scales, are difficult to fit on a screen. This may mean that the format may have to change (e.g. using a vertical arrangement) or the number of response items reduced. This in turn may affect the reliability or validity of a scale, if it was first designed for paper-and-pencil use.

Online surveys are much more flexible than those delivered by e-mail. This opens up many more options for designers, but also means that they must be aware of other factors that can influence the response rate. Dillman et al.'s (2014) recommendations for this mode of administration include:

1. *Use a welcome screen.* The first page, like the covering letter on a mailed questionnaire, should provide motivation for the person to continue. It should also emphasize the ease of responding, and instruct the respondent how to proceed. Because space on a computer screen is limited, the message should be short. Logos take up valuable space and should be limited in size and number, and instructions regarding how to answer should be left for the following pages.

2. *Provide a PIN to limit access.* As we mentioned earlier in discussing increasing the response rate, most online surveys are first introduced to potential respondents in an e-mail message. This should include a prominently-displayed PIN with which the person can get access to the questionnaire itself. This limits respondents to only those on the researcher's list, which is necessary to estimate the response rate, and to prevent people with strong opinions from answering two or three times.

3. *Start with a simple, interesting question.* This is similar to point 7 under e-mail surveys. In addition, the answering options should be simple and obvious. Not everyone is comfortable with these formats, so drop-down menus and scrolling should be avoided. As with paper-and-pencil questionnaires, demographic information should be placed at the very end, not on the first page.

4. *Use a format similar to that of self-administered, paper-and-pencil questionnaires.* All too often, online scales do not number the items—this is poor design. Also, don't forget that it is often impossible for respondents to scroll to the last page, so they have no idea how long it is. Our own recommendation is to have some indication

of how much of the questionnaire remains to be completed. This can be as simple as giving the number of remaining items, or, as we mentioned in #9 above, a progress bar showing the percentage that has been done. The layout of the page is also important. We normally begin reading in the upper left corner, so do not clutter that area with logos or other page clutter.

5. *Be restrained with the use of colour.* The ease with which colour can be incorporated into Web pages is seductive, but like many seductions, the thrill quickly fades. The figure-ground combination should be easy to read and consistent from one page to the next, with no very bright areas that draw the eye away from the item. Contrasting colours should be used only to highlight something other than the questions and answers themselves, such as instructions.

6. *Provide clear instructions how to answer the questions.* Online questionnaires offer many options for completing items: radio buttons, that force a choice among options; check boxes that allow multiple responses; drop-down menus; boxes for entering textual information; and so on. People with limited computer skills are likely unaware of the subtleties that a circle means only one response and a box means many, or that a down-pointing arrow means to choose among pre-selected options. We ourselves have become extremely frustrated when, after entering a long string of numbers, we received an error message saying that there should be no spaces or to omit the brackets around the area code of a telephone number. These, and other instructions, should be made explicit before the person enters a response. People may not realize that it is necessary to press Return or Enter after certain responses, and may sit waiting for the computer to present the next item, until they quit in frustration.

7. *Use drop-down boxes sparingly and carefully.* Drop-down boxes, like colour, are helpful when used well, and introduce bias when used poorly. Their major advantage is the ability to present many options without cluttering the page. But, they should be avoided when there are only a few options (e.g. Yes/No), because they require more key strokes than simply clicking on the answer. Another misuse is to have one of the options visible and the others available only after clicking the arrow; people may select the visible answer inadvertently.

8. *Allow people to omit an item.* One of the purported advantages of online questionnaires is that people cannot proceed to the next item until the current one has been answered, which eliminates missing data. As with other advances that we have discussed, this can be a mixed blessing. From an ethical perspective, respondents should have the option of omitting any item they find intrusive or offensive, by being able to choose 'I prefer not to say' or words to that effect. We have had the experience of receiving a questionnaire from a credit card company that included items such as 'This credit card makes me feel proud'. Because there was no way to avoid these asinine items with inappropriate descriptors, it was abandoned and never submitted. The problem is that while people can omit an item in a paper-and-pencil questionnaire, or tell a telephone interviewer that they do not want to answer a specific item, this is not spelled out explicitly. Doing so on an online survey may alter how people respond; data regarding this do not yet exist. It's a good idea,

though, to have a pop-up screen come up with a message such as, 'Did you mean to omit this question?' One study found that it virtually eliminated inadvertently omitted items (O'Rourke et al. 2013).

9. *Allow people to scroll through the items.* Many surveys present one item at a time. The advantage is that it reduces distraction. The other side of the coin, though, is that the person cannot see how one item relates to others, as would be possible with paper-and-pencil questionnaires. If the respondents have to leave the questionnaire and return to it later, it may be difficult for them to recapture where they were and how they had answered earlier items. A related issue is that people should be able to back up to previous items and modify their responses, as they can with paper-and-pencil questionnaires.

10. *Use incentives.* Not surprisingly, incentives are as important for online surveys as for mailed ones. Bosnjak and Tuten (2003) found that neither prepaid nor promised monetary incentives were as effective as having one's name put into a pool for a chance to win a prize; and being told immediately whether one has won was better than delayed notification (Tuten et al. 2004), but cold, hard cash ($5.00) sent by mail trumped even gift certificate codes sent with the survey (Birnholtz et al. 2004).

Dillman et al.'s (2014) book has many other suggestions and examples. It should be a primary reference for anyone contemplating e-mail or online surveys. See also Norman et al. (1982).

Artificial intelligence and bots

Before concluding this section, it is important to note some additional considerations. First, as we were completing this edition of the book, open-source artificial intelligence chatbots, most notably ChatGPT, were launched. Since then, universities have been playing catch-up, struggling to find the right balance for the use of these technologies in both learning and assessment. You can ask a chatbot to do just about anything, including writing a novel, computer code, and yes, survey items, and it will do so. Like anything else, the more you interact and instruct these programs, the better the quality of the output. Obviously, we could caution against blindly using any technology. Knowledge of content is still an absolute requirement before one can even begin to assess the accuracy of the items generated. Nevertheless, as this technology grows in both sophistication and application, we anticipate we will see more and more of its use in this field.

Survey bots have been around for some time. (A 'bot' is an automated software application that is programmed to do certain tasks.) If you have ever visited a website and a prompt suddenly appeared (often with a human or cartoon image asking you, 'Can I help?'), you have interacted with a bot. Bots can be designed to ask questions, such as how satisfied a customer might have been with a service or product. These survey bots can perform many of the same functions of an interviewer, but are rarely used outside of asking a few basic items, and usually for commercial purposes. Survey bots have limited capacity for handling open-ended responses and usually eventually push a respondent towards interacting with a human. The process of waiting can be frustrating and increase non-completion. Of course, bots can be programmed to not only ask questions, but also answer them. This has created a significant problem for online surveys, especially as the programs or scripts have become more sophisticated. Systems such as REDCap have devised 'diagnostics' to identify possible bot-derived responses. For example, often the e-mail addresses of fake respondents give away that the 'person' is a bot. Designers can also take steps to prevent bot-generated responses. For example, time stamps that include when a survey was started and completed provide one method for identifying bot- driven responses—typically the response time is in milliseconds, making it highly unlikely that a real person actually completed the survey. Lisa Hallberg from the University of Kentucky Life Span Institute identified a number of prevention and detection strategies for those who like a practical guide to dealing with this problem <https://lifespan.ku.edu/online-surveys-and-data-collect ion-tools>.

Smart phones

The multifunctional capacity of the smart phone makes it a powerful data -gathering device. Because it can be programmed, its screen can be used to display a visual ana- logue scale (albeit shorter than the conventional 10 cm), or to present scales, one item at a time. Further, it is equipped with wireless technology, so the data that are gathered can be downloaded to the researcher's computer automatically and on a regular basis. This ensures that data will not be missing because the subject forgot to mail in the form (although it does raise the spectre of data being lost because of equipment failure). It also does away with the necessity of having to enter the data into the computer by hand, eliminating a potential source of error.

There are two other attributes that increase its usefulness: signalling and time stamps. Auditory reminders can be programmed to sound an alarm at specified times to remind the subject to fill out the form, which has been found to enhance compli- ance (Stone and Shiffman 2002). The drawback is that the alarm may go off at in- convenient times. The second advantage is that the subject's responses can be 'time stamped' by the phone's internal clock. In studies of arthritis, for example (Stinson et al. 2006), it is common to have the person complete a pain scale upon awakening, in the middle of the day, and after dinner. The time stamp allows the researcher to de- termine if there was 'diary hoarding', in which the person backfills the forms to make it appear as if they were compliant with the instructions. One study (Stone et al. 2002) used photocells to determine when a paper diary was opened: 75 per cent of patients turned in completed pages for days on which the diary had not been opened; and 45 per cent 'forward-filled' the diary at least once, indicating what their pain would be the following day (although 82 per cent of people indicated that they were 'very' or 'extremely' compliant with the instructions). Either the phone can be programmed to prevent back- or forward-filling, or time stamping can let the researcher know that it has occurred.

However, there are costs associated with the use of smart phones, and they can be steep. Although prices for basic models may be low, the prices for high-end models seem to increase every year, and they require a yearly (or longer) contract. This may be prohibitive for large surveys. The second cost, shared with other automated techniques, is associated with developing an application to display the scale, branch to appropriate questions if required, and send the data back to the research office. Respondents may also need to be trained how to respond on the screen, and to ensure that the phone is kept charged at all times. Furthermore, the programmed displays and the necessity to step through a series of screens can be a significant deterrent. In one study (Norman et al. 2008), medical students in the experimental group were to have assessments completed on a personal data assistant (PDAs; a now obsolete technology); in the control group, assessments were to be done on paper. The study was abandoned because only 4 per cent of students in the experimental arm complied. Their reasons for non-compliance centred on the inconvenience of downloading software, stepping through multiple screens, and uploading the results.

The positive properties of PDAs and now smart phones have greatly facilitated a data-gathering technique called *ecological momentary assessment*, or EMA (Stone and Shiffman 1994). There are three key elements of EMA. The first is that the assessment is done within the natural environment (e.g. at work or at school) rather than in the researcher's lab or at home in the evening, thus enhancing the ecological validity of the data (Hufford et al. 2001). Second, the data are gathered as the events occur, minimizing the problems associated with recall (Palermo et al. 2004; Stone and Shiffman 2002). Third, EMA usually involves multiple assessments over time, which could be as short as every few hours for disorders such as arthritis (e.g. Stinson et al. 2006), or every week for conditions that change more slowly, such as bipolar affective disorders (Biller 2005). This allows the researcher to track disorders that vary over time.

Some events, such as migraine headaches or panic attacks, may be missed if data are recorded only at pre-specified times. To allow for this, data gathering can be modified so that it is contingent on the occurrence of symptoms. It is almost impossible to specify a priori how many data points must be gathered, or over what period of time. This depends very much on how much and how often symptoms vary. Jensen and McFarland (1993) found that reliable (alpha = 0.96) and valid (0.97) estimates of chronic pain in patients with arthritis could be obtained with three measures per day for 4 days; increasing this to 2 weeks did not significantly improve the quality of the data, and led to decreased compliance during the second week (Stinson et al. 2006). Another factor to bear in mind when considering designing forms for smart phones is scheduling reminders so that they are appropriate for the attribute being assessed. Other issues are discussed by Piasecki et al. (2007); these were written for PDAs but are easily modified to be applicable for smart phones.

In summary, there is no one method of administration that is ideal in all circumstances. Factors such as cost, completion rate, and the type of question asked must all be taken into account. The final decision will, to some degree, be a compromise, in that the disadvantages of the technique that is chosen are outweighed by the positive elements.

Mailed questionnaires

One issue facing us in this revision of the book was whether to keep this section on mailed questionnaires or to delete it entirely. The reality is that the use of 'snail mail' has dropped precipitously over the past decade. In 2012, the United States Postal Service

(USPS) handled nearly 160 billion pieces of mail; 8 years later, this had dropped to fewer than 130 billion pieces (USPS 2020), and it is most probable that this trend will only become more pronounced over time. Paralleling this decline, and arguably causing it, has been an even more dramatic use of the Internet, not only for e-mail but also as a method for administering questionnaires and surveys, as we have described. In the end, we decided to keep it for two reasons. First, there may still be some people who will use mailed surveys because Internet connectivity is still problematic in poorer countries and even in remote areas of developed ones. Second, many of the recommendations are readily transferrable to the online environment.

Advantages

Mailing questionnaires to respondents is by far cheaper than face-to-face or telephone interviewing; in Siemiatycki's study (1979), the average cost was $6.08, as opposed to $7.10 for telephone interviewing and $16.10 for home interviewing. While today these figures could easily be doubled or tripled owing to inflation, it is still true that the cost of home interviewing is easily more than double the cost of telephone or mailed surveys. Indeed, this would be a conservative estimate of relative cost differences. In the past, the major drawback has been a relatively low response rate, jeopardizing the generalizability of the results. Over the years, various techniques have been developed which have resulted in higher rates of return. Dillman (1978, 2007), one of the most ardent spokesmen for this interviewing method, has combined many of them into what he calls the *Total Design Method*. He believes that response rates of over 75 per cent are possible with a general mailing to a heterogeneous population, and of 90 per cent to a targeted group, such as family practitioners. However, these estimates are likely inflated by today's standard, given the reduction in use of mail noted earlier.

As with telephone interviews, mailed questionnaires can be coordinated from one central office, even for national or international studies. In contrast, personal interviews usually require an office in each major city, greatly increasing the expense. Further, since there is no interviewer present, either in person or at the other end of a telephone line, social desirability bias tends to be minimized.

Disadvantages

However, there are a number of drawbacks with this method of administration. First, if a subject does not return the questionnaire, it is almost impossible to get any demographic information, obviating the possibility of comparing responders with non-responders. Second, subjects may omit some of the items; it is quite common to find statements in articles to the effect that 5–10 per cent of the returned questionnaires were unusable due to omitted, illegible, or invalid responses (e.g. Nelson et al. 1986). Third, while great care may have been taken by the investigator with regard to the sequence of the items, there is no assurance that the subjects read them in order. Some people may skip to the end first; or go back and change their response in light of a later question; or delay answering some questions because they have difficulty interpreting them.

A fourth difficulty is that, to ensure a high response rate (over 80 per cent), it is often necessary to send out two or three mailings to some subjects. If the identity of the respondent is known, then this necessitates some form of bookkeeping system, to record who has returned the questionnaire and who should be sent a reminder. If anonymity is desired, then reminders and additional copies must be sent to all subjects, increasing the cost of the study. Fifth, there may be a delay of up to 3 months until all the questionnaires that will be returned have been received. Last, there is always the possibility that some or all of the questionnaires may be delayed by a postal strike.

Increasing the return rate

Many techniques have been proposed to increase the rate of return of mailed questionnaires, although not all have proven to be effective. These have included:

1. *A covering letter.* Perhaps the most important part of a mailed questionnaire is the letter accompanying it. It will determine if the form will be looked at or thrown away, and the attitude with which the respondent will complete it. A detailed description of letters and their contents is given by Dillman (2007), who stresses their importance. The letter should begin with a statement that emphasizes two points: why the study is important; and why that person's responses are necessary to make the results interpretable, in that order. Common mistakes are to indicate in the opening paragraph that a questionnaire (a word he says is to be avoided) is enclosed; that it is part of a survey (another 'forbidden' word); identifying who the researcher is before stating why the research is being done; or under whose auspices (again, best left for later in the letter). Other points that should be included in the letter are a promise of confidentiality, a description of how the results will be used, and a mention of any incentive. The letter should be signed by hand, with the name block under the signature indicating the person's title and affiliation. Since subjects are more likely to respond if the research is being carried out by a university or some other respected organization, its letterhead should be used whenever it is appropriate. Bear in mind, though, that the letterhead itself may affect the answers, as it influences respondents' inferences regarding what the questionnaire developer is interested in. Norenzayan and Schwarz (1999), for example, asked respondents about the motivations of mass murderers. When the letterhead said 'Institute of Personality Research', the answers focused on personality factors; when it said 'Institute of Social Research', they stressed social-contextual ones. The letter itself should fit onto one page; coloured paper may look more impressive, but does not appear to influence the response rate.

   Based on a meta-analysis of 292 randomized trials, Edwards et al. (2002) state that mentioning a university affiliation has an odds ratio (OR) for increasing the response rate of 1.31; and the meta-analysis by Fox et al. (1988) found it to be the most powerful factor affecting response rate. Using coloured ink had an OR of 1.39 (Edwards et al. 2002). However, there were no effects of stressing the benefit to the respondent, to the sponsor, or to society. Other factors that did not influence the response rate were giving a deadline (Edwards et al. 2002; Fox et al. 1988; Henley

1976) and having instructions. Giving the respondent an option to opt out of the study significantly decreased the response rate (OR = 0.76).

2. *Advance warning that the questionnaire will be coming.* A letter is seen as less of an intrusion than a form that has to be completed, especially one that arrives unannounced. The introductory letter thus prepares the respondent for the questionnaire, and helps differentiate it from junk mail. Edwards et al. (2002) report an OR of 1.54 for increased return rate with pre-contact, and that it does not matter if the contact is by letter or telephone, and Fox et al. (1988) found it to be one of the strongest factors in increasing response rate. In fact, Trussell and Lavrakas (2004) found that having people agree to participate in a survey during an initial telephone contact was more effective than even monetary incentives for increasing the completion rate. With the near-universal adoption of smart phones, some researchers have used short text messages as either pre-notification or post-notification reminders. However, the limited research would indicate that the small increase in response rates is not worth the effort (Keding et al. 2016).

   Unfortunately for the researcher, many 'give away' offers now use the same technique: an official-looking letter announcing the imminent arrival of a packet of chances to win millions of dollars. This makes the wording of the covering letter even more critical, in order to overcome the scepticism that often greets such unsolicited arrivals.

3. *Giving a token of appreciation.* The use of an incentive is predicated on 'social exchange theory', which states that even small incentives are effective because they inculcate a sense of social obligation on the respondent. Most often, this is a sum of money, which significantly increases the return rate (Edwards et al. 2002; Fox et al. 1988; Yammarino et al. 1991). However, the relationship between the amount of the incentive and the return rate flattens out quite quickly; amounts as low as $0.50 or $1.00 doubles it, but $15.00 increases the return rate only 2.5 times (Edwards et al. 2002).

   In a meta-analysis of 69 studies involving nearly 29,000 subjects, Edwards et al. (2006) found a sharp increase in the odds of return up to $1.00, then a smaller increase until $5.00, and no further increase after that. Thus, the conclusion seems to be that it doesn't make sense for financial incentives to exceed $5.00, and even $1.00 is sufficient in many cases. (If we translate 2006 dollars into 2022 based on inflation, then incentives should not exceed $7.50, and $1.50 is likely sufficient at the low end.) The explanation for this somewhat paradoxical result is that when the value of the incentive starts approaching the actual value of the task, then 'social exchange' becomes more like an 'economic exchange', and the person feels less of a social obligation to reciprocate (Dillman 2007; Trussell and Lavrakas 2004).

   A cost-effective method is to send cheques rather than cash, as James and Bolstein (1992) found that only 69 per cent of cheques for $5 were actually cashed. The promise of an incentive when the questionnaire is returned, as expected, has a much smaller effect, and some have said that it does not improve the response rate at all (Church 1993). For example, James and Bolstein (1992) found that the promise of $50 did not result in any increase in response rate. Other incentives that have been used with varying degrees of success have included lottery tickets, a chance to win a savings bond or a prize, pens or pencils (a favourite among census bureaus), tie clips, unused stamps, diaries, donations to charity, key rings, golf balls, and letter openers, but these seem to be much less powerful than cold, hard cash (Blomberg and Sandell 1996; Edwards et al. 2002; Warriner et al. 1996; Yammarino et al. 1991).

4. *Anonymity.* The literature on the effect of anonymity on response rate is contradictory. If the person is identifiable on questionnaires that ask for confidential information, such as income, sexual practices, or illegal acts, then the response rate is definitely jeopardized. In a meta-analysis by Singer et al. (1995) of 113 studies, assurances of confidentiality improved response rates to sensitive information. However, promises of confidentiality for non-sensitive material do not increase compliance. In fact, when the data are not sensitive, such assurances may make people more suspicious and result in an increased refusal rate (Singer et al. 1992), although they may be required by the research ethics board. If it is necessary to identify the respondent, in order to link the responses to other information or to determine who should receive follow-up reminders, then the purpose of the identification should be stated, along with guarantees that the person's name will be thrown away when it is no longer needed, and kept under lock and key in the meantime; and that in the final report, no subject will be identifiable.

5. *Personalization.* Envelopes addressed to 'Occupant' are often regarded as junk mail, and are either discarded unopened or read in a cursory manner; the same may be true of the salutation on the letter itself. However, some people see a personalized greeting using their name as an invasion of privacy and a threat to anonymity. This problem can be handled in a number of ways. First, the letter can be addressed to a group, such as 'Dear Colleague', 'Resident of ... Neighbourhood', or 'Member of ...'; the personalization is given with a handwritten signature. Maheux et al. (1989) found that adding a handwritten 'thank you' note at the bottom of the covering letter increased the response rate by 41 per cent. (Again, with the wide use by politicians and advertisers of machines that produce signatures which resemble handwriting, this may become less effective with time.) Another method to balance anonymity and personalization is to have the covering letter personalized, and to stress the fact that the questionnaire itself has no identifying information on it. Although there is a vast literature on personalization, the conclusions are confusing, to say the least. One meta-analysis found that the combination of the recipient's name and a hand-written signature increased the odds of responding by 50 per cent (Scott and Edwards 2006); while a study of nearly 40,000 participants found only a minimal effect of personalization (Luitten 2011). Be aware, though, that personalization may have some detrimental effects on questionnaires and surveys sent by e-mail or over the Internet.

Other aspects of personalization include typed addresses rather than labels, stamps rather than metered envelopes, and regular envelopes rather than business reply ones. The latter alternatives are usually associated with junk mail, and the former with important letters. Based on their meta-analysis of 34 published and unpublished studies, Armstrong and Lusk (1987) found that stamped, first-class mail had a return rate on average of 9.2 per cent higher than when business replies were used. Interestingly, using a number of small-denomination stamps on the envelope yielded slightly better results (by 3.5 per cent) than using one stamp with the correct postage. Overall, though, the difference between using stamps as opposed to metered postage is small and may not be worth the effort (Fox et al. 1988).

6. *Enclosing a stamped, self-addressed envelope.* Asking the respondents to complete the questionnaire is an imposition on their time; asking them to also find and address a return envelope and pay for the postage is a further imposition, guaranteed to lead to a high rate of non-compliance. In what appears to be the only empirical study of this, Ferriss (1951) obtained a response rate of 90.1 per cent with an enclosed stamped return envelope; this dropped to 25.8 per cent when the envelope was omitted. Surprisingly, the 'active ingredient' seems to be the envelope itself, rather than the stamp. Armstrong and Lusk (1987), after reviewing six articles comparing stamped versus unstamped return envelopes, found a difference of only 3 per cent in favour of using stamps; and the meta-analyses by Edwards et al. (2002) and Yammarino et al. (1991) similarly found non-significant increases in the return rate by putting a stamp on the return envelope.

7. *Length of the questionnaire.* It seems logical that shorter questionnaires should lead to higher rates of return than longer ones. However, the research is mixed and contradictory in this regard. Yu and Cooper (1983) showed that length is a relatively weak factor affecting return rate in comparison to others, but Edwards et al. (2002) found an OR of 1.86—that is, the odds of a response to a single -page questionnaire is almost twice that for a 3-page questionnaire—and Yammarino et al.'s meta-analysis (1991) concluded that response rates were significantly lower with questionnaires over 4 pages as compared to those with fewer pages. When the questionnaire is long (over roughly 100 items or 10 pages), each additional page reduces the response rate by about 0.4 per cent. Up to that point, the content of the questionnaire is a far more potent factor affecting whether or not the person will complete it (Goyder 1982; Heberlein and Baumgartner 1978). In fact, there is some evidence that lengthening the questionnaire by adding interesting questions may actually increase compliance and lead to more valid answers (Burchell and Marsh 1992; Dillman 1978). Thus, it seems that once a person has been persuaded to fill out the form, its length is of secondary importance. However, questions towards the end of long questionnaires are more prone to satisficing, resulting in answers like 'don't know' (Krosnick et al. 2002), or to having the same response to all questions (Herzog and Bachman 1981).

8. *Pre-coding the questions.* Although this does not appear to appreciably increase compliance, pre-coding does serve a number of useful purposes. First, open-ended questions must at some point be coded for analysis; in other words, coding must take place at one time or another. Second, subjects are more likely to check a box rather than write out a long explanation. Last, handwritten responses may be illegible or ambiguous. On the other hand, subjects may feel that they want to explain their answers, or indicate why none of the alternatives applies (a sign of a poorly designed

question). The questionnaire can make provisions for this, having optional sections after each section or at the end for the respondent to add comments.

9. *Follow-ups.* As important as the letter introducing the study is the follow-up to maximize returns. Dillman (1978) outlines a four-step process:

   a) 7–10 days after the first mailing, a postcard should be sent, thanking those who have returned the questionnaire and reminding the others of the study's importance. The card should also indicate to those who have mislaid the original where they can get another copy of the questionnaire.

   b) 2–3 weeks later, a second letter is sent, again emphasizing why that person's responses are necessary for this important study. Also included are another questionnaire and return envelope. This can lead to a problem, though, if it is sent to all subjects, irrespective of whether or not they are sent in the first form; very compliant or forgetful subjects may complete two of them.

   c) The third step, which is not possible in all countries, is to send yet another letter, questionnaire, and envelope via registered or special delivery mail. The former alternative is less expensive, but some people may resent having to make a special trip to the post office for something of no direct importance to them.

   d) The last step, often omitted because of the expense, is to call those who have not responded to the previous three reminders. This may be impractical for studies that span the entire country, but may be feasible for more local ones.

   Some researchers have maintained that while the individual effect of each of these procedures may be slight (with the exception of the initial letter, return envelope, and follow-up, where major effects are seen), their cumulative effect is powerful. An extremely thorough Cochrane review of factors that do and do not affect response rate of mailed and electronic surveys was done by Edwards et al. (2009).

The necessity of persistence

We would all want the response rate to a survey, no matter how it was administered, to be as high as possible. The problem is that no one knows how high is high enough. Johnson and Wislar (2012) state that the minimum threshold is usually regarded as 60 per cent, but add that this is only a rule of thumb, and that 'there is no scientifically proven minimally acceptable response rate'. Where there is consensus is that response rates have been dropping at a somewhat precipitous rate over the past few decades in most countries (Cull et al. 2005). Even when all the techniques are used to maximize the return rate of a mailed questionnaire or to talk to the designated respondent on the telephone, the initial response rate is usually too low to permit accurate conclusions to be drawn. Consequently, most surveys call for follow-up mailings or calls in order to contact most of the subjects. The experience of one typical telephone survey is presented in Fig. 13.1, based on data from Traugott (1987). After three follow-up calls, about two-thirds of the respondents were contacted; one particularly elusive person required a total of 30 calls before he was reached.

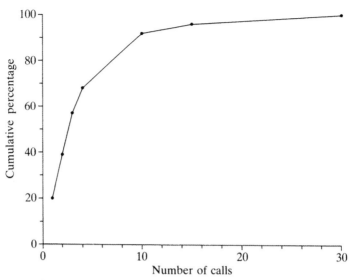

Fig. 13.1 Cumulative contact rate as a function of the number of telephone calls.
Source: data from Traugott, M.W., The importance of persistence in respondent selection for preelection surveys, *Public Opinion Quarterly*, Volume 51, Issue 1, pp. 48–57, Copyright © 1987 by the American Association for Public Opinion Research.

The necessity of persistence in follow-up has been demonstrated in a number of studies, which have shown that people who are easier to contact are different in some important ways from those who are more difficult to find or who require more reminders before they return a questionnaire. Traugott (1987) found that during the 1984 Presidential campaign, Democrats were more accessible than Republicans. As Fig. 13.2 shows, people who were found after one telephone call favoured Reagan by 3 per cent; the lead increased to nine points when the sample included people who were reached after three calls; and the total sample gave Reagan a 13-point advantage. He concluded that 'through persistence, the sample became younger and more male' (p. 53). Similar results were found in the health field by Fowler et al. (2002). An initial mailed survey to people enrolled in a health plan yielded a 46 per cent return rate. Phoning the non-responders raised this to 66 per cent. Of the 24 comparisons between those who responded by mail and those who were later contacted by telephone, 21 were significantly different. The former group was older, had a greater proportion of women, consistently reported more health problems, were more likely to have been hospitalized and to have seen a physician two or more times, took more prescription medication, and used more medical services than those who did not return the survey. In the same vein, Stallard (1995) found that non-respondents to a psychotherapy follow-up survey were more likely to have dropped out of therapy, and were more dissatisfied with the process than survey responders. Rao (1983) and Converse and Traugott (1986) summarize a number of characteristics which are different between early and late responders.

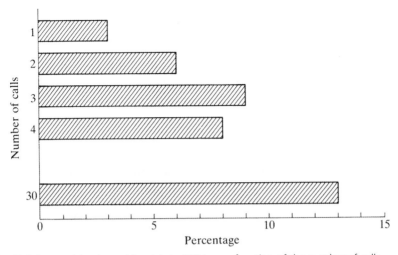

Fig. 13.2 Reagan's lead over Mondale in 1984, as a function of the number of calls required to reach the respondent.

Source: data from Traugott, M.W., The importance of persistence in respondent selection for preelection surveys, *Public Opinion Quarterly*, Volume 51, Issue 1, pp. 48–57, Copyright © 1987 by the American Association for Public Opinion Research.

Heerwegh et al. (2007) were able to compare answers to survey questions to a 'gold standard'. There were nearly twice as many people who refused to cooperate (16.7 per cent) as who were unable to be contacted (8.8 per cent). However, the error in the estimated values due to an inability to contact the person was 2.6 times higher than that due to refusal, indicating that these likely represent two different populations: re-fusers are more similar to those who complete surveys than are those who, for various reasons, cannot be reached.

However, Keeter et al. (2000) found that while the demographic characteristics of the sample changed with more 'rigorous' attempts to contact people, the results of a survey focusing on engagement in politics, social and political attitudes, and social trust and connectedness were roughly the same for those easier and harder to find. Similarly, Siemiatycki and Campbell (1984) found relatively few differences between those who responded to initial mail and telephone surveys and those who needed further follow-up before they responded, and little evidence of non-response bias. There have been other studies that have also failed to find differences in the prevalence of various disorders between those who needed few versus many reminders (Hardie et al. 2003; Wang et al. 2002), or differences in answers to survey questions among completers, refusers, and non-responders (Heerwegh et al. 2007; McFarlane et al. 2007). Consequently, it is difficult to come to any definitive conclusion regarding the need for aggressive follow-up. Perhaps the most prudent course would be to balance the desirability of a high response rate with the increasing costs for each additional wave of reminders. The results of Heerwegh et al. (2007) would also suggest that more effort should be placed in trying to trace people who cannot be contacted than in repeatedly contacting those who simply do not respond.

From administration to content: the impact of technology on scale construction

Up to this point, the discussion has focused on the use of technologies (computers, smart phones) in relation to test administration. We would be remiss, however, not to point out that this same technology offers the possibility of changing the very way in which we design tests, affecting content as well as administration.

Often implicit in discussions of scale construction, we would argue, is the assumption that questionnaires follow pencil and paper format: questions (sentences/phrases) or statements are provided and respondents select from pre-determined response categories. Through technology, we can substitute screens, touchpads, and keyboards for pencil and paper without fundamentally altering the structure of the tests we create.

This format, regardless of whether the measure is administered electronically or not, is entirely dependent on written language. Considerable space in this book has already been devoted to issues related to dependence on written language, and the potential this dependency can have on results. Simply put, relying solely on the written word to communicate complex ideas or concepts is a significant challenge for test constructors.

Electronic formats, however, offer us the possibility to use multimedia to convey information and communicate ideas. Pictures (still images), video, sound, even touch and smell, instead of words alone, can be incorporated. While these media are not immune to problems related to response bias, they do allow the test constructor to potentially address limitations, particularly in relation to interpretation, associated with word-only formats. Here are a few specific examples.

In the area of child development, parents are often asked to assess their child in relation in other children, in domains such as motor behaviour. The challenge is that most parents (for that matter, most teachers, physicians, and psychologists as well) are not comfortable evaluating motor ability in children. Consider the following items, taken from a measure used to assess motor coordination problems in children: 'Your child throws a ball in a controlled and accurate fashion' and 'Your child learns new motor tasks (e.g. swimming, rollerblading) easily and does not require more practice or time than other children to achieve the same level of skill' (Wilson et al. 2009). In addition to the fact that these items have other problems we have previously discussed (e.g. 'controlled *and* accurate' is a definite no-no is double-barrelled with ambiguous words; see Chapter 3), they may be difficult for some parents to answer because of lack of knowledge or familiarity with the behaviour in the context of motor development. What exactly does a controlled throw look like when the subject is a 5-year-old child? With video, however, a film of a child throwing a ball, with a narrator describing what the viewer is seeing (commenting on what to observe and why), could overcome the problem of trying to evaluate a behaviour (controlled and accurate ball throwing); this, clearly, would benefit from a visual, rather than written, presentation. At the opposite end of the age spectrum, Balachandran et al. (2016) developed a video-based questionnaire to assess physical function in older adults. They watched a video of a person performing various activities of daily living, such as standing up from a sitting position and balancing on one leg, and then used a slider to indicate the degree to which they could perform the task. This gave the respondents a clear indication of what was meant by each item.

Another example comes from social psychology, and the use of vignettes to study attitudes and perceptions (Rossi 1979). In medicine, this method has been used, for example, to study medical decision-making (e.g. Bachman et al. 2008). Vignettes are short descriptions (a paragraph or two), describing a specific scenario or situation where the researcher will vary specific details, such as the gender or age of the characters, to assess how changing these aspects of the narrative influences the response of the subject. In doing so, underlying values, attitudes, and preferences can be elicited. Among the many challenges associated with the method, reading a short story (or a series of short stories) and answering questions is a cognitively demanding task. Again, the use of video could enhance the presentation of information, allowing the test constructor to control many different aspects of the narrative, while minimizing demand on the test-taker. Indeed, video-taped scenarios have been used before with general practitioners (McKinley et al. 1997) and even for medical school admissions (Dore et al. 2009).

These examples only scratch the surface of potential uses of technology in this regard. With the wide spread use of new technologies, perhaps it is time to begin to think beyond the two-dimensional, written page, and further explore the use of multimedia, multimodal sensory applications to the challenges of measurement design.

Reporting response rates

The plethora of methods of administering scales—face-to-face interviews, mailed questionnaires, over the telephone, using the Web—has been a boon to researchers. At the same time, though, it has made it far more difficult to report response rates, because there are now a wider range of reasons for non-completion: randomly dialled telephone numbers can be disconnected, or lead to a business office or a fax machine at the other end, for example; and it is hard to know how many people may actually receive a questionnaire that was posted at a website.

To try to bring some order to this chaos, the American Association for Public Opinion Research (AAPOR) has issued standard definitions that can—and should—be used to record the final disposition of attempts to contact people, and how to determine outcome rates for surveys administered in four different ways: (1) random digit dialling, (2) in-person household surveys, (3) mail surveys of specifically named people, and (4) Internet surveys of specifically named people (American Association for Public Opinion Research 2006). Their Final Disposition Codes are probably far too detailed for any except very large surveys. There are four major categories of disposition for each of the survey types—interview; eligible, non-interview; unknown eligibility, non-interview; and not eligible—which are subdivided into as many as 37 different reasons. However, for even small, research surveys, it is well worthwhile using a shortened list of dispositions.

Box 13.1 Disposition categories

I = Complete interviews

P = Partial interviews (e.g. part of the questionnaire is left blank, or the person terminates the interview before its completion)

R = Refusal

NC = Non-contact

O = Other

UH = Unknown if household occupied

UO = Unknown, other.

One major contribution of these standards is that they define a number of different response and cooperation rates, rather than just one of each. This allows for a more complete and accurate picture of how many people did and did not respond. First, the dispositions are counted in a number of different categories (Box 13.1).

The minimal response rate, R_1, is the number of complete interviews divided by all attempts at contact:

$$R_1 = \frac{I}{(I+P)+(R+NC+O)+(UH+UO)}$$

and R_2 (complete and partial interviews) is slightly less conservative, in that it counts partial interviews as respondents:

$$R_2 = \frac{(I+P)}{(I+P)+(R+NC+O)+(UH+UO)}$$

There are a number of other response rates, which require some estimate of the proportion of cases of unknown eligibility (UH and UO) that are eligible.

Somewhat different from the response rate is the *cooperation rate*, which is based only on the number of people (or households) that were actually contacted. The minimum cooperation rate is:

$$COOP_1 = \frac{I}{(I+P)+R+O}$$

and, analogously to R_2, there is a less conservative rate that includes partial interviews as responders:

$$COOP_2 = \frac{(I+P)}{(I+P)+R+O}$$

Even more liberally, $COOP_3$ and $COOP_4$ delete from the denominator those people who are incapable of cooperating (people captured in the O category); $COOP_3$ uses I in the numerator, and $COOP_4$ uses $(I + P)$.

Missing from these formulae is the response or cooperation rates for Internet surveys that are not targeted to specific individuals: because the target population is unknown, there is no way to estimate the denominator. Consequently, the results cannot be generalized beyond the respondents with any degree of confidence.

Further reading

Dillman, D.A., Smyth, J.D., and Christian, L.M. (2014). *Internet, phone, mail, and mixed-mode surveys: The tailored design method* (4th edn). Wiley, New York.

International Test Commission (2006). International guidelines on computer-based and internet delivered testing. *International Journal of Testing*, **6**, 143–71.

Kaye, B.K. and Johnson, T.J. (1999). Research methodology: Taming the cyber frontier. *Social Science Computer Review*, **17**, 323–37.

Kosinski, M., Matz, S.C., Gosling, S.D., Popov, V., and Stillwell, D. (2015). Facebook as a research tool for the social sciences: Opportunities, challenges, ethical considerations, and practical guidelines. *American Psychologist*, **70**, 543–56.

References

American Association for Public Opinion Research (2006). *Standard definitions: Final disposition of case codes and outcome rates for surveys* (4th edn). AAPOR, Lenexa, KS.

American Psychiatric Association (2013). *Diagnostic and statistical manual of mental disorders: 5th Edition—DSM-5*. APA, Arlington, VA.

Aneshensel, C.S., Frerichs, R.R., Clark, V.A., and Yokopenic, P.A. (1982). Measuring depression in the community: A comparison of telephone and personal interviews. *Public Opinion Quarterly*, **46**, 110–21.

Armstrong, J.S. and Lusk, E.J. (1987). Return postage in mail surveys: A meta-analysis. *Public Opinion Quarterly*, **51**, 233–48.

Bachman, L.M., Mühleisen, A., Bock, A., ter Riet, G., Held, U., and Kessels, A.G.H. (2008). Vignette studies of medical choice and judgement to study caregivers' medical decision behaviour: Systematic review. *BMC Medical Research Methodology*, **8**, 50.

Backlinko (n.d.). Social network usage & growth. Available at: https://backlinko.com/social-media-users. Accessed 2 March 2022.

Backstrom, C.H. and Hursh-Cesar, G. (1981). *Survey research* (2nd edn). Wiley, New York.

Balachandran, A., Verduin, C.N., Potiaumpai, M., Ni, M., and Signorile, J.F. (2016). Validity and reliability of a video questionnaire to assess physical function in older adults. *Experimental Gerontology*, **81**, 76–82.

Barron, M. and Khare, M. (2008). Manipulating caller ID for higher survey response in RDD surveys. *Proceedings of the Survey Research Methods Section*. 62nd annual conference of the American Association for Public Opinion Research, pp. 3957–62. American Statistical Association, Alexandria, VA.

Ben-Porath, Y.S., Slutske, W.S., and Butcher, J.N. (1989). A real-data simulation of computerized administration of the MMPI. *Psychological Assessment*, **1**, 18–22.

Biller, B.A. (2005). Examining the utility of ecological momentary assessment with individuals diagnosed with depressive disorder. *Dissertation Abstracts International: Section B: The Sciences and Engineering*, **65**(8-B), 4274.

Birnholtz, J.P., Horn, D.B., Finholt, T.A., and Bae, S.J. (2004). The effects of cash, electronic, and paper gift certificates as respondent incentives for a Web-based survey of technologically sophisticated respondents. *Social Science Computing Review*, **22**, 355–62.

Blomberg, J. and Sandell, R. (1996). Does a material incentive affect response on a psychotherapy follow-up questionnaire? *Psychotherapy Research*, **6**, 155–63.

Blumberg, S.J. and Luke, J.V. (2021). *Wireless substitution: Early release of estimates from the National Health Interview Survey, January–June 2021*. National Center for Health Statistics, Hyattsville, MD.

Bosnjak, M. and Tuten, T.L. (2003). Prepaid and promised incentives in Web surveys. *Social Science Computer Reviews*, **21**, 208–17.

Bradley, N. (1999). Sampling for Internet surveys: An examination of respondent selection for Internet research. *Journal of the Market Research Society*, **41**, 387–95.

Burchell, B. and Marsh, C. (1992). The effect of questionnaire length on survey response. *Quality and Quantity*, **26**, 233–44.

Callegaro, M., McCutcheon, A.L., and Ludwig, J. (2010). Who's calling? The impact of caller ID on telephone survey response. *Field Methods*, **22**, 175–91.

Church, A.H. (1993). Estimating the effect of incentives on mail survey response rates: A meta-analysis. *Public Opinion Quarterly*, **57**, 62–79.

Cinà, C. and Clase, C.M. (1999). The Illness Intrusiveness Rating Scale: A measure of severity in individuals with hyperhidrosis. *Quality of Life Research*, **8**, 693–8.

Colombotos, J., Elinson, J., and Loewenstein, R. (1968). Effect of interviewers' sex on interview responses. *Public Health Reports*, **83**, 685–90.

Converse, P.E. and Traugott, M.W. (1986). Assessing the accuracy of polls and surveys. *Science*, **234**, 1094–8.

Cull, W.L., O'Connor, K.G., Sharp, S., and Tang, S.F. (2005). Response rates and response bias for 50 surveys of pediatricians. *Health Services Research*, **40**, 213–26.

DeAngelo, T.I. and Feng, B. (2019). From inbox reception to compliance: A field experiment examining the effects of e-mail address and subject line on response and compliance rates in initial e-mail encounters. *Social Science Computer Review*, **38**, 766–78.

Devins, G.M., Binik, Y.M., Hutchinson, T.A., Hollomby, D.J., Barre, P.E., and Guttmann, R.D. (1983–1984). The emotional impact of end-stage renal disease: Importance of patients' perception of intrusiveness and control. *International Journal of Psychiatry and Medicine*, **13**, 327–43.

Dhalla, I.A., Kwong, J.C., Streiner, D.L., Baddour, R.E., Waddell, A.E., and Johnson, I.L. (2002). Characteristics of first-year students in Canadian medical schools. *Canadian Medical Association Journal*, **166**, 1029–35.

Dillman, D.A. (1978). *Mail and telephone surveys: The total design method*. Wiley, New York.

Dillman, D.A. (2002). Navigating the rapids of change: Some observations on survey methodology in the early twenty-first century. *Public Opinion Quarterly*, **66**, 473–94.

Dillman, D.A. (2007). *Mail and internet surveys: The tailored design method* (2nd edn). Wiley, New York.

Dillman, D.A., Smyth, J.D., and Christian, L.M. (2014). *Internet, phone, mail, and mixed-mode surveys: The tailored design method* (4th edn). Wiley, New York.

Dore, K.L., Reiter, H.I., Eva, K.W., Krueger, S., Scriven, E., Siu, E., *et al.* (2009). Extending the interview to all medical school candidates—Computer Based Sample Evaluation of Non-cognitive Skills (CMSENS). *Academic Medicine*, **84**, S9–12.

Edwards, P., Roberts, I., Clarke, M., DiGuiseppi, C., Pratap, S., Wentz, R., *et al.* (2002). Increasing response rate to postal questionnaires: Systematic review. *BMJ*, **324**, 1183–5.

Edwards, P., Cooper, R., Roberts, I., and Frost, C. (2006). Meta-analysis of randomized trials of monetary incentives and response to mailed questionnaires. *Journal of Epidemiology and Community Health*, **59**, 987–99.

Edwards, P.J., Roberts, I., Clarke, M.J., DiGuiseppi, C., Wentz, R., Kwan, I., *et al.* (2009). Methods to increase response to postal and electronic questionnaires. *Cochrane Database of Systematic Reviews*, **3**, Article MR000008.

Eley, S. (1999). Nutritional research using electronic mail. *British Journal of Nutrition*, **81**, 413–16.

Eysenbach, G. (2004). Improving the quality of web surveys: The Checklist for Reporting Results of Internet E-Surveys (CHERRIES). *Journal of Medical Internet Research*, **6**, e34.

Ferriss, A.L. (1951). A note on stimulating response to questionnaires. *American Sociological Review*, **16**, 247–9.

Finkel, S.E., Guterbock, T.M., and Borg, M.J. (1991). Race-of-interviewer effects in a pre-election poll: Virginia 1989. *Public Opinion Quarterly*, **55**, 313–30.

Finkelman, M.D., Lowe, S.R., Kim, W., Gruebner, O., Smits, N., and Galea, S. (2018). Item ordering and computerized classification tests with cluster-based scoring: An investigation of the countdown method. *Psychological Assessment*, **30**, 204–19.

Fishman, K.D. (1981). *The computer establishment*. Harper and Row, New York.

Forbey, J.D. and Ben-Porath, Y.S. (2007). Computerized adaptive personality testing: A review and illustration with the MMPI-2 computerized adaptive version. *Psychological Assessment*, **19**, 14–24.

Fowler, F.J., Gallagher, P.M., Stringfellow, V.L., Zaslavsky, A.M., Thompson, J.W., and Cleary, P.D. (2002). Using telephone interviews to reduce nonresponse bias to mail surveys of health plan members. *Medical Care*, **40**, 190–200.

Fox, R.J., Crask, M.R., and Kim, J. (1988). Mail survey response rate: A meta-analysis of selected techniques for inducing response. *Public Opinion Quarterly*, **52**, 467–91.

Galesic, M. and Bosnjak, M. (2009). Effects of questionnaire length on participation and indicators of response quality in a Web survey. *Public Opinion Quarterly*, **73**, 349–60.

Glassmeyer, D.M. and Dibbs, R.-A. (2012). Researching from a distance: Using live web conferencing to mediate data collection. *International Journal of Qualitative Methods*, **11**, 292–302.

Goering, P.N., Streiner, D.L., Adair, C., Aubrey, T., Barker, J., Distasio, J., *et al.* (2011). The At Home/Chez Soi trial protocol: A pragmatic, multi-site, randomized controlled trial of Housing First intervention for homeless mentally ill in five Canadian cities. *BMJ Open*, **1**, e000323.

Goyder, J.C. (1982). Further evidence on factors affecting response rate to mailed questionnaires. *American Sociological Review*, **47**, 550–3.

Granello, D.H. and Wheaton, J.E. (2004). Online data collection: Strategies for research. *Journal of Counseling and Development*, **82**, 387–93.

Groves, R.M. and Fultz, N.H. (1985). Gender effects among telephone interviewers in a survey of economic attitudes. *Sociological Methods and Research*, **14**, 31–52.

Hardie, J.A., Bakke, P.S., and Mørkve, O. (2003). Non-response bias in a postal questionnaire survey on respiratory health in the old and very old. *Scandinavian Journal of Public Health*, **31**, 411–17.

Hartford, K., Carey, R., and Mendonca, J. (2007). Sampling bias in an international internet survey of diversion programs in the criminal justice system. *Evaluation & the Health Professions*, **30**, 35–46.

Heberlein, T.A. and Baumgartner, R. (1978). Factors affecting response rate to mailed questionnaires: A quantitative analysis of the published literature. *American Sociological Review*, **43**, 447–62.

Heerwegh, D. (2005). Effects of personal salutations in e-mail invitations to participate in a web survey. *Public Opinion Quarterly*, **69**, 588–98.

Heerwegh, D. and Loosveldt, G. (2006). Personalizing e-mail contacts: Its influence on web survey response rate and social desirability response bias. *International Journal of Public Opinion Research*, **19**, 258–68.

Heerwegh, D. and Loosveldt, G. (2008). Face-to-face versus web surveying in a high-internet-coverage population. *Public Opinion Quarterly*, **72**, 836–46.

Heerwegh, D., Vanhove, T., Matthijs, K., and Loosveldt, G. (2005). The effect of personalization on response rates and data quality in web surveys. *International Journal of Social Research Methodology: Theory and Practice*, **8**, 85–99.

Heerwegh, D., Abts, K., and Loosveldt, G. (2007). Minimizing survey refusal and noncontact rates: Do our efforts pay off? *Survey Research Methods*, **1**, 3–10.

Henley, J. (1976). Response rate to mail questionnaires with a return deadline. *Public Opinion Quarterly*, **40**, 374–5.

Herzog, A.R. and Bachman, J.G. (1981). Effects of questionnaire length on response quality. *Public Opinion Quarterly*, **45**, 549–59.

Holbrook, A.L., Green, M.C., and Krosnick, J.A. (2003). Telephone versus face-to-face interviewing of national probability samples with long questionnaires: Comparisons of respondent satisficing and social desirability bias. *Public Opinion Quarterly*, **67**, 79–125.

Hornik, J. (1982). Impact of pre-call request form and gender interaction on response to a mail survey. *Journal of Marketing Research*, **19**, 144–51.

Huff, C. and Tingley, D. (2015). "Who are these people?": Evaluating the demographic characteristics and political preferences of MTurk survey respondents. *Research and Politics*, **2**, 1–12.

Hufford, M.R., Shiffman, S., Paty, J., and Stone, A.A. (2001). Ecological momentary assessment: Real-world, real-time measurement of patient experience. In *Progress in ambulatory assessment: Computer-assisted psychological and psychophysiological methods in monitoring and field studies* (eds. J. Fahrenberg and M. Myrtek), pp. 69–92. Hogrefe & Huber, Seattle, WA.

Hutchinson, K.L. and Wegge, D.G. (1991). The effects of interviewer gender upon response in telephone survey research. *Journal of Social Behavior and Personality*, **6**, 573–84.

Hyman, H.H., Cobb, W.J., Feldman, J.J., Hart, C.W., and Stember, C.H. (1954). *Interviewing in social research*. University of Chicago Press, Chicago, IL.

James, J.M. and Bolstein, R. (1992). Large monetary incentives and their effects on mail survey response rates. *Public Opinion Quarterly*, **56**, 442–53.

Jamnik, M.R. and Lane, D.J. (2017). The use of Reddit as an inexpensive source for high-quality data. *Practical Assessment, Research, and Evaluation*, **22**, Article 5.

Jensen, M.P. and McFarland, C.A. (1993). Increasing the reliability and validity of pain intensity measurement in chronic pain patients. *Pain*, **55**, 195–203.

Johnson, D.R., Scheitle, C.P., and Ecklund, E.H. (2019). Beyond the in-person interview? How interview quality varies across in-person, telephone, and Skype interviews. *Social Science Computer Review*, **39**, 1142–58.

Johnson, T.P. and Wislar, J.S. (2012). Response rates and nonresponse errors in surveys. *JAMA*, **307**, 1805–6.

Joinson, A.N., Woodley, A., and Reips, U.-D. (2007). Personalization, authentication and self-disclosure in self-administered Internet surveys. *Computers in Human Behavior*, **23**, 275–85.

Jones, R. and Pitt, N. (1999). Health surveys in the workplace: Comparison of postal, email and World Wide Web methods. *Occupational Medicine (Oxford)*, **49**, 556–8.

Kaye, B.K. and Johnson, T.J. (1999). Research methodology: Taming the cyber frontier. *Social Science Computer Review*, **17**, 323–37.

Keding, A., Brabyn, S., MacPherson, H., Richmond, S.J., and Torgerson, D.J. (2016). Text message reminders to improve questionnaire response rate. *Journal of Clinical Epidemiology*, **79**, 90–5.

Keeter, S. (1995). Estimating telephone noncoverage bias in a telephone survey. *Public Opinion Quarterly*, **59**, 196–217.

Keeter, S., Miller, C., Kohut, A., Groves, R.M., and Presser, S. (2000). Consequences of reducing nonresponse in a national telephone survey. *Public Opinion Quarterly*, **64**, 125–48.

Kennedy, C., McGeeney, K., Keeter, S., Patten, E., Perrin, A., Lee, A., *et al.* (2018). Implications of moving public opinion surveys to a single-frame cell-phone random-digit-dial design. *Public Opinion Quarterly*, **82**, 279–99.

Kessler, R.C. and Üstün, T.B. (2004). The World Mental Health (WMH) Survey Initiative Version of the World Health Organization (WHO) Composite International Diagnostic Interview (CIDI). *International Journal of Methods in Psychiatric Research*, **13**, 93–121.

King, D.B., O'Rourke, N., and DeLongis, A. (2014). Social media recruitment and online data collection: A beginner's guide and best practices for accessing low-prevalence and hard-to-reach populations. *Canadian Psychology*, **55**, 240–9.

Kosinski, M., Matz, S.C., Gosling, S.D., Popov, V., and Stillwell, D. (2015). Facebook as a research tool for the social sciences: Opportunities, challenges, ethical considerations, and practical guidelines. *American Psychologist*, **70**, 543–56.

Krosnick, J.A., Holbrook, A.L., Berent, M.K., Carson, R.T., Hanemann, W.M., Kopp, R.J., *et al.* (2002). The impact of 'no opinion' response options on data quality: Non-attitude reduction or an invitation to satisfice? *Public Opinion Quarterly*, **66**, 371–403.

Kwong, J.C., Dhalla, I.A., Streiner, D.L., Baddour, R.E., Waddell, A.E., and Johnson, I.L. (2002). Effects of rising tuition fees on medical school class composition and financial outlook. *Canadian Medical Association Journal*, **166**, 1023–8.

Lazar, J. and Preece, J. (1999). Designing and implementing Web-based surveys. *Journal of Computer Information Systems*, **39**, 63–7.

Levay, K.E., Freese, J., and Druckman, J.N. (2016). The demographic and political composition of Mechanical Turk samples. *SAGE Open*, **6**, 1–17.

Lobe, B., Morgan, D., and Hoffman, K.A. (2020). Qualitative data collection in an era of social distancing. *International Journal of Qualitative Methods*, **19**.

Locander, W.B. and Burton, J.P. (1976). The effect of question form on gathering income data by telephone. *Journal of Marketing Research*, **13**, 189–92.

Lucas, R.W., Mullin, P.J., Luna, C.B.X., and McInroy, D.C. (1977). Psychiatrists and a computer as interrogators of patients with alcohol-related illness: A comparison. *British Journal of Psychiatry*, **131**, 160–7.

Luitten, A. (2011). Personalisation in advance letters does not always increase response rates: Demographic correlates in a large scale experiment. *Survey Research Methods*, **5**, 11–20.

Lusk, C., Delclos, G.L., Burau, K., Drawhorn, D.D., and Aday, L.A. (2007). Mail versus internet surveys: Determinants of method of response preferences among health professionals. *Evaluation & the Health Professions*, **30**, 186–201.

MacInnis, B., Krosnick, J.A., Ho, A.S., and Cho, M.J. (2018). The accuracy of measurements with probability and nonprobability survey samples: Replication and extension. *Public Opinion Quarterly*, **82**, 707–44.

Maheux, B., Legault, C., and Lambert, J. (1989). Increasing response rates in physicians' mail surveys: An experimental study. *American Journal of Public Health*, **79**, 638–9.

McFarlane, E., Olmsted, M.G., Murphy, J., and Hill, C.A. (2007). Nonresponse bias in a mail survey of physicians. *Evaluation & the Health Professions*, **30**, 170–85.

McKinlay, J.B., Burns, R.B., Durante, R., Feldman, H.A., Freund, K.M., Harrow, B.S., *et al.* (1997). Patient, physician and presentational influences on clinical decision making for breast cancer: Results from a factorial experiment. *Journal of Evaluation in Clinical Practice*, **3**, 23–57.

McMorris, B.J., Petrie, R. S., Catalano, R.F., Fleming, C.B., Haggerty, K.P., and Abbott, R.D. (2009). Use of Web and in-person survey modes to gather data from young adults on sex and drug use: An evaluation of cost, time, and survey error based on a randomized mixed-mode design. *Evaluation Review*, **33**, 138–58.

Meislin, R. (1987). Racial divisions seen in poll on Howard Beach attack. *New York Times*, 8 January.

Merten, T. and Ruch, W. (1996). A comparison of computerized and conventional administration of the German versions of the Eysenck Personality Questionnaire and the Carroll Rating Scale for Depression. *Personality and Individual Differences*, **20**, 281–91.

Miller, J. (2006). Online marketing research. In *The handbook of marketing research: Uses, abuses, and future advances* (eds. R. Grover and M. Vriens), pp. 110–31. Sage, Thousand Oaks, CA.

Monsees, M.L. and Massey, J.T. (1979). Adapting a procedure for collecting demographic data in a personal interview to a telephone interview. *Proceedings of the American Statistical Association, Social Statistics Section*, 130–5.

Mortensen, K. and Hughes, T.L. (2018). Comparing Amazon's Mechanical Turk platform to conventional data collection methods in the health and medical research literature. *Journal of General Internal Medicine*, **33**, 533–8.

Mullinix, K.J., Leeper, T.J., Freese, J., and Druckman, J.N. (2015). The generalizability of survey experiments. *Journal of Experimental Political Science*, **2**, 109–38.

Nelson, N., Rosenthal, R., and Rosnow, R.L. (1986). Interpretation of significance levels and effect sizes by psychological researchers. *American Psychologist*, **41**, 1299–301.

Nicolaas, G. and Lynn, P. (2002). Random-digit dialling in the UK: Viability revisited. *Journal of the Royal Statistical Society, A*, **165**(Part 2), 297–316.

Norenzayan, A. and Schwarz, N. (1999). Telling what they want to know: Participants tailor causal attributions to researchers' interests. *European Journal of Social Psychology*, **29**, 1011–20.

Norman, G.R., McFarlane, A.H., Streiner, D.L., and Kneale, K.A. (1982). Health diaries: Strategies for compliance and relation to other measures. *Medical Care*, **20**, 623–9.

Norman, G.R., Oppenheimer, L., and Keane, D.R. (2008). Compliance of medical students with voluntary use of personal data assistants for clerkship assessments. *Teaching and Learning in Medicine*, **20**, 295–301.

O'Rourke, N., Carmel, S., Chaudhury, H., Polchenko, N., and Bachner, Y.G. (2013). A cross-national comparison of reminiscence functions between Canadian and Israeli older adults. *Journal of Gerontology: Series B. Psychological Sciences and Social Sciences*, **68**, 184–92.

Palermo, T.M., Witherspoon, D., Valenzuela, D., and Drotar, D.D. (2004). Development and validation of the Child Activity Limitations Interview: A measure of pain-related functional impairment in school-age children and adolescents. *Pain*, **109**, 461–70.

Pettigrew, T.F. (1964). *A profile of the Negro American*. Van Nostrand, Princeton, NJ.

Pettit, F.A. (2002). A comparison of World-Wide Web and paper-and-pencil personality questionnaires. *Behavior Research Methods, Instruments, & Computers*, **34**, 50–4.

Piasecki, T.M., Hufford, M.R., Solhan, M., and Trull, T.J. (2007). Assessing clients in their natural environments with electronic diaries: Rationale, benefits, limitations, and barriers. *Psychological Assessment*, **19**, 25–43.

Pignata, S., Lushington, K., Sloan, J., and Buchanan, F. (2015). Employees' perceptions of email communication, volume and management strategies in an Australian university. *Journal of Higher Education Policy and Management*, **37**, 159–71.

Pinsoneault, T.B. (1996). Equivalency of computer-assisted and paper-and-pencil administered versions of the Minnesota Multiphasic Personality Inventory-2. *Computers in Human Behavior*, **12**, 291–300.

Pollner, M. (1998). The effects of interviewer gender in mental health interviews. *Journal of Nervous and Mental Disease*, **186**, 369–73.

Quagan, B., Woods, S.W., and Powers, A.R. (2021). Navigating the benefits and pitfalls of online psychiatric data collection. *JAMA Psychiatry*, **78**, 1185–6.

Quine, S. (1985). 'Does the mode matter?': A comparison of three modes of questionnaire completion. *Community Health Studies*, **9**, 151–6.

Rao, P.S.R.S. (1983). Callbacks, follow-ups, and repeated telephone calls. In *Incomplete data in sample surveys. Vol. 2: Theory and bibliographies* (eds. W.G. Madow, I. Olkin, and D.B. Rubin), pp. 33–44. Academic Press, New York.

Raziano, D.B., Jayadevappa, R., Valenzula, D., Weiner, M., and Lavizzo-Mourey, R. (2001). E-mail versus conventional postal mail survey of geriatric chiefs. *The Gerontologist*, **41**, 799–804.

Rice, S.A. (1929). Contagious bias in the interview. *American Journal of Sociology*, **35**, 420–3.

Rogers, E.M. and Bhowmik, D.K. (1970). Homophily-heterophily: Relational concepts for communication research. *Public Opinion Quarterly*, **34**, 523–38.

Roper, B.L., Ben-Porath, Y.S., and Butcher, J.N. (1995). Comparability and validity of computerized adaptive testing with the MMPI-2. *Journal of Personality Assessment*, **65**, 358–71.

Rossi, P.H. (1979). Vignette analysis: Uncovering the normative structure of complex judgments. In *Qualitative and quantitative social research: Papers in honor of Paul*

F. Lazarsfeld (eds. R.K. Merton, J.S. Coleman, and P.H. Rossi), pp. 176–86. Free Press, New York.

Saltier, J. (1970). Racial 'experimenter effects' in experimentation, interviewing and psychotherapy. *Psychological Bulletin*, **73**, 137–60.

Scott, P. and Edwards, P. (2006). Personally addressed hand-signed letters increase questionnaire response: A meta-analysis of randomised controlled trials. *BMC Health Services Research*, **6**, 111.

Siemiatycki, J. and Campbell, S. (1984). Nonresponse bias and early versus all responders in mail and telephone surveys. *American Journal of Epidemiology*, **120**, 291–301.

Singer, E., Hippler, H.J., and Schwarz, N. (1992). Confidentiality assurances in surveys: Reassurance or threat? *International Journal of Public Opinion Research*, **4**, 256–68.

Singer, E., von Thurn, D.R., and Miller, E.R. (1995). Confidentiality assurances and response: A quantitative review of the experimental literature. *Public Opinion Quarterly*, **59**, 66–75.

Skinner, H.A. and Allen, B.A. (1983). Does the computer make a difference? Computerized versus face-to-face versus self-report assessment of alcohol, drug, and tobacco use. *Journal of Consulting and Clinical Psychology*, **51**, 267–75.

Stallard, P. (1995). Parental satisfaction with intervention: Differences between respondents and non-respondents to a postal questionnaire. *British Journal of Clinical Psychology*, **34**, 397–405.

Statistics Canada (2006). The daily, 5 April 2006. Statistics Canada, Ottawa.

Statistics Canada (2019). Landline and cellular telephone use by province, 2019. Statistics Canada, Ottawa.

Stein, S.J. (1987). Computer-assisted diagnosis for children and adolescents. In *Computerized psychological assessment* (ed. J.N. Butcher), pp. 145–58. Basic Books, New York.

Stinson, J.N., Petroz, G., Tait, G., Feldman, B., Streiner, D.L., McGrath, P.J, *et al.* (2006). E-Ouch: Usability testing of an electronic chronic pain diary for adolescents with arthritis. *Clinical Journal of Pain*, **22**, 295–305.

Stone, A.A. and Shiffman, S. (1994). Ecological momentary assessment: Measuring real world processes in behavioral medicine. *Annals of Behavioral Medicine*, **16**, 199–202.

Stone, A.A. and Shiffman, S. (2002). Capturing momentary, self-report data: A proposal for reporting guidelines. *Annals of Behavioral Medicine*, **24**, 236–43.

Stone, A.A., Shiffman, S., Schwartz, J.E., Broderick, J.E., and Hufford, M.R. (2002). Patient non-compliance with paper diaries. *BMJ*, **324**, 1193–4.

Thornberry, O.T. (1987). An experimental comparison of telephone and personal health interview surveys. *Vital and Health Statistics. Series 2. Data evaluation and methods research*, **106**, 1–6.

Tourangeau, R. (2004). Survey research and societal change. *Annual Review of Psychology*, **55**, 775–801.

Traugott, M.W. (1987). The importance of persistence in respondent selection for preelection surveys. *Public Opinion Quarterly*, **51**, 48–57.

Trussell, N. and Lavrakas, P.J. (2004). The influence of incremental increases in token cash incentives on mail survey response: Is there an optimal amount? *Public Opinion Quarterly*, **68**, 349–67.

Tucker, C., Brick, J.M., and Meekins, B. (2007). Household telephone service and usage patterns in the United States in 2004: Implications for telephone samples. *Public Opinion Quarterly*, **71**, 3–22.

Tuten, T.L., Galesic, M., and Bosnjak, M. (2004). Effects of immediate versus delayed notification of prize draw results on response behavior in Web surveys: An experiment. *Social Science Computer Review*, **22**, 377–84.

Wang, P.S., Beck, A.L., McKenas, D.K., Meneades, L.M., Pronk, N.P., Saylor, J.S., *et al.* (2002). Effects of efforts to increase response rates on a workplace chronic condition screening survey. *Medical Care*, **40**, 752–60.

Warriner, K., Goyder, J., Gjertsen, H., Hohner, P., and McSpurren, K. (1996). Charities, no; lotteries, no; cash, yes. *Public Opinion Quarterly*, **60**, 542–62.

Watson, C.G., Manifold, V., Klett, W.G., Brown, J., Thomas, D., and Anderson, D. (1990). Comparability of computer- and booklet-administered Minnesota Multiphasic Personality Inventories among primarily chemically dependent patients. *Psychological Assessment*, **2**, 276–80.

Weinman, L. (1996). *Designing web graphics*. New Riders, Indianapolis, IN.

Weiss, C.H. (1975). Interviewing in evaluation research. In *Handbook of evaluation research*, Vol. 1 (eds. E.L. Struening and M. Guttentag), pp. 355–95. Sage, Beverly Hills, CA.

Wilson, B.N., Crawford, S.G., Green, D., Roberts, G., Aylott, A., and Kaplan, B. (2009). Psychometric properties of the revised developmental coordination disorder questionnaire. *Physical & Occupational Therapy in Pediatrics*, **29**, 182–202.

Yammarino, F.J., Skinner, S.J., and Childers, T.L. (1991). Understanding mail survey response behavior. *Public Opinion Quarterly*, **55**, 613–39.

Yu, J. and Cooper, H. (1983). A quantitative review of research design effects on response rates to questionnaires. *Journal of Marketing Research*, **20**, 36–44.

Zhang, C., Antoun, C., Yan, H.Y., and Conrad, F.G. (2019). Professional respondents in opt-in online panels: What do we really know? *Social Science Computer Review*, **38**, 703–19.

Zukin, C. (2015, June 21). What's wrong with polling? *New York Times*

Chapter 14

Ethical considerations

Introduction to ethical considerations

For the most part, ethical discussions concerning the development and administration of scales and tests have centred around assessments conducted within clinical, educational, or employment settings, and where the results would directly affect the person being evaluated. These situations would include, for example, intelligence, achievement, and aptitude testing in schools; personality and neurocognitive evaluations of patients; and ability testing of job applicants.

Initially, the major focus of the professional organizations was on establishing standards for the tests themselves. In 1895, the American Psychological Association (APA) began looking at the feasibility of standardizing 'mental' and physical tests (Novick 1981). The first formal set of guidelines appeared in 1954—the *Technical Recommendations for Psychological Tests and Diagnostic Techniques*, published by the APA—and these were followed a year later by the *Technical Recommendations for Achievement Tests*, prepared by the American Educational Research Association (AERA) and the National Council on Measurement in Education (NCME) (1954). These two sets of recommendations set standards for the assessment and reporting of the psychometric properties of tests, and for the first time set forth the requirements for reliability and validity testing. Later revisions modernized the definitions of reliability and validity, and put greater emphasis on the qualifications of the test user.

Tests that are used only for research purposes, however, are usually considered to be exempt from these standards. This does not mean that there are no ethical problems in devising and using instruments for primarily research questions. Consider the following situations:

Example A. While filling out a questionnaire enquiring about various mood states, one respondent writes in the margin of the answer sheet that they are feeling very despondent and have recently been thinking of taking their own life. Another subject, while not as explicit about their suicidal thoughts, scores in a range indicative of severe emotional turmoil.

Example B. You are developing a test of marital relationships and have assured the respondents that their answers will remain confidential, especially since some of the items tap issues of infidelity. One year later, the spouse of one of the respondents files for a divorce, and subpoenas the questionnaire to be used as evidence in court.

Example C. In order to validate a self-report measure of medical utilization, you need to examine the charts of subjects to see how much use they make of various hospital services. In order to ensure that the results are not biased by those who refused to participate in the study, you want to pull their charts to obtain some basic demographic information about them, and to determine their use of medical services.

Example D. Your aim is to develop a measure of self-esteem. One validity study would involve testing two groups of students before and after they make an oral presentation. Subjects in one group are told that they did very well, and those in the other group that they had done very badly and had made fools of themselves, irrespective of how they actually had performed. The students were enrolled in an Introductory Psychology class, and were required to participate in three studies as part of the course requirements.

Example E. In order to develop a test of abstract reasoning ability, it is necessary to administer it to people ranging in age from 5 to 75 years, and to psychiatric patients who may exhibit problems in this area, such as schizophrenics and those with brain injuries.

Example F. You have developed a new scale of parenting ability. It appears to show that those from a specific minority group have much poorer skills.

Example G. You develop a test to measure motor coordination in children, which involves a number of tasks related to balance, ball skills, and fine motor skills (e.g. tracing with a pen, threading beads onto a string). The test is difficult for children with poor motor co-ordination and can cause anxiety, anger, and frustration.

These situations illustrate a number of ethical considerations which may be encountered, such as the use of deception, confidentiality, free and informed consent, the proper balance between the researcher's need for data and the individual's right to privacy, the potential anxiety-inducing nature of the testing situation, and the consequences of the test's results. In this chapter, we will discuss these and other issues, and see how they affect scale development. As with many aspects of ethics, there are few right or wrong answers. Rather, there are general considerations which must be weighed and balanced against each other, and the 'correct' approach may vary from one situation and institution to another.

The primary consideration in all discussions of ethics is *respect for the individual's autonomy*. This means that we treat people in such a way that they can decide for themselves whether or not to participate in a study. At first glance, this principle may seem so self-evident that one wonders why it is even mentioned; it appears as if it should be understood and accepted by everyone, both researchers and subjects. However, the implementation of the principle of autonomy can lead to some thorny issues.

Informed consent

To begin with, people cannot exercise autonomy unless they know what it is that they are agreeing to. This means that there must be *informed consent*; that is, the subjects must be told:

1. that they are participating in a research study
2. what the study is about
3. what they are being called upon to do.

In studies done for the purpose of scale development, these requirements are most often easy to meet and present no difficulties.

Deception

Example D, though, involves deception, in that the subjects are not told that the feedback about their performance is fallacious. Indeed, it could be argued that the study would be impossible if the students were told its true nature. Wilson and Donnerstein (1976) give examples of at least eight types of studies in which they feel deception was a necessary and integral part. This may be as innocuous as giving a deceptive title to a scale, to the more extreme example cited here, of inducing stress by giving false feedback. Some professional organizations—mainly medical ones, which have little experience with psychosocial research methods—have a blanket prohibition against all studies that involve deception. Ortman and Hertwig (1997), for example, have said that deception should never be used because it taints all of research; and some people have argued that it is always possible to substitute observational procedures, which do not involve deception, for experiments which do (e.g. Shipley 1977). Others, such as the APA and the Canadian Institute of Health Research (CIHR), discourage its use, but recognize that there are some situations where it is required. If no alternative research strategy is possible, then the APA and CIHR state that:

1. the subjects must be told of the deception after their participation; and
2. the researcher must be able to cope with any possible psychological sequelae that may result from the deception (American Psychological Association 2017; Canadian Institutes of Health Research et al. 2018).

The process of debriefing after deception is well described in the Tri-Council Policy Statement (Canadian Institutes of Health Research et al. 2018). It says (p. 38):

> Often, debriefing can be a simple and straightforward candid disclosure. In sensitive cases, researchers should also provide a full explanation of why participants were temporarily led to believe that the research, or some aspect of it, had a different purpose, or why participants received less than full disclosure. The researchers should give details about the importance of the research, the necessity of having to use partial disclosure or deception, and express their concerns about the welfare of the participants. They should also seek to remove any misconceptions that may have arisen and to re-establish any trust that may have been lost, by explaining why these research procedures were necessary to obtain scientifically valid findings.

Vulnerable populations

A different problem with free and informed consent is raised in Examples E and G. How 'informed' can the consent be from minors or those whose cognitive processes are compromised because of some innate or acquired disorder? Some ethicists have argued that those who are unable to fully comprehend the nature of the study and their right to refuse to participate should never be used in research studies unless they benefit directly from their participation; even parents or legal guardians should not be able to give surrogate consent for their children. Adoption of this extreme view, though, would result in 'research orphans': groups on whom no research can be done, even if it may result in potential benefit to other members of that group. This is not an issue when developing a self-report scale, because if a person cannot understand the nature of the consent, it is unlikely they can read and understand the instrument. It is a concern, though, in trying to develop a scale based on observation of the child, or using children over the age of 8 or so, who are able to read to some degree, or scales intended to be completed by proxy (on behalf of) others.

Although few people adhere to such an extreme position, it is widely recognized that special precautions must be taken with these vulnerable groups. For those who are legally minors (the age of majority varies between 16 and 18, depending on the jurisdiction), the consent of at least one parent is mandatory. Increasingly over the years, there has been legal recognition of a grey zone between the age of majority and some vaguely defined point where the child is capable of understanding that they are part of a study. Within this age frame, the child's *assent* is required in addition to the parent's consent. This means that the child must not object to being in the study, although actively saying 'I agree' is not necessary. If they do object, this overrides the consent of the parent. Unfortunately for the investigator, the lower age of this zone is rarely explicitly stated, in recognition of the fact that children mature at different rates; it is left to the judgement of the researcher to determine if the child is cognitively capable of understanding.

A rational guideline for what can be done with children is provided by the guidelines of the Medical Research Council of Canada (1987). They state that (p. 29):

> society and parents should not expose children to greater risks, for the sake of pure medical research, than the children take in their everyday lives ... Parents may consent to inspection of their children's medical records for research.

Psychiatric patients pose a different set of problems. Having a diagnosed disorder, such as schizophrenia, does not necessarily mean that the person is incompetent and unable to give consent (or to deny it). Some institutions have taken the position that a mental health worker who does not have a vested interest in the research should sign a portion of the consent form indicating that, in their opinion, the patient was able to understand what was being asked. In cases where the patient has been judged to be incompetent (e.g. suffering from some severe psychiatric disorders, Alzheimer's disease, mental retardation, and the like), consent is gained from the legal guardian or next of kin, such as a spouse, child, or parent.

Written consent

In most studies, the participant must read and sign a consent form, summarizing what the study is about, what the person will be asked to do, the right of withdrawal, and so forth. All too many researchers, though, equate the consent *form* with the *process* of gaining consent, and they are not the same. The form exists for two purposes: so that the participants have a record of what they consented to (although this is rarely an issue when they complete a scale immediately after signing the form); and to keep the institution's lawyers and 'risk management' people happy. The most important point is that the participants understand their involvement, not that they sign a piece of paper. This has a number of implications.

The first is that the form is not always sufficient. Especially with children and those with limited cognitive ability, a verbal explanation is usually far superior to having them read a description of the study. The second implication is that written consent may not always be necessary. If the scale and the instructions are mailed or e-mailed to potential participants, the very fact that they did not throw these out or hit the 'delete' key is an indication of implied consent. Having to also sign a form is superfluous, likely insisted upon by the same lawyers and risk managers who are more concerned about protecting the institution's collective rear-ends against the unlikely lawsuit than the rights of the participants. Not all ethics boards take this enlightened stance, and the researcher should always check beforehand.

If the ethics board decides that a written consent form is required, it usually contains the following information:

1. Identification of the researcher and (if appropriate) the research institution.

2. Why the research is being carried out, that is, a brief description of its aims, and, if appropriate, whether it is a thesis project.

3. Identification of any risks. This most often does not apply, but should mention if the questionnaire will delve into sensitive topics.

4. A statement that the research is voluntary and that the person can omit any question, and can withdraw at any time.

5. That the data will by anonymized and no identifying information will appear in any publication

6. The approximate time it will take to complete the questionnaire.

7. A contact number if any issues arise. Most often, this will be the researcher themself, or the thesis supervisor. Some boards may require the name and telephone number of an ombudsman, who is a member of the institution but not on the research team.

Freedom of consent

The other aspect of autonomy, in addition to the informed part, is *freedom to not participate in* or to *withdraw from* the study (hence, it is often referred to as 'free and informed consent'). This component of consent can be violated in ways which range from the blatantly obvious to the sublimely subtle. Since flagrant violations are easy to detect and are usually patently unethical, we will devote most of the discussion to the less obvious situations, where researchers may not even be aware of the fact that they are trespassing on dangerous territory.

Having Introductory Psychology students participate in studies as a requirement of the course or for extra marks has been a long, if not hallowed, tradition. (Indeed, as far back as 1946, McNemar referred to psychology as 'the science of the behavior of sophomores'. We would add white rats to the list also.) However, this clearly obviates the freedom to withdraw, since to do so would result in a lower mark or perhaps even a failing grade. Many universities have banned this practice entirely, or allow the student to perform some other activity, such as writing a paper, as an alternative to serving as a research subject (American Psychological Association 2017).

A more subtle form of coercion may exist when a clinician recruits their patients to be research subjects. Some subjects may agree to participate because they are concerned that, if they do not, they will not receive the same level of care, despite assurances to the contrary. At one level, they are probably correct. Even if the clinician does not intend to withdraw services or to perform them in a more perfunctory manner, it is natural to assume that their attitude towards the patient may be affected by the latter's cooperation or refusal. Other patients may agree to participate out of a sense of gratitude, as a way of saying 'Thank you' for the treatment received. There is considerable debate whether this is a mild form of coercion, capitalizing on the patient's sense of obligation, or a very legitimate form of quid pro quo, allowing the patient to repay a perceived debt. Perhaps the safest course to take is for consent to be sought by a person not directly involved in the patient's care: a research assistant, teaching fellow, or another, disinterested clinician. Many ethics boards expressly prohibit clinicians from recruiting their patients.

Another consideration, which can give rise to subtle forms of coercion, is the time frame of the study. If the participant has to complete a survey only once, there is little concern regarding consent and freedom to withdraw because the consent process is usually quite close in time to participation in the study. For participants enrolled in longitudinal or cohort studies, however, which could last months or even years, it is important to remind participants that they can withdraw at any time for any reason, even if they have consented and previously participated in earlier waves of the study. Often this reminder occurs when participants are scheduled to participate in follow-ups. Some research ethics boards do not always require formal re-consent, unless the original study has concluded and the research team is seeking to continue to follow participants; whereas other boards state that consent is valid for only a limited period of time (6 or 12 months) and must be sought again after this period.

Confidentiality

The use of hospital or agency charts without the express permission of the patient is another area in which there is no consensus of opinion. The most stringent interpretation of the principle of consent is that in the absence of it, the researcher is prohibited from opening them. This would ban access to patient charts in such circumstances as:

1. gathering information to determine if those who refused to participate in a study differed in terms of demographic information from those who took part

2. wanting to correlate test data with clinical information, such as the number of times a patient presented at the emergency room or at an outpatient clinic

3. even finding a group of patients who should later be approached to participate in a study (e.g. those with specific disorders, those who make frequent use of clinical services, or who have certain demographic characteristics).

It is obvious that this strict interpretation of consent would make some forms of research impossible, or at least extremely costly. A more liberal view is held by people such as Berg (1954), who states that (p. 109):

> If the persons concerned are not harmed by the use of their records and their identities are not publicly revealed, there is no problem and their consent for the professional use of their records is not necessary.

Most research ethics committees take an intermediate position, exemplified by the Ethical Principles of Research of the British Psychological Society (1977). It states that when there is any 'encroachment upon privacy', the 'investigator should seek the opinion of experienced and disinterested colleagues', a role that is usually played now by the ethics committees of various institutions themselves. The Council for International Organizations of Medical Sciences (CIOMS 2012) adopts a similar position, explicitly stating that the review must be done by an ethical review committee, and further adds the stipulation that 'access ... must be supervised by a person who is fully aware of the confidentiality requirements'.

This confidentiality of records continues after the data have been collected. The research guidelines of all psychological organizations have emphasized this point for both clinical and research findings (cf. Schuler 1982). Whenever possible, forms should be completed anonymously. However, this is not always feasible; it is sometimes necessary for the purposes of validity testing to link the results of the scale under development to other data or, when test–retest reliability is being determined, to scores on the same measure completed at some later date. When this is the case, then:

1. the data should be kept in a locked storage cabinet, to which only the researcher has access
2. the names should be removed and replaced by identification numbers as soon as possible.

The limits of confidentiality

Even when these precautions are taken, there may be circumstances (albeit admittedly rare) in which confidentiality cannot be maintained. In Example B, the data have been subpoenaed by a court. If the names have already been removed, and no key linking the names with the ID numbers exists, then there is no problem; the data are irretrievable in a form which can be linked to a specific individual. However, if the individual people are still identifiable because the data must be linked, then the test developer is legally obligated to provide the information, and can be cited for contempt of court if they do not. The rule of privileged communication does not apply in this case for a number of reasons. First, the researcher is most often not in a fiduciary or therapeutic relationship with the subject. Indeed, they may never have met the subject previously, and the contact was usually made at the researcher's initiative and for their purposes. Second, the rule is not universal, and rarely extends beyond lawyers and the clergy; psychologists, physicians, and other health providers are usually not protected.

Finally, there are situations where confidentiality must be violated by the researcher. These involve cases where the investigator believes that the subject is in imminent danger of harming themselves or other people (see Example A). The person should be offered help and encouraged to seek professional advice. If the researcher feels that the danger is acute, and that the person is unwilling to be helped, then the 'duty to warn' supersedes the rules of confidentiality; this is called the Tarasoff rule, following the case of *Tarasoff v Regents of University of California* (Supreme Court of California 1974). Even if the test is not yet validated, so that the researcher is not sure that a high score truly reflects emotional disturbance, it is often better to err on the side of intervening than simply dismissing the test as 'under development'.

Consequential validation

Example F, in which some groups (e.g. ethnic or marginalized populations) score higher or lower on a scale than respondents from the white middle class, raises a different type of ethical issue: that scores on a scale may have consequences. This was discussed briefly in Chapter 10 when we looked at consequential validation. As a brief review, the term was introduced by Messick (1980, 1988) to mean that scale developers must investigate the consequences—intended and unintended, positive and negative—of any inferences based on the scores. Although some have argued that it should not be considered to be a part of validity, the point remains that it is an aspect of scale development that needs to be considered from an ethical perspective when developing a measure. These groups may be stigmatized by 'poor' scores on the measure, even if the scale is intended solely for research purposes.

A group's scores may deviate from those of the majority population for a number of reasons (Streiner 2013):

1. *Differing interpretation of the items.* As one example, a colleague in China told us that he was getting an unusual pattern of responses on a scale of activities of daily living. It turned out that people were interpreting the item 'I am able to climb a flight of stairs' not as a reflection of physical ability but as an index of wealth: 'I am rich enough to be able to afford a second storey on my house'. They were similarly over-stating the number of cigarettes they smoked each day, also as a reflection of their ability to buy them.
2. *Differing manifestations of the construct.* Many psychological states are experienced differently in non-Western cultures. Pang (1995), for example, found that older Korean immigrants did not state that they felt depressed; rather, they reported feelings of loneliness and somatic symptoms.
3. *Differing cultural norms regarding what is acceptable behaviour.* We mentioned in Chapter 3 that an American scale of child abuse was not appropriate in Chile, where corporal punishment is more accepted as a method of discipline. Similar problems exist with other behaviours that are sanctioned by middle-class North American mores, such as alcohol use, disobeying the police, or avoiding taxes.
4. *Differing educational levels.* Minority groups and immigrants may have had less formal education than the norm, leading to difficulties understanding the items.

It is important to determine whether differences among groups are due to factors such as these which may distort the meaning of the scores.

Summary

In conclusion, the major issue confronting the scale developer is that of the autonomy of the subject. If the person is seen as an autonomous individual, who has the right to privacy and to not participate in the study irrespective of the difficulties this may pose for the researcher, then most problems should be avoidable.

Further reading

Streiner, D.L. (2013). Ethical issues in measurement studies. In *Life quality outcomes in children and young people with neurological and developmental conditions* (eds. G.M. Ronen and P.L. Rosenbaum), pp. 249–61. Mac Keith Press, London.

References

American Educational Research Association, National Council on Measurement in Education (1955). *Technical recommendations for achievement tests.* American Psychological Association, Washington, DC.

American Psychological Association (1954). *Technical recommendations for psychological tests and diagnostic techniques.* American Psychological Association, Washington, DC.

American Psychological Association (2017). Ethical principles of psychologists and code of conduct. American Psychological Association, Washington, DC.

Berg, I.A. (1954). The use of human subjects in psychological research. *American Psychologist*, **9**, 108–11.

British Psychological Society, Scientific Affairs Board (1977). Ethics of investigations with human subjects: A set of principles proposed by the Scientific Affairs Board. *Bulletin of the British Psychological Society*, **30**, 25–6.

Canadian Institutes of Health Research, Natural Sciences and Engineering Research Council of Canada, and Social Sciences and Humanities Research Council of Canada (2018). *Tri-Council Policy Statement: Ethical Conduct for Research Involving Humans—TCPS 2.* Canadian Institutes of Health Research, Ottawa, ON.

Council for International Organizations of Medical Sciences (2012). International ethical guidelines for biomedical research involving human subjects. *Bulletin of Medical Ethics*, **182**, 17–23.

McNemar, Q. (1946). Opinion-attitude methodology. *Psychological Bulletin*, **43**, 289–374.

Medical Research Council of Canada (1987). *Guidelines on research involving human subjects: 1987.* Medical Research Council of Canada, Ottawa, ON.

Messick, S. (1980). Test validity and the ethics of assessment. *American Psychologist*, **35**, 1012–27.

Messick, S. (1988). The once and future issues of validity. Assessing the meaning and consequences of measurement. In *Test validity* (eds. H. Wainer and H. Braun), pp. 33–45. Lawrence Erlbaum, Mahwah, NJ.

Novick, M.R. (1981). Federal guidelines and professional standards. *American Psychologist*, **36**, 1035–46.

Ortman, A. and Hertwig, R. (1997). Is deception acceptable? *American Psychologist*, **52**, 746–7.

Pang, K.Y. (1995). A cross-cultural understanding of depression among elderly Korean immigrants: Prevalence, symptoms and diagnosis. *Clinical Gerontologist*, **15**, 3–20.

Schuler, H. (1982). *Ethical problems in psychological research* (Trans. M.S. Woodruff and R.A. Wicklund). Academic Press, New York.

Shipley, T. (1977). Misinformed consent: An enigma in modern social science research. *Ethics in Science and Medicine*, **4**, 93–106.

Streiner, D.L. (2013). Ethical issues in measurement studies. In *Life quality outcomes in children and young people with neurological and developmental conditions* (eds. G.M. Ronen and P.L. Rosenbaum), pp. 249–61. Mac Keith Press, London.

Supreme Court of California (1976). *Tarasoff v Regents of the University of California*, **131** Cal. Rptr. 14, 551 P 2d 334.

Wilson, D.W. and Donnerstein, E. (1976). Legal and ethical aspects of nonreactive social psychological research. *American Psychologist*, **31**, 765–73.

Chapter 15

Reporting test results

Introduction to reporting test results

After performing all the studies necessary to develop a test—devising and evaluating the items, estimating the reliabilities, performing some preliminary validity assessments—you are naturally eager to get your results into print. What, though, should be reported, and how? Until recently, the answer to this question was 'Whatever you want and the journal editor asks for'. However, there are now many sets of guidelines relating to the reporting of test results: the *Standards for Educational and Psychological Testing* (American Educational Research Association et al. 2014), the *STARD* initiative (*Standards for Reporting of Diagnostic Accuracy*; Bossuyt et al. 2015), the *Guidelines for Reporting Reliability and Agreement Studies* (GRRAS; Kottner et al. 2011), the *Quality Assessment of Diagnostic Accuracy Studies* (QUADAS; Whiting et al. 2003), the *Quality Appraisal of Diagnostic Reliability Checklist* (QAREL; Lucas et al. 2010), the *Consensus-Based Standards for the Selection of Health Status Measurement Instruments* (COSMIN; Mokkink et al. 2018), and likely many others by the time this book will have been printed. Some of these are aimed at authors reporting on tests they have developed—the *Standards*, STARD, and GRRAS. The others—QUADAS, QAREL, and COSMIN—are meant for those who want to evaluate scales in meta-analyses, although it is obvious that their points to be evaluated can easily be interpreted as points to be reported. Because there is considerable overlap amongst these guidelines, only a few will be reviewed here.

The most comprehensive of these are the *Standards*, which is currently the fifth edition of a fairly hefty monograph (230 pages) that has been updated periodically since its inception as the *Technical recommendations for psychological tests and diagnostic techniques* over half a century ago (American Psychological Association 1954). The newest version is based on over 4,000 comments sent to the Joint Commission regarding suggested changes from the previous version. There are 240 standards (although some are duplicates) that are now more than merely recommendations; they have been used numerous times in legal disputes to criticize or justify the use of tests for placement purposes (Eignor 2001). Its thoroughness is due to the fact that it covers tests used in psychology and education, both those that are developed for research purposes and commercially produced and high-stakes ones. The *Standards* are divided into three sections: Foundations (covering validity, reliability/measurement error, and fairness in testing); Operations (test design and development, scores, norms, and cut scores, reporting and interpretation, supporting documents, and rights and responsibilities of test takers and users); and Testing Applications (which covers the use of tests diagnostically, in the workplace, and in education). It is freely available at <https://www.testingstandards.net/uploads/7/6/6/4/76643089/9780935302356.pdf>.

STARD is an outgrowth of the Consolidated Standards of Reporting Trials (CONSORT) initiative (Altman et al. 2001) and, as the name implies, is more limited in scope than the American Educational Research Association, American Psychological Association, and National Council on Measurement in Education's *Standards*, dealing only with diagnostic tests. It consists of a checklist, a flow chart, and a more detailed explanation (available at <http://www.consort-statement.org/stardstatement.htm>). Many of the leading biomedical journals that publish reports of diagnostic tests, such as the *Annals of Internal Medicine*, *JAMA*, *Radiology*, *The Lancet*, *BMJ*, and *Clinical Chemistry and Laboratory Medicine*, have adopted STARD, and they are being joined by journals in psychology such as the *Journal of Personality Assessment*. This means that, fairly soon, all submitted articles that deal with the development of diagnostic tests must adhere to these guidelines. As the name implies, the GRRAS is narrower than the *Standards*, addressing only studies that look at the reliability of scales. In this chapter, we have abstracted only parts of the *Standards*, assuming that, for the most part, readers of this book will be developing non-commercial scales to be used solely for research purposes. However, STARD, GRRAS, and to an even greater extent the *Standards* are required reading for anyone who is considering a commercial application of a test, or for an instrument that is to be used for decision-making about individuals, whether the test is published or not. Examples of possible commercial applications would include acceptance into or placement in an educational programme; as part of an evaluation of competency as a professional, or to have custody of a child, or to retain a driver's license; or as a component of a diagnostic work-up, for example—in other words, any time a decision is made about an individual that may affect their life and that consequently may lead to litigation (what also has been referred to as 'high-stakes' situations).

Standards for educational and psychological testing

The parts of the *Standards* that have been omitted from this chapter deal with aspects of test development that deal primarily with high-stake instruments (e.g. those that will be used to determine admission into a programme or that will be used clinically), as well as aspects dealing with fairness in testing and issues of cultural sensitivity. We are leaving them out, not because they are not important, but because we believe that readers of this book will rarely face these issues.

Test development

1. The purpose of the test must be clearly stated, with a definition of the construct being measured (e.g. 'This is a scale to measure quality of life, which is defined as …'). There are two implications of this standard: first, that the rationale for the scale must be given; and second, that if an instrument is used in a new way (e.g. to measure change, rather than to simply describe a group), evidence must be provided to show that the scale is valid for that purpose.

2. Specifications about the normative or standardization sample must be given. As appropriate, this would include the participants' age, gender, ethnic background, how they were recruited, whether they are clinic patients or volunteers from the community, and so forth. The reader should be able to judge how similar these people are to those in their sample in order to determine whether the results are applicable.

STANDARDS FOR TESTING | **399**

3. The items and response formats should be reviewed by a panel of experts, whose qualifications should be specified. These people may include content experts (e.g. clinicians) and/or people who are representative of those with whom the scale will ultimately be used, who would be better able to make judgements about such matters as understandability, the use of jargon, and so forth.

4. Any pilot testing should be described, including characteristics of the sample(s) tested. These sample(s) should be representative of the intended population for which the scale is designed.

5. The criteria for keeping and rejecting items, whether based on judgement, classical test theory, or item response theory (or some combination of these), must be given (e.g. 'Items were dropped if fewer than four of the five content experts rated them above 3 on a 5-point scale of relevance'; 'Factorially complex items, or those that did not load on any of the first three factors were eliminated'; or 'Items whose residuals were over 2 were discarded').

6. If the items are selected on the basis of empirical relationships (e.g. factor analysis, item-total correlations) rather than on theoretical grounds, then there should be at least one cross-validational study to confirm the results. Any discrepancies between the results of the studies should be documented.

7. Some evidence should be given regarding the content coverage of the scale. This may be provided by a panel of expert judges, for example, or by using focus groups of patients.

8. If the items are weighted, a rationale (either statistical or theoretical) should be given for the weights.

9. If scoring involves more than simply adding up the responses (e.g. making judgements about the adequacy of the answers), then detailed instructions should be given, including any training that is required of the raters or scorers.

10. If a scale is used only for research purposes, this should be clearly stated to the test taker.

11. If a short form of a test is developed, then two things must be specified: the procedures or criteria by which items were selected for deletion, and how the short form's psychometric properties compare against the original (e.g. reliability, validity).

12. If, due to research or theory, the definition of the domain has changed significantly from the time the instrument was originally developed, then the scale should be modified to reflect this.

Reliability

1. The reliability and standard error of measurement (SEM) must be reported for the total score. If the instrument has subscales, then this information must also be given.

2. When difference scores are interpreted (e.g. differences between groups or changes over time), the reliabilities and SEMs of the difference scores should be reported.

3. The sample must be described in sufficient detail to allow the readers to determine if the data apply to their groups.

4. The procedures that were used must be explained (e.g. the test–retest interval, any training given to the raters, etc.).

5. If the reliability coefficients were adjusted for restriction in range, then both adjusted and unadjusted values should be reported.

6. If there is reason to believe that the reliability may vary with age, or with different groups (e.g. males versus females, those from different cultures), then the reliabilities and SEMs should be reported separately for these groups, as soon as sufficient data are available.

Validity

1. Because no test is valid for all people and in all situations, the population for which the test is appropriate (i.e. data on validity exist for them) should be clearly stated, including relevant socio-demographic information.

2. If the scale is to be used in a novel way (e.g. with different populations, or predictively rather than descriptively), validity data must be gathered to support this new use.

3. A rationale should be given for the domains covered or not covered in the content validation phase of development.

4. When any phase of development depends on the opinions of experts, raters, or judges (e.g. delineation of the domains, checks for content coverage, or readability), the qualifications of these people should be given, as well as any training or instructions they may have received.

5. Sufficient details should be reported about any validational studies to allow users to judge the relevance of the findings to their local conditions.

6. When the validational studies involve relating of the new scale to other measures (that is, criterion validation), the rationale and psychometric properties of the other measures (e.g. reliability and validity) must be given. The developer should also guard against spurious sources of correlations among the variables, such as both measures being completed by the same person using the same response format (i.e. common method variance).

7. If adjustments have been made for restriction in the range of scores, both adjusted and unadjusted coefficients should be reported.

The STARD initiative

The STARD initiative was developed by a group of 25 experts within the medical community, and their statement was published simultaneously in a number of prominent medical journals. As mentioned earlier, it is beginning to be adopted by psychological and educational journals, and some minor modifications have been made to the checklist by Meyer (2003) and by us, primarily to incorporate key words used by the PsycLit (as opposed to the MeSH key words used by Medline) database and to reflect the words that are more commonly used in psychometrics, such as 'reliability' rather than 'reproducibility' (Streiner and Norman 2006).

Because its scope is more limited and there are many areas of overlap between STARD and the *Standards*, we will not go into much detail. As with the *Standards*, it calls for sufficient information about the process of checking for reliability and validity so that the reader and potential user can judge the adequacy of the process and

Table 15.1 STARD checklist for the reporting of studies on diagnostic accuracy

Section and topic	Item description
Title or Abstract	1. The article is a study on diagnostic accuracy (recommend MeSH heading 'sensitivity and specificity'; 'diagnostic efficiency' for PsycLit)
Abstract	2. Structured summary of design, methods, results, and conclusions
Introduction	3. Background, including intended use and clinical role of the instrument
	4. Study objectives and hypotheses
Methods	
Study design	5. Were the participants identified and data collected before the index test(s) and reference standards were performed (prospective study) or after (retrospective study)?
Participants	6. Eligibility criteria
	7. How potential participants were identified (e.g. symptoms, results from previous tests, a registry)
	8. Setting, location, and dates of where eligible participants were identified
	9. Whether participants were consecutive, random, or convenience sample
Test methods	10a. Index test, in sufficient detail to allow replication
	10b. Reference standard, in sufficient detail to allow replication
	11. If alternatives exist, rationale for choosing reference standard
	12a. Definition and rationale for the units, cut-offs, and/or categories of the results of the index test
	12b. The same for the reference standard
	13a. Whether clinical information and reference standard results were available to those who assessed the index test
	13b. Whether clinical information and index test results were available to those who assessed the reference standard
Analysis	14. Methods for estimating or comparing measures of diagnostic accuracy
	15. How indeterminate scores on index or reference test were handled
	16. How missing data were handled
	17. Any analyses of variability in diagnostic accuracy
	18. Sample size, and how it was determined
Results	
Participants	19. Flow of participants, using a diagram
	20. Baseline demographic and clinical characteristics of participants
	21a. Distribution of severity of disease in those with target condition
	21b. Distribution of alternative diagnoses in those without target condition
	22. Time interval and any clinical interventions between index test and reference standard

Table 15.1 (continued) STARD checklist for the reporting of studies on diagnostic accuracy

Section and topic	Item description
Test results	23. Cross tabulation (or distribution) of index test results by results of reference standard
	24. Estimates of diagnostic accuracy and their precision (e.g. 95% CIs)
	25. Any adverse events from performing the index test or reference standard
Discussion	
	26. Study limitations, including sources of potential bias, statistical uncertainty, and generalizability
	27. Implications for practice, including the intended use and clinical role of the index test
Other information	
	28. Registration number and name of registry
	29. Where full study protocol can be accessed
	30. Sources of funding and other support; role of funders

Adapted with permission from Bossuyt, Patrick M.; for the STARD Group, STARD 2015: An Updated List of Essential Items for Reporting Diagnostic Accuracy Studies, *Clinical Chemistry*, 2015, 61, 12, pp. 1446 –52, by permission of American Association for Clinical Chemistry and Oxford University Press.

the applicability of the results for their samples. The checklist, which is reproduced in Table 15.1, is intended to be a cover sheet accompanying the article when it is submitted. In the original (which is freely available), the author is to indicate next to each item where the details are to be found in the text, both ensuring that all aspects of diagnostic test development are covered and aiding the reviewer in evaluating the article. On the other hand, the flow chart (Fig. 15.1) is meant to be a general example, which would be modified to suit the particulars of the study and presented within the text of the article.

As can be seen from both the flow chart and the checklist, the STARD recommendations are oriented towards tests that yield dichotomous (present/absent) or trichotomous (present/absent/inconclusive) outcomes, and less towards scales that result in a continuous measure, such as quality of life or degree of symptomatology. In the latter case, it is sufficient to show, either in a flow chart or in the text, how many people were eligible and the reasons why some may have been excluded.

GRRAS

The eight authors of the GRRAS came primarily from the health and social sciences—instrument development and evaluation, reliability and agreement estimations, and systematic reviews of reliability studies—and used a nominal group technique to arrive at the guidelines. As would be expected, there is considerable overlap with the STARD initiative, but the explanations and elaborations of the various points are appropriate

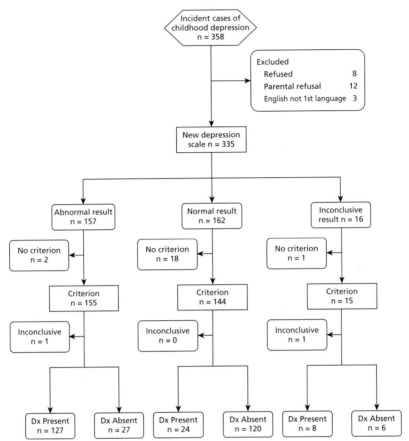

Fig. 15.1 The STARD flow chart applied to a new diagnostic test for depression. Adapted with permission from Bossuyt, Patrick M.; for the STARD Group, STARD 2015: An Updated List of Essential Items for Reporting Diagnostic Accuracy Studies, *Clinical Chemistry*, 2015, 61, 12, pp. 1446–52, by permission of American Association for Clinical Chemistry and Oxford University Press.

for those developing scales that have a continuous, as well as a dichotomous, outcome. For example, it discusses using the intraclass correlation to measure reliability in addition to kappa. Because its table is similar to that of STARD, we will not reproduce it here, but would strongly recommend that scale developers read the entire article (see Kottner et al. 2011).

Summary

STARD, GRRAS, and the *Standards* are meant to be descriptive as well as prescriptive. Because of their adoption by leading organizations and journals in the area of test development, it will become increasingly difficult to publish articles that do not adhere to them. This, we believe, is most definitely a very positive step. These statements reflect what is now called 'best practices' in the field of psychometrics, and do not propose anything that is an unnecessary burden on test developers. We can only hope (most probably futilely) that it may result in fewer poorly executed studies cluttering the literature.

Further reading

Altman, D.G., Schulz, K.F., Moher, D., Egger, M., Davidoff, F., Elbourne, D., *et al.* (2001). The revised CONSORT statement for reporting randomised trials: Explanation and elaboration. *Annals of Internal Medicine*, **134**, 663–94.

American Educational Research Association, American Psychological Association, and National Council on Measurement in Education (2014). *Standards for educational and psychological testing*. American Educational Research Association, Lanham, MD.

Association of Test Publishers (2001). *Guidelines for computer-based testing and the internet*. Association of Test Publishers, Washington, DC.

Joint Committee on Testing Practices (2004). *Code of fair testing practices in education*. Joint Committee on Testing Practices, Washington, DC.

Kottner, J., Audigé, L., Brorson, S., Donner, A., Gajewski, B.J., Hrøbjartsson, A., *et al.* (2011). Guidelines for Reporting Reliability and Agreement Studies (GRRAS) were proposed. *Journal of Clinical Epidemiology*, **64**, 96–106.

National Commission for Certifying Agencies (2004). *Standards for the accreditation of certification programs*. National Organization for Competency Assurance, Washington, DC.

Society for Industrial and Organizational Psychology (2003). *Principles for the validation and use of personnel selection procedures*. Society for Industrial and Organizational Psychology, College Park, MD.

References

Altman, D.G., Schulz, K.F., Moher, D., Egger, M., Davidoff, F., Elbourne, D., *et al.* (2001). The revised CONSORT statement for reporting randomized trials: Explanation and elaboration. *Annals of Internal Medicine*, **134**, 663–94.

American Educational Research Association, American Psychological Association, and National Council on Measurement in Education (2014). *Standards for educational and psychological testing*. American Educational Research Association, Lanham, MD.

American Psychological Association (1954). *Technical recommendations for psychological tests and diagnostic techniques*. American Psychological Association, Washington, DC.

Bossuyt, P.M., Reitsma, J.B., Bruns, D.E., Gatsonis, C.A., Glasziou, P.P., Irwig, L.M., et al. (2015). STARD 2015: An updated list of essential items for reporting diagnostic accuracy studies. *Clinical Chemistry*, **61**, 1446–1452.

Eignor, D.R. (2001). Standards for the development and use of tests: The *Standards for Educational and Psychological Testing*. *European Journal of Psychological Assessment*, **17**, 157–63.

Kottner, J., Audigé, L., Brorson, S., Donner, A., Gajewski, B. J., Hrøbjartsson, A., *et al.* (2011). Guidelines for Reporting Reliability and Agreement Studies (GRRAS) were proposed. *Journal of Clinical Epidemiology*, **64**, 96–106.

Lucas, N.P., Macaskill, P., Irwig, L., and Bogduk, N. (2010). The development of a quality appraisal tool for studies of diagnostic reliability (QAREL). *Journal of Clinical Epidemiology*, **63**, 854–61.

Meyer, G.J. (2003). Guidelines for reporting information in studies of diagnostic accuracy: The STARD initiative. *Journal of Personality Assessment*, **81**, 191–3.

Mokkink, L.B., deVet, H.C.W., Prinsen, C.A.C., Patrick, D.L., Alonso, J., Bouter, L.M., *et al.* (2018). COSMIN Risk of Bias checklist for systematic reviews of patient-reported outcome studies. *Quality of Life Research*, **27**, 1171–9.

Streiner, D.L. and Norman, G.R. (2006). "Precision" and "accuracy": Two terms that are neither. *Journal of Clinical Epidemiology*, **59**, 327–30.

Whiting, P., Rutjes, A.W., Reitsma, J.B., Bossuyt, P.M., and Kleijnen, J. (2003) The development of QUADAS: A tool for the quality assessment of studies of diagnostic accuracy included in systematic reviews. *BMC Medical Research Methodology*, **3**, Article 25.

Appendix A

Where to find tests

Introduction to where to find tests

As mentioned in Chapter 3, a very useful place to find questions is to look at what others have done. It is also useful to have objective evaluations of scales that can be adopted for research studies. A partial listing of books and articles that are compendia of information about published and unpublished scales follows. We give a brief description of the books and articles we have been able to look at ; others are just listed. We have not given references for educational, intellectual, achievement, or diagnostic tests.

Guide to this section

A. General
B. Online sources
C. Social and attitudinal scales
D. Personality and behaviour
E. Child, family, and marriage (see also I)
F. Health and clinical conditions (see also E)
G. Substance abuse problems (see also B, E, and J)
H. Quality of life (see also B, E, F, I, and K)
I. Pain (see also E, F, and K)
J. Gerontology
K. Nursing and patient education
L. Sex and gender
M. Work
N. Violence
O. Special populations
P. Miscellaneous

A. General

1. Piotrowski, C. and Perdue, B. (1999). Reference sources on psychological tests: A contemporary review. *Behavioral & Social Sciences Librarian*, **17**, 47–58.

A guide to print, online, and electronic reference sources, and gives examples of searches to find specific tests.

2. *Mental measurements yearbook (MMY) series.* Buros Center for Testing, Lincoln, NE .

The first eight editions of the *MMY* were edited by Oscar Buros, and the set is often referred to as 'Buros'. After his death, there have been various editors of this excellent series. The latest volume, the 21st in the series, is edited by Carlson, Geisinger, and Jonson. Only published tests are listed, and most are reviewed by two or more experts in the field. The articles also include a fairly comprehensive list of published articles and dissertations about the instruments. The yearbooks, which are published every three years despite the title, are cumulative: tests reviewed in one edition are not reviewed in subsequent ones. There are over 7,500 reviews, which are also available online at <http://www.buros.unl.edu/buros/jsp/search.jsp> at a cost of US $15 per title.

The group has also brought out more focused indices: *Reading tests and reviews*, *Tests in print*, and *Personality tests*. The latter two volumes do not have reviews, but are keyed back to the *MMY*.

3. Keyser, D.J. and Sweetland, R.C. *Test critiques*. Test Corporation of America, Kansas City, MO.

As of the date of writing this chapter, there were 11 volumes in this series of critical evaluations of published tests; there do not appear to have been any additions since 2005. Unlike the *MMY*, there is only one review per test, and the reference list is representative rather than exhaustive. However, the reviews are considerably longer and more detailed, and follow a common format: introduction, practical applications and uses, technical aspects, and critique.

4. Maddox, T. (2008). *Tests: A comprehensive reference for assessment in psychology, education, and business* (6th edn). PRO-ED, Austin, TX.

This is the latest version of the book, first authored by Sweetland and Keyser, and is similar to *Tests in print*. It gives a brief description of published tests: their purpose, format, description, appropriate population, approximate time to complete them, and where to order them.

5. *Directory of unpublished experimental mental measures*. American Psychological Association, Washington, DC.

In addition to *HaPI* (see section B), this is one of the few comprehensive sources of scales that have appeared in journals but have not been issued commercially. There are nine volumes in the set, with various authors for each. Over 10,000 tests are described, with one or two key articles cited for each; there are no reviews, although psychometric information is given when available, and the scales themselves are not printed. There are 24 categories, and, for each scale, its purpose and format are given. Each volume has a cumulative index, covering earlier volumes.

B. **Online sources**

1. Behavioral Measurement Database Services. *Health and psychological instruments database* (HaPI). BRS Retrieval Service. Available at: < https://www.bmdshapi.com/>.

This is an online, computerized database, similar to Medline or PsycLit, containing over 200,000 documents (as of the time this chapter was written) about unpublished scales. It covers health, social sciences, organizational behaviour, and human resources, with approximately two-thirds in the area of medicine and nursing (e.g. pain, quality of life (QOL), drug efficacy). Coverage has been comprehensive since 1985, with many earlier measures included on a haphazard basis. It consists of abstracts and bibliographies about the scales, but not the scales themselves. Individual subscriptions can be purchased, but university libraries may have access to it through Ovid.

2. National Library of Medicine. *Health Services and Sciences Research Resources*. Available at: <http://www.nlm.nih.gov/nichsr/hsrr_search/>.

This database covers a very large number of scales in the areas of health services research, the behavioural and social sciences, and public health. It describes each one, summarizing psychometric data when available, and gives a hyperlink to it. For many, the actual scale can be downloaded.

3. Mapi Research Trust. *PROQOLID* (Patient-Reported Outcome and Quality of Life Instrument Database). Available at: <http://proqolid.org/>.

Covers QOL and patient-reported outcomes; as of when this was written, there are 641 instruments, approximately 500 reviews, and nearly 1,000 translations, with descriptions of 80 databases that have used the tools. Free access gives basic information about the scales. Advanced access (which costs US $710 or €500 per year for individual academics) gives psychometric properties, reviews, and, when available, copies of the instruments and the user manual.

4. American Psychological Association. *PsycTESTS*. Available at: http://www.apa.org/pubs/databases/psyctests

This is described as 'a research database that provides access to published and unpublished psychological tests, measures, scales, surveys, and other assessments as well as descriptive information about the test and its development and administration'. It contains records of over 20,000 actual tests or test items, and is updated monthly. A permissions field alerts users to the tests they can use for research or teaching without formal permission. Other options include contacting the author and/or the publisher. The majority of tests in the database can be used without formal permission. Institutional access is available through APA PsycNET, OvidSP, and the EBSCO*host* platform and to individuals who subscribe to APA PsycNET.

C. **Social and attitudinal scales**

1. Bearden, W.O., Netemeyer, R.G., and Haws, K.L. (2010). *Handbook of marketing scales* (3rd edn). Sage, Thousand Oaks, CA.

The focus of the book is on consumer behaviour and marketing research. However, it also covers tests of individual traits which may have a role in such behaviours, such as values, susceptibility to peer pressure, materialism, and the like.

Number of scales: 197   *Psychometric properties:* Yes   *Scales given:* Yes

2. Bonjean, C.M., Hill, R.J., and McLemore, S.D. (1967). *Sociological measurement: An inventory of scales and indices.* Chandler, San Francisco, CA.

Lists and describes every scale used in four sociology journals between 1954 and 1965. There are about 80 different areas covered, including achievement, aspirations, family, marital roles, and others of interest to sociologists.

Number of scales: 200+ *References:* Yes   *Scales given:* For 25

3. Heitzman, C.A. and Kaplan, R.M. (1988). Assessment of methods for measuring social support. *Health Psychology*, 7, 75–109.

Critically reviews some of the more widely used social support scales, with excellent assessments.

Number of scales: 24   *Psychometrics:* Yes   *Scales given:* No

4. Lester, P.E., Inman, D., and Bishop, L.K. (2014). *Handbook of tests and measurement in education and the social sciences* (3rd edn). Rowman & Littlefield, Lanham, MD.

In addition to covering scales of dogmatism, self-efficacy, self-esteem, and gender identification, the book lists scales appropriate for the workplace (e.g. honesty, conflict management, decision making); it excludes psychology and personality.

Number of scales: 130+ *Psychometrics:* Yes   *Scales given:* Yes

5. Miller, D.C. and Salkind, N.J. (eds) (2002). *Handbook of research design and social measurement* (6th edn). Sage, Thousand Oaks, CA.

Covers areas of social status, group structure and dynamics, morale, job satisfaction, leadership, supervisory behaviour, alienation, and anomie.

Number of scales: 36   *Psychometrics:* Yes   *Scales given:* Portions

6. Robinson, J.P., Shaver, P.R., and Wrightsman, L.S. (eds) (1998) (rev edn). *Measures of social political attitudes.* Institute for Social Research, Ann Arbor, MI.

7. Robinson, J.P., Shaver, P.R., and Wrightsman, L.S. (eds) (1991). *Measures of personality and social psychological attitudes.* Academic Press, San Diego, CA.

8. Robinson, J.P., Shaver, P.R., and Wrightsman, L.S. (eds) (1999). *Measures of political attitudes.* Academic Press, San Diego, CA.
    Number of scales: 30–90 each   *Psychometrics:* Yes   *Scales given:* Yes

9. Shaw, M.E. and Wright, J.M. (1967). *Scales for the measurement of attitudes.* McGraw-Hill, New York.

Covers areas such as international and social issues, social practices and problems, and political and religious attitudes .

Number of scales: 176   *Psychometrics:* Yes   *Scales given:* Yes

D. **Personality and behaviour**

1. Andrulis, R.S. (1977). *Adult assessment: A source book of tests and measures of human behavior.* Thomas, Springfield, IL.

   Number of scales: 155   *Psychometrics:* Yes   *Scales given:* No

2. Burn, B. and Payment, M. (2000). *Assessments A to Z: A collection of 50 question-naires, instruments, and inventories.* Jossey-Bass/Pfeiffer, San Francisco, CA.

   Covers areas such as assertiveness, problem solving, risk taking, and stress management.

   Number of scales: 50   *Psychometrics:* Yes   *Scales given:* Yes

3. Burns, R.B. (1979). *The self concept in theory, measurement, development, and be-haviour.* Longman, New York.

   Some instruments are included.

4. Byrne, B.M. (1996). *Measuring self-concept across the lifespan: Methodology and instrumentation for research and practice.* American Psychological Association, Washington, DC.

   Discusses scales of self-concept applicable to a variety of areas, such as academic and physical appearance, and for a number of different groups. The focus is on scales that are psychometrically sound, have a strong theoretical base, and have demonstrated utility.

   Number of scales: ?   *Psychometrics:* Yes   *Scales given:* No

5. Chéné, H. (1986). *Index de variables mesurées par les tests de personnalité* (2nd edn). Les Presses de l'Université Laval, Laval, Quebec.

   Brief, non-evaluative descriptions in French of primarily published tests. The book has been translated into English.

6. Chun, K.-T., Cobb, S., and French, J.R.P., Jr. (1975). *Measures for psychological as-sessment: A guide to 3,000 original sources and their applications.* Institute for Social Research, Ann Arbor, MI.

   A listing of 3,000 articles about unpublished or experimental measures derived from 26 journals in psychology and sociology between 1960 and 1970. The 'Applications' section lists over 6,600 additional studies about additional uses of these tests. It is very useful for describing these scales, but is outdated.

   Number of scales: 3,000   *Psychometrics:* Yes   *Scales given:* No

7. Gallagher, M.W. and Lopez, S.J. (eds) (2019). *Positive psychological assessment: A handbook of models and measures* (2nd edn). American Psychological Association, Washington, DC.

   Covers areas such as optimism, self-efficacy, courage, wisdom, forgiveness, gratitude, and other positive aspects of personality.

   Number of scales: 19   *Psychometrics:* Yes   *Scales given:* Yes

8. Lake, D.G., Miles, M., and Earle, R. (1973). *Measuring human behavior.* Teachers College Press, New York.

   Covers areas such as personal attributes, and interpersonal and organizational relationships .

Number of scales: 84   *Psychometrics:* Yes   *Scales given:* No

9. Shaw, M.E. and Wright, J.M. (1967). *Scales for the measurement of attitudes.* McGraw-Hill, New York.

Covers social practices, religion, ethnic and national groups, etc.
Number of scales: 176   *Psychometrics:* Yes   *Scales given:* Yes

10. Simon, A. and Boyer, E.G. (eds) (1974). *Mirrors for behavior. III: An anthology of observational instruments.* Communications Materials Center, Wyncote, PA.

Number of scales: 99   *Psychometrics:* Yes   *Scales given:* Yes

E. Child, family, and marriage

1. Alderfer, M.A., Fiese, B.H., Gold, J.I., Cutuli, J.J., Holmbeck, G.N., Goldbeck, L., *et al.* (2008). Evidence-based assessment in pediatric psychology: Family measures. *Journal of Pediatric Psychology,* **33**, 1046–61.

Covers family functioning, dyadic family relationships, and family functioning in the context of childhood chronic health conditions.
Number of scales: 29   *Psychometrics:* Yes   *Scales given*: No

2. Blount, R.L., Simons, L.E., Devine, K.A., Jaaniste, T., Cohen, L.L., Chambers, C.T., *et al.* (2008). Evidence-based assessment of coping and stress in pediatric psychology. *Journal of Pediatric Psychology,* **33**, 1021–45.

Number of scales: 15   *Psychometrics:* Yes   *Scales given*: No

3. Campbell, J.M., Brown, R.T., Cavanagh, S.E., Vess, S.F., and Segall, M.J. (2008). Evidence-based assessment of cognitive functioning in pediatric psychology. *Journal of Pediatric Psychology,* **33**, 999–1014.

Number of scales: 27   *Psychometrics:* Yes   *Scales given*: No

4. Child Trends (2003). *Conceptualizing and measuring 'healthy marriages' for empirical research and evaluation studies: A compendium of measures—Part II.* Child Trends, Washington, DC.

Number of scales: 104   *Psychometrics:* ?   *Scales given:* Yes

5. Filsinger, E.E. (1983). *Marriage and family assessment: A sourcebook for family therapy.* Sage, Thousand Oaks, CA.

Number of scales: 6   *Psychometrics:* Yes   *Scales given:* Yes

6. Fischer, J., Corcoran, K.J., and Springer, D.W. (2020). *Measures for clinical practice: A sourcebook. Volume 1* (6th edn). Oxford University Press, New York.

The first volume of this excellent set has scales that can be used with children, couples, and families. For each scale, there is one page describing its norms, scoring system, psychometrics, and availability.
Number of scales: 120   *Psychometrics:* Yes   *Scales given:* Yes

7. Friedman, N. and Sherman, R. (1987). *Handbook of measurements for marriage and family therapy.* Brunner/Mazel, New York.

Covers satisfaction and adjustment (nine scales), communication and intimacy (seven scales), special family assessment (eight scales), and the Minnesota Family Inventories (seven scales).

Number of scales: 31   *Psychometrics:* Yes   *Scales given:* Yes

8. Grisso, T., Vincent, G., and Seagrave, D. (eds) (2005). *Mental health screening and assessment in juvenile justice.* Guilford, Hingham, MA.

Discusses scales tapping areas such as substance abuse, trauma, risk of violence, competence, and other topics of relevance to forensics.

Number of scales: Many   *Psychometrics:* Yes   *Scales given:* No

9. Grotevant, H.D. and Carlson, C.I. (1989). *Family assessment: A guide to methods and measures.* Guilford, New York.

Covers family interaction, global rating of family processes, and self-reports of family functioning.

Number of scales: ?   *Psychometrics:* Yes   *Scales given:* No

10. Holmbeck, G.N., Thill, A.W., Bachanas, P., Garber, J., Miller, K.B., Abad, M., *et al.* (2008). Evidence-based assessment of pediatric psychology: Measures of psychosocial adjustment and psychopathology. *Journal of Pediatric Psychology*, **33**, 958–80.

Number of scales: 37   *Psychometrics:* Yes   *Scales given:* No

11. Johnson, O.G. (1976). *Tests and measurements in child development: Handbooks I and II.* Jossey-Bass, San Francisco, CA.

This is an update of Johnson and Dommarito's earlier book, which was subtitled simply *A handbook.* The two volumes cover non-commercial tests for those under 19 years of age. A wide variety of areas are covered.

Number of scales: c.1,200   *Psychometrics:* Yes   *Scales given:* No

12. Kelley, M.L., Noell, G.H., and Reitman, D. (eds) (2003). *Practitioner's guide to empirically based measures of school behavior.* Guilford, Hingham, MA.

Discusses the psychometric properties of scales in areas such as externalizing behaviours, instructional needs, and attentional problems.

Number of scales: ?   *Psychometrics:* Yes   *Scales given:* No

13. L'Abate, L. and Bagarozzi, D. A. (1993). *Sourcebook of marriage and family evaluation.* Brunner/Mazel, New York.

Number of scales: ?   *Psychometrics:* Yes   *Scales given:* No

14. Levy, P. and Goldstein, H. (eds) (1984). *Tests in education: A book of critical reviews.* Academic Press, London.

Similar in design and intent to the *MMY* and *Test critiques*, this volume is oriented towards published tests available in England, which do not need to be administered by a psychologist, and which cover children from nursery school through secondary school. It covers areas such as early development, language, personality, and counselling .

Number of scales: 38   *Psychometrics:* Yes   *Scales given:* No

15. McCubbin, H.I., Thompson, A.I., and McCubbin, M.A. (eds) (1996). *Family assessment: Resiliency, coping and adaptation: Inventories for research and practice.* University of Wisconsin, Madison, WI.

    Number of scales: 28   *Psychometrics:* Yes   *Scales given:* Yes

16. Naar-King, D.A., Ellis, M.A., and Frey, M.L. (2003). *Assessing children's well-being: A handbook of measures.* Lawrence Erlbaum, Mahwah, NJ.

Covers health status, quality of life, adherence, pain management, behaviour, development, coping, cognitions, attitudes, environment, and satisfaction.

    Number of scales: 20   *Psychometrics:* Yes   *Scales given:* Yes

17. Orvaschel, H., Sholomskas, D., and Weissman, M. M. (1980). *The assessment of psychopathology and behavioral problems in children: A review of scales suitable for epidemiological and clinical research (1967–1979).* NIMH, Rockville, MD.

18. Orvaschel, H. and Walsh, G. (1984). *The assessment of adaptive functioning in children: A review of existing measures suitable for epidemiological and clinical services research.* NIMH, Rockville, MD.

These two monographs list and critique unpublished scales that can be used with children under the age of 18.

    Number of scales: 44/?   *Psychometrics:* Yes   *Scales given:* No

19. Palermo, T.M., Long, A.C., Lewandowski, A.S., Drotar, D., Quittner, A.L., and Walker, L.S. (2008). Evidence-based assessment of health-related quality of life and functional impairment in pediatric psychology. *Journal of Pediatric Psychology,* **33**, 983 –96.

    Number of scales: 16   *Psychometrics:* Yes   *Scales given:* No

20. Quittner, A.L., Modi, A.C., Lemanek, K.L., Ievers-Landis, C.E., and Rapoff, M.A. (2008). Evidence-based assessment of adherence to medical treatments in pediatric psychology. *Journal of Pediatric Psychology,* **33**, 916 –36.

Reviews self-reports, diaries, and electronic monitors as measures of adherence, based on strict criteria.

    Number of scales: 18   *Psychometrics:* Yes   *Scales given:* No

21. Rodrique, J.R., Geffken, G.R., and Streisand, R.M. (2000). *Child health assessment: A handbook of measurement techniques.* Allyn & Bacon, Boston, MA.

Domains covered include stress and coping, attitudes and beliefs, pain, quality of life, and health-related knowledge .

    Number of scales: 100 +   *Psychometrics:* Yes   *Scales given:* No

22. Sperry, L. (ed.) (2019). *Couple and family assessment: Contemporary and cutting edge strategies* (3rd edn). Routledge, London.

    Number of scales: 130 +   *Psychometrics:* Yes   *Scales given:* No

23. Straus, M.A. and Brown, B.W. (1978). *Family measurement techniques: Abstracts of published instruments, 1935–1974* (rev edn). University of Minnesota Press, Minneapolis, MN.

Contains descriptions of family behaviour measures culled from journals in psychology, education, and sociology, and covering husband–wife, parent–child, and sibling interactions, sex, and premarital relations.

Number of scales: 318   *Psychometrics:* Yes   *Scales given:* No

24. Touliatos, J., Perlmutter, B.F., Straus, M.A., and Holden, G.W. (eds) (2001). *Handbook of family measurement techniques* (3 volumes). Sage, Thousand Oaks, CA.

Extensive bibliography regarding tests of various aspects of family functioning, such as family and marital interaction, intimacy and family values, parenthood, roles and power, and adjustment.

Number of scales: 976   *Psychometrics:* Yes   *Scales given:* For 189

25. Tzeng, O.C.S. (1993). *Measurement of love and intimate relations: Theories, scales, and applications for love development, maintenance, and dissolution.* Praeger, Westport, CN.

Number of scales: 28   *Psychometrics:* Yes   *Scales given:* Yes

26. Verhulst, F.C. and van der Ende, J. (2006). *Assessment scales in child and adolescent psychiatry.* Informa, Oxon.

Covers areas of general rating scales, specific symptoms, and impairment. Both published and unpublished instruments are covered.

Number of scales: 94   *Psychometrics:* Yes   *Scales given:* Yes

27. Walker, D.K. (1973). *Socioemotional measures for preschool and kindergarten children.* Jossey-Bass, San Francisco, CA.

Covers published and unpublished, copyrighted and freely available tests for children between the ages of 3 and 6.

Number of scales: 143   *Psychometrics:* Yes   *Scales given:* No

F. Health and clinical conditions

1. Allison, D.B. and Baskin, M.L. (eds) (1995). *Handbook of assessment methods for eating behaviors and weight related problems: Measures, theory, and research* (2nd edn). Sage, Thousand Oaks, CA.

Contains chapters on assessment of personality, quality of life, body image, restrained eating, physical activity and exercise, food intake, binge eating and purging, body composition, and energy expenditure.

Number of scales: 45 +   *Psychometrics:* Yes   *Scales given:* Some

2. American Physical Therapy Association (1995). *Patient satisfaction instruments: A compendium.* APTA, Alexandria, VA.

Number of scales: 36   *Psychometrics:* Yes   *Scales given:* Yes

3. Antony, M.M., Orsillo, S.M., and Roemer, L. (2001). *Practitioner's guide to empirically based measures of anxiety.* Guilford, Hingham, MA.

Number of scales: 200 +   *Psychometrics:* Yes   *Scales given:* For 77

4. Bech, P. (1993). *Rating scales for psychopathology, health status, and quality of life: A compendium on documentation in accordance with the DSM-III-R and WHO systems.* Springer, New York.

Covers psychopathological states, mental disorders, personality disorders, somatic disorders, psychosocial stressors, social functioning and coping, quality of life, and adverse drug reactions. Although superseded by later versions of the DSM and ICD, still a valuable source of items.

Number of scales: ? *Psychometrics:* No *Scales given:* Yes

5. Bowers, A.C. and Thompson, J.M. (1992). *Clinical manual of health assessment* (4th edn). Mosby-Year Book, St. Louis, MO.

Aimed primarily at nurses.

Number of scales: 14 *Psychometrics:* Yes *Scales given:* Yes

6. Cohen, S., Kessler, R.C., and Gordon, L.U. (eds) (1995). *Measuring stress: A guide for health and social scientists.* Oxford University Press, Oxford.

Discusses and assesses stress questionnaires in such areas as life events, chronic stressors, and stress appraisal.

Number of scales: ? *Psychometrics:* Yes *Scales given:* No

7. Comrey, A. L., Backer, T. E., and Glaser, E. M. (1973). *A sourcebook for mental health measures.* Human Interaction Research Institute, Los Angeles, CA.

Discusses unpublished questionnaires, surveys, rating scales, and inventories in the areas of mental health, marriage and family, social relationships, and education.

Number of scales: 1,100 *Psychometrics:* Yes *Scales given:* No

8. Dittmer, S.S. and Gresham, G.E. (eds) (1997). *Functional assessment and outcome measures for the rehabilitation health professional.* Aspen Publishers, Gaitherburgs, MD.

The appendix of this book has 30 scales measuring disability and six assessing social limitations.

Number of scales: 36 *Psychometrics:* Yes *Scales given:* Yes

9. Finch, E., Brooks, D., Stratford, P. W., and Mayo, N. E. (2002). *Physical rehabilitation outcome measures: A guide to enhanced clinical decision making* (2nd edn). B.C. Decker, Hamilton, ON.

Published under the auspices of the Canadian Physiotherapy Association, this book lists scales grouped by outcome (e.g. development, dyspnoea, pain, QOL) and patient population (e.g. paediatric, respiratory, rheumatology). Of these, 15 are given in full on an accompanying CD, and web links to the others are given when available. Psychometric properties of all of the scales are described.

Number of scales: 75 *Psychometrics:* Yes *Scales given:* Some

10. Fischer, J., Corcoran, K. J., and Springer, D.W. (2020). *Measures for clinical practice: A sourcebook. Volume 2* (6th edn). Oxford University Press, New York.

The second volume of this two volume set has scales for adults. For each scale, there is one page describing its norms, scoring system, psychometrics, and availability.

Number of scales: 302 *Psychometrics:* Yes *Scales given:* Yes

11. Frank-Stromborg, M. and Olsen S. J. (2004). *Instruments for clinical health-care research* (3rd edn). Jones and Bartlett, Sudbury, MA.

Covers areas such as measurement and assessment of health and function, outcomes of care, and clinical problems (e.g. anxiety, depression, sleep, body image), as well as coping, hope, and other positive attributes.

Number of scales: ?   *Psychometrics:* Yes   *Scales given:* No

12. Herndon, R.M. (ed.) (2006). *Handbook of neurologic rating scales* (2nd edn). Demos Medical Publishing, New York.

Oriented towards neurologists, it covers areas of generic and general use (e.g. affective lability, quality of life), paediatric development and rehabilitation, movement disorders, ageing and dementia, stroke, headache, and other specific disorders.

Number of scales: 110   *Psychometrics:* Yes   *Scales given:* Some

13. Hersen, M. and Bellack, A. S. (eds) (2002). *Dictionary of behavioral assessment techniques* (2nd edn). Percheron Press, Clinton Corners, NY.

Covers many different techniques to measure attributes such as anxiety, assertiveness, beliefs, and skills. Some of the techniques are scales, while others are structured tasks or even pieces of electronic equipment.

Number of scales: c. 300   *Psychometrics:* Yes   *Scales given:* No

14. Jenkinson, C. (ed.) (1994). *Measuring health and medical outcomes.* UCL Press, London.

Number of scales: ?   *Psychometrics:* Yes   *Scales given:* 4

15. Larson, J.S. (1991). *The measurement of health: Concepts and indicators.* Greenwood Press, NY.

Focuses primarily on indicators of population health, morbidity, and disability.

Number of scales: 8   *Psychometrics:* Yes   *Scales given:* Yes

16. McDowell, I. (2006). *Measuring health* (3rd edn). Oxford University Press, Oxford.

The scales cover physical disability, psychological well-being, social health, depression, pain, general health and quality of life, and mental status. An excellent guide.

Number of scales: 104   *Psychometrics:* Yes   *Scales given:* Yes

17. Nezu, A.M., McClure, K.S., Ronan, G.F., and Meadows, E.A. (2000). *Practitioner's guide to empirically-based measures of depression.* Guilford, Hingham, MA.

Number of scales: 94   *Psychometrics:* Yes   *Scales given:* 25

18. Perlman, C.M., Neufeld, E., Martin, L., Goy, M., and Hirdes, J.P. (2011). Suicide risk assessment guide: A resource for health care organizations. Ontario Hospital Association and Canadian Patient Safety Institute, Toronto, ON. Available at: <https://www.patientsafetyinstitute.ca/en/toolsresources/suiciderisk/documents/suicide%20risk%20assessment%20guide.pdf>.

Covers the assessment of suicidal risk.

Number of scales: 15   *Psychometrics:* Yes   *Scales given:* No

19. Reeder, L. G., Ramacher, L., and Gorelnik, S. (1976). *Handbook of scales and indices of health behavior.* Goodyear Publishing, Pacific Palisades, CA.

Covers health behaviour, health status, and utilization.

Number of scales: ? *Psychometrics:* Yes *Scales given:* Yes

20. Rush, A.J., First, M.B., and Blacker, D. (eds) (2008). *Handbook of psychiatric measures* (2nd edn). American Psychiatric Association, Washington, DC.

Covers areas such as mental health status, disorders of childhood and adolescence, functioning, disabilities, quality of life, adverse events, perceptions of care, stress, and family and relational issues .

Number of scales: 275 + *Psychometrics:* Yes *Scales given:* Some (*c.* 150 on CD)

21. Sajatovic, M. and Ramirez, L.F. (2012). *Rating scales in mental health* (3rd edn). Johns Hopkins University Press, Baltimore, MD.

Covers anxiety, disability, fear, social anxiety, depression, obsessionality, mania, etc.

Number of scales: 120 *Psychometrics:* Yes *Scales given:* For some

22. Sartorius, N. and Ban, T.A. (eds) (1986). *Assessment of depression.* Springer , New York.

Number of scales: 13 *Psychometrics:* Yes *Scales given:* Yes

23. Schutte, N. and Malouff, J.M. (1996). *Sourcebook of adult assessment strategies.* Plenum Press, New York.

Covers depression, delirium, symptoms of psychotic conditions, various fear and anxiety scales, and so forth.

Number of scales: 75 *Psychometrics:* Yes *Scales given:* Yes

24. Stamm, B.H. (ed.) (1996). *Measurement of stress, trauma, and adaptation.* Sidran Press, Baltimore, MD.

25. Stewart, A.L. and Ware, J.E. (eds) (1992). *Measuring functioning and well-being: The Medical Outcomes Study approach.* Duke University Press, Durham, NC.

Focuses on the tests used in a very large study, the Medical Outcomes Study, primarily the MOS-36 (also called the SF-36). Within this limited scope, it provides useful information on some of the indices for social and role functioning, psychological distress, pain, sleep, and the like.

26. Thompson, J.K., Heinberg, L.J., Altabe, M., and Tanleff, D.S. (1999). *Exacting beauty: Theory, assessment, and treatment of body image disturbance.* American Psychological Association, Washington, DC.

Number of scales: 36 *Psychometrics:* Yes *Scales given:* Yes

27. Wilkin, D., Hallam, L., and Doggett, M.A. (1992). *Measures of need and outcome for primary health care.* Oxford University Press, Oxford.

Covers tests in seven areas: functioning, mental health and illness, social support, patient satisfaction, disease-specific questionnaires, multi-dimensional tests, and miscellaneous. A number of tests in each area are reviewed.

Number of scales: 40 *Psychometrics:* Yes *Scales given:* 35

28. Zalaquett, C.P. and Wood, R.J. (eds) (1997). *Evaluating stress: A book of resources* (Vols 1 –2). Scarecrow, Lanham, MD.

Number of scales: 40   *Psychometrics:* Yes   *Scales given:* 20

G. Substance abuse problems

1. Allen, J.P. and Wilson, V.B. (eds) (2003). *Assessing alcohol problems: A guide for clinicians and researchers* (2nd edn). NIAA Treatment Handbook Series 4. US Department of Health and Human Services, National Institutes of Health, Washington, DC.

Covers scales in the areas of screening, diagnosis, assessment of drinking behaviour, adolescent assessment, treatment planning, treatment and process assessment, and outcome evaluation.

Number of scales: 78 *Psychometrics:* Yes   *Scales given:* For 53

2. Lettieri, D. J., Nelson, J. E., and Sayers, M. A. (1985). *Alcoholism treatment assessment research instruments.* NIAA, Rockville, MD.

Number of scales: 50   *Psychometrics:* Yes   *Scales given:* Yes

3. Nehemkis, A., Macari, M.A., and Lettieri, D.J. (eds) (1976). *Drug abuse instrument handbook: Selected items for psychosocial drug research.* NIDA, Washington, DC.

Number of scales: 42   *Psychometrics:* Yes   *Scales given:* Yes

4. Perkinson, R.R. (2021). *Chemical dependency counseling: A practical guide* (6th edn). Sage, Thousand Oaks, CA.

Number of scales: 34 +   *Psychometrics:* Yes   *Scales given:* Yes

5. Perkinson, R.R. (2004). *Treating alcoholism: Helping your clients find the road to recovery.* Wiley, Hoboken, NJ.

Number of scales: 33   *Psychometrics:* Yes   *Scales given:* Yes

6. University of Washington, Alcohol and Drug Abuse Institute. *Substance use & screening assessment instruments database.* Available at: <http://lib.adai.washington.edu/instrumentsearch.htm>.

An online resource. Links are provided to the source of the instrument or to the publisher if it is a commercial scale.

Number of scales: 515   *Psychometrics*: Yes   *Scales given*: No

H. Quality of life

1. Bowling, A. (2001). *Measuring disease: A review of disease-specific quality of life measurement scales* (2nd edn). Open University Press, Philadelphia, PA.

Number of scales: ~200   *Psychometrics:* Yes   *Scales given:* Some

Covers many disease-specific and generic instruments, in areas such as cancer, and respiratory and neurological conditions . It also provides a discussion of the theoretical and practical problems involved in measuring these conditions. An excellent resource.

2. Bowling, A. (2017). *Measuring health: A review of subjective health, well-being and quality of life measurement scales* (4th edn). Open University Press, Philadelphia, PA.

Covers functional ability, health status, well-being, social networks and support, and so forth. A companion book to *Measuring disease.*

Number of scales: 78   *Psychometrics:* Yes   *Scales given:* Some

3. Drotar, D. (ed.) (1998). *Measuring health-related quality of life in children and adolescents: Implications for research and practice.* Lawrence Erlbaum, Mahwah, NJ.

Number of scales: 4   *Psychometrics:* ?   *Scales given:* Yes

4. Fayers, P.M. and Machin, D. (2016). *Quality of life: The assessment, analysis, and reporting of patient-reported outcomes* (3rd edn). Wiley, New York.

Number of scales: 15   *Psychometrics:* Yes   *Scales given:* Yes

5. Salek, S. (1998). *Compendium of quality of life instruments* (Volumes 1–6). Wiley, Chichester.

Includes CDs, so high-quality versions of the scales can be printed. However, priced at over £8,000, so look for it in a library.

Number of scales: 221   *Psychometrics:* Yes   *Scales given:* Yes

6. Spilker, B. (ed.) (1996). *Quality of life and pharmacoeconomics in clinical trials* (2nd edn). Lippincott-Raven Press, New York.

The first edition of this book was called *Quality of life assessments in clinical trials.*

Number of scales: ?   *Psychometrics:* Yes   *Scales given:* No

I. Pain

1. Bush, J.P. and Harkins, S.W. (eds) (1991). *Children in pain: Clinical and research issues from a developmental perspective.* Springer, New York.

Number of scales: 4   *Psychometrics:* ?   *Scales given:* Yes

2. Cohen, L.L., Lemanek, K., Blount, R.L., Dahlquist, L.M., Lim, C.S., Palermo, T.M., *et al.* (2008). Evidence-based assessment of pediatric pain. *Journal of Pediatric Psychology,* **33**, 939–55.

Evaluates scales as 'well-established', 'approaching well-established', or 'promising' according to established criteria.

Number of scales: 17   *Psychometrics:* Yes   *Scales given:* No

3. McGrath, P.A. (1990). *Pain in children: Nature, assessment, treatment.* Guilford Press, New York.

Number of scales: 20   *Psychometrics:* Yes   *Scales given:* Yes

4. Turk, D.C. and Melzak, R. (eds) (2010). *Handbook of pain assessment* (3rd edn). Guil ford Press, New York.

Covers self-reports, assessments by others, special populations (children and older people), and specific pain conditions.

Number of scales: Many   *Psychometrics:* Yes   *Scales given:* 5

5. Tyler, D.C. and Krane, E.J. (1990). *Pediatric pain: Advances in pain research and therapy*. Raven Press, New York.

   Number of scales: ?   *Psychometrics:* Yes   *Scales given:* 5

J. Gerontology

1. Burns, A., Lawlor, B., and Craig, S. (2004). *Assessment scales in old age psychiatry* (2nd edn). Martin Dunitz, London.

Covers areas such as depression, activities of daily living, quality of life, care-giver assessments, and cognitive assessment.

   Number of scales: 241   *Psychometrics:* Yes   *Scales given:* No

2. Eliopoulos, C. (1990). *Health assessment of the older adult* (2nd edn). Addison-Wesley, Menlo Park, CA.

   Number of scales: ?   *Psychometrics:* ?   *Scales given:* 9

3. Gallo, J.J., Bogner, H.R., Fulmer, T., and Paveza, G.J. (eds.) (2006). *Handbook of geriatric assessment* (4th edn). Aspen, Gaithersburg, MD.

Covers substance use and abuse, abuse and neglect of older people, depression, social assessment, driving, assessment of daily living, adherence to medical treatment, and so forth.

   Number of scales: ?   *Psychometrics:* No   *Scales given:* No

4. Israël, L., Kozarevic, D., and Sartorius, N. (1984). *Source book of geriatric assessment* (Volumes 1–2). S. Karger, Basel.

   Number of scales: 126   *Psychometrics:* ?   *Scales given:* Yes

5. Kane, R.A. and Kane, R.L. (1981). *Assess the elderly: A practical guide to measurement*. Lexington Books, Lexington, MA.

   Number of scales: 33   *Psychometrics:* Yes   *Scales given:* Yes

6. Mangen, D.J. and Peterson, W.A. (eds) (1982). *Research instruments in social gerontology: Vol. 1. Clinical and social psychology*. University of Minnesota Press, Minneapolis, MI.

7. Mangen, D.J. and Peterson, W.A. (eds) (1982). *Research instruments in social gerontology: Vol. 2. Social roles and social participation*. University of Minnesota Press, Minneapolis, MI.

8. Mangen, D.J. and Peterson, W.A. (eds) (1984). *Research instruments in social gerontology: Vol. 3 Health, program evaluation, and demography*. University of Minnesota Press, Minneapolis, MI.

   Number of scales: 400 +   *Psychometrics:* Yes   *Scales given:* Some

9. McKeith, I., Cummings, J., Lovestone, S., Harvey, R., and Wilkinson, D. (eds) (1999). *Outcome measures in Alzheimer's disease*. Martin Dunitz, London.

   Number of scales: ?   *Psychometrics:* No   *Scales given:* No

K. Nursing and patient education

1. Beaton, S.R. and Voge, S.A. (1998). *Measurements for long-term care: A guidebook for nurses.* Sage, Thousand Oaks, CA.

   Number of scales: 100 +   *Psychometrics:* No   *Scales given:* Sample items

2. Blattner, B. (1981). *Holistic nursing.* Prentice Hall, Englewood Cliffs, NJ.

   Number of scales: 22   *Psychometrics:* ?   *Scales given:* Yes

3. Block, G. J. and Nolan, J. W. (1986). *Health assessment for professional nursing: A developmental approach* (2nd edn). Appleton-Century-Crofts, Norwalk, CT.

   Number of scales: 7   *Psychometrics:* ?   *Scales given:* Yes

4. Frank-Stromborg, M. and Olsen, S. (eds) (2004). *Instruments for clinical nursing research* (3rd edn). Jones & Bartlett, Boston, MA.

Each of the book's chapters covers a different functional area or clinical problem, such as quality of life, sleep, dyspnoea, pain, or spirituality. Numerous scales are mentioned within each chapter, and most get only one or two paragraphs. A good source of tests, but weak on evaluation.

   Number of scales: ?   *Psychometrics:* Some   *Scales given:* No

5. Guzzetta, C.E., Bunton, S.D., Prinkey, L.A., Sherer, A.P, and Seifert, P.C. (1989). *Clinical assessment tools for use with nursing diagnoses.* C.V. Mosby, St. Louis, MO.

   Number of scales: 26   *Psychometrics:* No   *Scales given:* Yes

6. Joint Commission on Accreditation of Healthcare Organizations (1997). *Nursing practice and outcome measurement.* Oakbrook, Terrace, IL.

   Number of scales: 5   *Psychometrics:* ?   *Scales given:* Yes

7. Lorig, K. (2001). *Patient education: A practical approach* (3rd edn). Sage, Thousand Oaks, CA.

   Number of scales: ?   *Psychometrics:* ?   *Scales given:* 6

8. Lorig, K., Stewart, A., Ritter, P., Gonzalez, V.M., Laurent, D., and Lynch, J. (1996). *Outcome measures for health education and other health care interventions.* Sage, Thousand Oaks, CA.

   Number of scales: 25   *Psychometrics:* ?   *Scales given:* Yes

9. McDaniel, C. and Nash, J.G. (1990). Compendium of instruments measuring patient satisfaction with nursing care. *Quality Review Bulletin,* 16(5), 182 –8.

As the title states, this article describes scales measuring patient satisfaction with nursing care.

   Number of scales: 21   *Psychometrics:* Yes   *Scales given:* No

10. Redman, B.K. (2003). *Measurement tools in patient education* (2nd edn). Springer, New York.

Covers patient teaching tools that can be used for assessment of patients' educational needs, evaluation of teaching effectiveness, and improving quality of care. Includes areas such as diabetes self-management, asthma, stroke care, chronic pain, and osteo-porosis .

Number of scales: 89   *Psychometrics:* Yes   *Scales given:* Yes

11. Sitzman, K.L. and Watson, J. (2019). *Assessing and measuring caring in nursing and health sciences* (3rd edn). Springer, New York.

Number of scales: 22   *Psychometrics:* Yes   *Scales given:* Yes

12. Stanhope, M. and Knollmueller, R.N. (2000). *Handbook of community-based and home health nursing practice: Tools for assessment, intervention, and education* (3rd edn). Mosby, St. Louis, MO.

Primarily checklists for nursing interventions (e.g. catheter management), but also includes scales about eating, nutrition, pain, etc.

Number of scales: 287   *Psychometrics:* Yes   *Scales given:* Yes

13. Strickland, O.L. and Dilorio, C. (ed s) (2003). *Measurement of nursing outcomes: Vol. II. Client outcomes and quality of care* (2nd edn). Springer, New York.

Number of scales: c . 80   *Psychometrics:* Yes   *Scales given:* Yes

14. Strickland, O.L. and Dilorio, C. (eds) (2003). *Measurement of nursing outcomes: Vol. III. Self care and coping* (2nd edn). Springer, New York.

Number of scales: ?   *Psychometrics:* Yes   *Scales given:* Yes

15. Waltz, C.F. and Jenkins, L.S. (eds) (2001). *Measurement of nursing outcomes: Vol. I. Measuring nursing performance in practice, education, and research* (2nd edn). Springer, New York.

Covers areas such as decision-making, clinical judgement, performance appraisal, competence, educational outcomes, and professionalism.

Number of scales: 30   *Psychometrics:* Yes   *Scales given:* Most

16. Ward, M. J. and Fetler, M. E. (1979). *Instruments for use in nursing education research.* Western Interstate Commission for Higher Education, Boulder, CO.

A wide variety of instruments are discussed, ranging from achievement tests of nursing knowledge to attitudes towards nursing and towards various patient groups, learning style, and so forth.

Number of scales: 78   *Psychometrics:* Yes   *Scales given:* Yes

17. Ward, M.J. and Lindeman, C.A. (eds) (1979). *Instruments for measuring nursing practice and other health care variables* (Volumes 1–2). Bureau of Health Manpower, Division of Nursing, Hyattsville, MD.

These volumes cover 140 scales which measure psychosocial factors and 19 measuring physiological variables. They focus on nursing practice rather than education, and stress patient as opposed to nurse variables.

Number of scales: 159   *Psychometrics:* Yes   *Scales given:* No

L. Sex and gender

1. Beere, C.A. (1990). *Gender roles: A handbook of tests and measures.* Greenwood, Westport, CA.

   Number of scales: 211   *Psychometrics:* Yes   *Scales given:* No

2. Beere, C.A. (1990). *Sex and gender issues: A handbook of tests and measures.* Greenwood, Westport, CA.

Covers areas such as sexuality, contraception and abortion, perceptions about child-bearing, somatic issues, homosexuality, rape and sexual coercion, family violence, and body image .

   Number of scales: 197   *Psychometrics:* Yes   *Scales given:* No

3. Beere, C.A. (1979). *Women and women's issues: A handbook of tests and measures.* Jossey-Bass, San Francisco, CA.

Covers published and unpublished tests from 1920 to 1977, regarding 'variables pertinent to women's issues', such as sex roles, sex stereotypes, children's sex roles, gender knowledge, marital and parental roles, and employee roles .

   Number of scales: 235   *Psychometrics:* Yes   *Scales given:* No

4. Fischer, T.D., Davis, C.M., and Yarber, W.L. (eds) (2011). *Handbook of sexually-related measures* (3rd edn). Sage, Thousand Oaks, CA.

Covers sexual behaviour, beliefs, attitudes, and more.

   Number of scales: 218   *Psychometrics:* Yes   *Scales given:* For most

M. Work

1. Bearden, W.O., Netemeyer, R.G., and Haws, K.L. (2010). *Handbook of marketing scales: Multi-item measures for marketing and consumer behavior research* (3rd edn). Sage, Thousand Oaks, CA.

Includes scales of job behaviour (e.g. conflict, burnout, satisfaction, leadership) as well as measures of marketing and consumer behaviour.

   Number of scales: 150 +   *Psychometrics:* Yes   *Scales given:* Yes

2. Cook, J.D., Hepworth, S.J., Wall, T.D., and Warr, P.B. (1981). *The experience of work: A compendium and review of 249 measures and their use.* Academic Press, NY.

Covers areas such as leadership style, job satisfaction, work values, alienation, occupational mental health, job involvement, organizational climate, and commitment.

   Number of scales: 249   *Psychometrics:* Yes   *Scales given:* For 93

3. Fields, D.L. (2002). *Taking the measure of work: A guide to validated scales for organizational research and diagnosis.* Sage, Thousand Oaks, CA.

Covers areas such as organizational commitment, job characteristics, person–organization fit, work-family conflict, job satisfaction, and job roles.

   Number of scales: 136   *Psychometrics:* Yes   *Scales given:* Yes

4. Graham, E.E. and Mazer, J.P. (eds) (2000). *Communication research measures III: A sourcebook.* Rout ledge, New York.

Covers communication in a wide range of areas: organizations, family, sports, public relations, and so forth.

Number of scales: ?   *Psychometrics:* Yes   *Scales given:* ?

5. Price, J.M. and Mueller, C.W. (1986). *Handbook of organizational measurement.* Pitman, Marshfield, MA.

Although oriented towards people in businesses, also covers such topics as autonomy, communication, and satisfaction.

Number of scales: 30   *Psychometrics:* Yes   *Scales given:* For 26

6. Robinson, J.P., Athanasiou, R., and Head, H.B. (1969). *Measures of occupational attitudes and occupational characteristics.* Survey Research Center, Ann Arbor, MI.

This book, one of a series from the Institute for Social Research, covers measures of general job satisfaction as well as satisfaction with particular occupations, values, and attitudes, and of leadership styles.

Number of scales: 77   *Psychometrics:* Yes   *Scales given:* Yes

N. Violence

1. Brodsky, S.L. and Smitherman, H .O. (1983). *Handbook of scales for research in crime and delinquency.* Plenum Press, New York.

Covers scales in the areas of law enforcement and the police, courts and the law, corrections, delinquency, offenders, crime and criminality, and general scales; divided into attitude measures, behavioural ratings, personality assessment, milieu ratings, prediction, and descriptive scales.

Number of scales: 380 +   *Psychometrics:* Yes   *Scales given:* Some

2. Dahlberg, L.L., Toal, S.B., Swahn, M., and Behrens, C.B. (2005). *Measuring violence-related attitudes, beliefs and behaviors among youths: A compendium of assessment tools* (2nd edn). Centers for Disease Control and Prevention, Atlanta, GA.

This compendium is divided into four sections: attitude and belief assessments, psychosocial and cognitive assessments, behaviour assessments, and environmental assessments.

Number of scales: 170   *Psychometrics:* Yes   *Scales given:* Yes

3. Grisso, T. (2003). *Evaluating competencies* (2nd edn). Guilford, Hingham, MA.

Includes tests used in forensic psychology, covering competence to stand trial, waiver of rights to legal counsel and to remain silent, not guilty by reason of insanity, parenting capacity, guardianship, and competence to consent to treatment.

Number of scales: 36   *Psychometrics:* Yes   *Scales given:* No

4. Thompson, M.P., Basile, K.C., Hertz, M.F., and Sitterle, D. (2006). *Measuring intimate partner violence victimization and perpetration: A compendium of assessment tools.* Centers for Disease Control and Prevention, Atlanta, GA.

There are scales in the areas of physical, sexual, psychological/emotional, and stalking victimization; and equivalent scales for perpetration. The document is available at <http://www.cdc.gov/ncipc/dvp/compendium/ipv%20compendium.pdf>.

Number of scales: 20 +   *Psychometrics:* Yes   *Scales given:* Yes

O. Special populations

1. Antonak, R.F. and Livneh, H. (1998). *The measurement of attitudes toward people with disabilities: Methods, psychometrics and scales.* C.C. Thomas, Springfield, IL.

   Number of scales: 24   *Psychometrics:* Yes   *Scales given:* Yes

2. Jones, R.L. (ed.) (1996). *Handbook of tests and measurements for Black populations* (Volumes 1–2). Cobb & Henry, Hampton, VA.

Many of the scales are unpublished and not yet validated. Volume 1 covers measures for infants through adults, language assessment, parental attitudes, and family dynamics. Volume 2 includes measures of worldview, spirituality, acculturation, racial identity, mental health, and other areas.

   Number of scales: 82   *Psychometrics:* Some *Scales given:* Yes

3. Pontón, M.O. and Leon-Carrión, J. (eds) (2001). *Neuropsychology and the Hispanic patient: A clinical handbook.* Erlbaum, Mahwah, NJ.

P. Miscellaneous

1. Fetzer Institute (1999). *Multidimensional measurement of religiousness/ spirituality for use in health research.* Fetzer Institute, Kalamazoo, MI.

   Number of scales: 15   *Psychometrics:* ?   *Scales given:* ?

2. Hill, P.C. and Hood, R.W. (eds) (1999). *Measures of religiosity.* Religious Education Press, Birmingham, AL.

   Covers scales in areas such as religious belief and practices, religious orientation, religious development, and religious experience .

   Number of scales: 124   *Psychometrics:* Yes   *Scales given:* Yes

3. Kennedy, J.A. (2013). *Fundamentals of psychiatric treatment planning* (2nd edn). American Psychiatric Publishers, Washington, DC.

   Number of scales: 11   *Psychometrics:* Yes   *Scales given:* Yes

4. Kirby, R.F. (1991). *Kirby's guide to fitness and motor performance tests.* BenOak Publishing Co., Cape Girardeau, MO.

   Number of scales: 193   *Psychometrics:* Yes   *Scales given:* Yes

5. Ostrow, A.C. (1996). *Directory of psychological tests in the sport and exercise sciences* (2nd edn). Fitness Information Technology, Morgantown, WV.

Covers primarily non-commercial scales used for research.

   Number of scales: 314   *Psychometrics:* Yes   *Scales given:* No

6. Redman, B.K. (2002). *Measurement instruments in clinical ethics.* Sage, Thousand Oaks, CA.

Includes areas important in ethics, such as autonomy, comprehension, decisional capacity, information style, and desire for a role in decision-making.

   Number of scales: 65   *Psychometrics:* Yes   *Scales given:* Yes

A (very) brief introduction to factor analysis

Exploratory factor analysis

Assume you are developing a test to measure a person's level of anxiety. After following the steps in Chapter 3 ('Devising the items'), you come up with the following ten items:

1. I often avoid high places.

2. I worry a lot.

3. My hands often get sweaty.

4. I cross the street in order to avoid having to meet someone.

5. I have difficulty concentrating.

6. I can often feel my heart racing.

7. I find myself pacing when I'm under stress.

8. I frequently feel tense.

9. When I'm under stress, I tend to get headaches.

10. People tell me I have trouble letting go of an idea.

There are three hypotheses regarding the way these ten items are related. At the one extreme, the first hypothesis is that they are totally unrelated, and tap ten different, uncorrelated aspects of anxiety. The second, at the other extreme, is that they are all highly correlated with each other. The third hypothesis is somewhere in the middle: that there are groups of items that cluster together, with each cluster tapping a different aspect of anxiety. A natural place to begin is to look at the correlation matrix. If all of the correlations are high, it would favour the second hypothesis; while all low correlations would lead you to adopt the first; and groups of items that seem related to each other but uncorrelated with the other groups would support the last hypothesis. There are two problems, though, in simply examining a correlation matrix. First, it is unusual for correlations to be very close to 1.0 or to 0.0; most often, they fall in a more restricted range, making it more difficult to separate high correlations from low ones. Second, even with as few as ten items, there are 45 unique correlations to examine; if there are 30 items, which is more common when we are developing a test, there will be 435 correlations to look at (the number of unique correlations is $n(n-1)/2$) —far more than we can comfortably make sense of. However, we can turn to factor analysis to help us.

What factor analysis does with the correlation matrix is, as the name implies, to derive *factors*, which are weighted combinations of all of the variables. The first two factors will look like:

$$F_1 = w_{1,1}X_1 + w_{1,2}X_2 + ...w_{1,10}X_{10}$$
$$F_2 = w_{2,1}X_1 + w_{2,2}X_2 + ...w_{2,10}X_{10},$$

where the *F*s are the factors, the *X*s are the variables (in this case, the items), and the *w*s are weights. The first subscript for *w* indicates the factor number, and the second the variable, so that $w_{1,2}$ means the weight for Factor 1 and variable 2.

There are as many factors 'extracted' as there are variables, so that there would be ten in this case. It may seem as if we have only complicated matters at this point, because we now have ten factors, each of which is a weighted combination of the variables, rather than simply ten variables. However, the factors are extracted following definite rules. The weights for the first factor are chosen so that it *explains*, or *accounts for*, the maximum amount of the variability (referred to as the *variance*) among the scores across all of the subjects. The second factor is derived so that it:

1. explains the maximum amount of the variance that remains (i.e. that is left unaccounted for after Factor 1 has been extracted), and

2. is uncorrelated with (the technical term is *orthogonal to*) the first factor.

Each remaining factor is derived using these same two rules: account for the maximum amount of remaining variance, and be orthogonal to the previous factors. In order to completely capture all of the variance, we would need all ten factors. But, we hope that the first few factors will adequately explain most (ideally, somewhere above 70 per cent or so when the variables are scales, around 60 per cent when they are individual items) of the variance, and we can safely ignore the remaining ones with little loss of information. There are a number of criteria that can be used to determine how many factors to retain; these are described in more detail in Norman and Streiner (2003, 2014). At this point, the computer will print a table called the *factor loading matrix*, where there will be one row for each variable, one column for each retained factor, and where the cells will contain the *w*s. These weights are called the *factor loadings*, and are the correlations between the variables and the factors. After we have done this initial factor extraction, we usually find that:

1. the majority of the items 'load' on the first factor

2. a number of the items load on two or more factors

3. most of the factor loadings are between 0.3 and 0.7, and

4. each factor after the first has some items that have positive weights and other items with negative weights.

Mathematically, there is nothing wrong with any of these, but they make the interpretation of the factors quite difficult.

To try to overcome these four problems, the factors are *rotated*. In the best of cases, this results in:

1. a more uniform distribution of the items among the factors that have been retained

2. items loading on one and only one factor

3. loadings that are closer to either 1.0 or 0.0, and

4. all of the significant loadings on a factor having the same sign (assuming all of the items are scored in the same direction, which they should be).

A hypothetical example of a rotated factor matrix with three factors is seen in Table B.1.

Table B.1 An example of a rotated factor loading matrix for three factors and ten variables

Item	Factor 1	Factor 2	Factor 3
1	0.12	0.75	0.33
2	0.81	0.11	−0.02
3	0.03	0.22	0.71
4	0.40	0.45	0.27
5	0.74	0.29	0.15
6	0.23	0.31	0.55
7	0.22	0.71	0.32
8	0.86	−0.18	0.17
9	0.33	0.19	0.66
10	0.72	0.21	0.05
Eigenvalue	2.847	1.622	1.581

At the bottom of each column is a number called the *eigenvalue*, which is an index of the amount of variance accounted for by each factor. Its value is equal to the sum of the squares of all of the *w*s in the column, so for Factor 1, it is $(0.12^2 + 0.81^2 + \ldots + 0.72^2)$. Because all of the variables have been standardized to have a mean of zero and a standard deviation (and hence, a variance) of 1.0, the total amount of variance in the data set is equal to the number of variables —in this case, ten. Consequently, Factor 1 accounts for 2.847/10 = 28.47 per cent of the variance, and the three factors together account for (2.847 + 1.622 + 1.581)/10 = 6.050/10 = 60.5 per cent of the variance; this is typical when the variables are individual items, rather than scales.

The items that load highest on Factor 1 are 2, 5, 8, and 10, which appear to tap the *cognitive* aspect of anxiety. Similarly, Factor 2, composed of items 1, 4, and 7, reflects the *behavioural* component; and Factor 3, with items 3, 6, and 9, measures the *physiological* part of anxiety. Note also that, although item 4 loads most heavily on Factor 2, its loading on Factor 1 is nearly as high. This *factorially complex* item may warrant rewording in a revised version.

This is the older, more traditional form of factor analysis, and is generally what is meant when people use the term. Because a new form of factor analysis was later introduced (described in the next section on confirmatory factor analysis), a way had to be found to distinguish the two. Consequently, this is now referred to as *exploratory factor analysis* (EFA). This reflects the fact that we start with no a priori hypotheses about the correlations among the variables, and rely on the procedure to explore what relationships do exist. This example was also somewhat contrived, in that the rotated solution was easily interpreted, corresponded to existing theory about the nature of anxiety (Lang 1971), did not have too many factorially complex items, nor any items that did not load on any of the extracted factors, and there are three items per factor, which is the smallest number needed to mathematically define one. Reality is rarely so generous to us. More often, the results indicate that more items should be written or rewritten, others discarded, and there may be factors which defy explanation.

It cannot be emphasized too strongly that EFA should not be used with dichotomous items, and most likely not with ordered category (e.g. Likert scale) items either (which makes about 95 per cent of factor analyses inappropriate). The reason is that the correlation between two dichotomous items is not a Pearson correlation (r), but rather a phi (ϕ) coefficient. Unlike r, which can assume any value between −1.0 and +1.0, ϕ is constrained by the marginal totals. Table B.2 shows the proportions of people responding True or False to each of two items. The value of ϕ is quite small, only 0.09. However, because the marginal distribution of Item A deviates so much from a 50:50 split, the maximum possible value of ϕ is 0.29 and, compared with this, 0.09 is no longer negligible. Thus, EFA groups items that are similar in terms of the proportions of people endorsing them, rather than their content (Ferguson 1941). Special programs exist to factor analyse dichotomous or ordinal level data, which begin with different types of coefficients, called *tetrachoric correlations* in the case of dichotomous items, and *polychoric correlations* for ordered categories.

Confirmatory factor analysis

Confirmatory factor analysis (CFA) is a subset of a fairly advanced statistical technique called *structural equation modelling* (see Norman and Streiner (2003) for a basic introduction, and Norman and Streiner (2014) for a more complete one). Although it has been around for many years, the earlier statistical programs required a high degree of statistical sophistication. Since about the 1980s, though, a number of programs have appeared that have made the process considerably easier and available to more researchers.

We said in the previous section on exploratory factor analysis that EFA is a *hypothesis-generating* technique, used when we do not know beforehand what relationships exist among the variables. Thus, while it can be used to evaluate construct validity, the support is relatively weak because no hypotheses are stated a priori. As the name implies, though, CFA is a *hypothesis-testing* approach, used when we have some idea regarding which items belong to each factor. So, if we began with Lang's conceptualization of the structure of anxiety, and specifically wrote items to measure each of the three components, it would be better if we were to use CFA rather than EFA, and hypothesize which

Table B.2 Proportions of people answering True or False to two items

		Questions A		
		True	False	
Question B	True	0.40	0.03	0.43
	False	0.50	0.07	0.67
		0.90	0.10	

items should belong to which factor. At the simplest level, we can specify which items comprise each factor. If our hypotheses were better developed, or we had additional information, we can 'constrain' the loadings to be of a given magnitude: for example, that certain items will have a high loading and others a moderate one.

The technique is extremely useful when we are trying to compare two different versions of a scale (e.g. an original and a translated version), or to see if two different groups (e.g. men and women) react similarly to the items. We would begin by running an EFA on the target version in order to determine the characteristics of the items. Testing for equivalence could then be done in a stepwise fashion.

First, we would simply specify that the items on the second version (or with the second group of people) load on the same factors as the original. If this proves to be the case, we can make the test for equivalence more stringent, by using the factor loadings from the original as trial loadings in the second. If this more tightly specified model continues to fit the data we have from the second sample, we can proceed to the final step, where we see if the variances of each item are equivalent across versions. If all three steps are passed successfully, we can be confident that both versions of the test or both groups are equivalent. Various 'diagnostic tests' can tell us which items were specified correctly and which do not fit the hypothesized model. However, unlike EFA, CFA will not reassign an ill-fitting item to a different factor. Excellent guides to using CFA in this way are the books by Byrne (2009). We have listed the one using the program AMOS, but she has also written them for most other programs.

References

Byrne, B.M. (2009). *Structural equation modeling with AMOS: Basic concepts, applications, and programs* (2nd edn). Routledge, New York.

Ferguson, G.A. (1941). The factorial interpretation of test difficulty. *Psychometrika*, **6**, 323–9.

Lang, P.J. (1971). The application of psychophysiological methods. In *Handbook of psychotherapy and behavior change* (eds. S. Garfield and A. Bergin), pp. 75–125. Wiley, New York.

Norman, G.R. and Streiner, D.L. (2003). *PDQ Statistics* (3rd edn). PMPH USA, Shelton, CT.

Norman, G.R. and Streiner, D.L. (2014). *Biostatistics: The bare essentials* (4th edn). PMPH USA, Shelton, CT.

Some common examples of G studies

In this section, we have chosen some examples to illustrate common issues in designing G studies. We show how the facets are derived for some common measurement situations, and what the G coefficient formulae look like. For simplicity, we are only showing the Relative Error coefficients. More details, including the rules for devising G coefficients, can be found in the G_String manual.

Therapists rating patients on multiple occasions

Let us begin with the first simple extension of the essay example. Imagine a study where physiotherapists are rating the physical functioning of a group of respiratory rehabilitation patients. Suppose there are 20 patients in the programme, and two therapists are involved in the care of all patients. Each therapist rates each patient's functioning on a 10-point scale on four occasions—at the beginning of treatment, and after 2, 4, and 6 weeks of therapy.

Like the essay example, there are three factors in the design—Patient, Therapist, and Occasion, with 20, 2, and 4 levels, respectively. Exploring the basic definitional issues, since each therapist rates each patient on all four occasions, all factors are completely crossed (meaning all patients are assessed by all therapists at all occasions using the same 10-point scale) in this design. Patient is the facet of Differentiation. There are two facets in addition to Patient: Rater and Occasion.

The analysis resembles the ANOVA table (Table C.1, where df is the degrees of freedom for the particular main effect or interaction, SS the sum of squares, MS the mean square, and VC the computed variance component, and p, R, and O are Patient, Rater, and Occasion, respectively. As we might anticipate, the major source of variance, 1.41, is Patient. There is some error from Raters (P × R) = 0.129, but the major source of error is the three-way error term, 0.35. There is also a large effect of Occasion.

From these variance components, we can compute the inter-rater reliability. That is, Rater is the random facet of generalization and Occasion is the fixed facet of generalization. (For the relative error coefficient, this omits the main effects of Rater and Occasion from the numerator and denominator.)

$$G\left(Rater\right) = \frac{V\left(p\right) + V\left(pO\right)}{V\left(p\right) + V\left(pO\right) + V\left(pR\right) + V\left(OR\right) + V\left(pOR\right)} = \frac{1.45}{1.93} = 0.75.$$

Note that because Rater is random, the main effect R and the OR interaction are both considered error terms (but since V(OR) is negative it is set to zero). We can also

Table C.1 ANOVA table—example 1: physiotherapy ratings

Effect	df	SS	MS	VC
p	19	232.88	12.26	1.416
O	3	104.15	34.72	0.858
R	1	2.50	2.50	0.021
pO	57	23.35	0.41	0.029
pR	19	16.50	0.87	0.129
OR	3	0.95	0.32	−0.002
pOR	57	20.05	0.35	0.352

compute the inter-occasion (or test–retest) G coefficient, which makes O the random facet and Rater is fixed:

$$G(Occasion) = \frac{V(p) + V(pR)}{V(p) + V(pO) + V(pR) + V(OR) + V(pOR)} = \frac{1.55}{1.93} = 0.80.$$

We could do the equivalent of a D study, and compute a G coefficient corresponding to the average across all four occasions and both raters (rater and occasion are random facets):

$$G(OR, average) = \frac{V(p)}{V(p) + \dfrac{V(pO)}{4} + \dfrac{V(pR)}{2} + \dfrac{V(OR)}{8} + \dfrac{V(pOR)}{8}} = \frac{1.42}{1.50} = 0.95.$$

There is one final coefficient we will compute. This is a situation where we would hope to see improvement over time—what is called 'responsiveness' (see Chapters 10 and 11). Although, typically, responsiveness is expressed as an effect size, it could also be shown as a G coefficient. In the present example, the coefficient would look like:

$$G(pR) = \frac{V(O)}{V(O) + V(pO) + V(OR) + V(pOR)} = \frac{0.86}{1.24} = 0.69.$$

OSCE

The Objective Structured Clinical Examination or OSCE has become the mainstay of performance assessment in the health sciences. In an OSCE, each student rotates through a series of 'stations', each typically lasting 10–15 minutes, where they are required to demonstrate some aspect of clinical competence—performing a brief history or physical examination, counselling a patient, and so forth. The 'patient' is usually a 'standardized patient', a person trained to simulate a disorder.

Students may be scored with a station-specific checklist of things that should be done, or with global ratings, which are often common across stations. Scoring can be done by either the patient, after the encounter is over, or by a physician examiner.

OSCEs are almost always evaluated with G study methods. In this example, we have a highly nested design—the Raters are nested within Station, and if we use checklists, the Items are nested within Station (but not within Rater). If the study uses global ratings which are common to all stations, only Rater is nested; Item is crossed with Station.

The present example is a database derived from a special OSCE used for medical school admissions, called a Multiple Mini Interview or MMI (Eva et al. 2004). In this study we had 18 students, and six stations, each with two raters, and four rating scales common to all stations. So there are four facets in the design: Participant (p) with 18 levels, Station (s) with six, Rater:Station (r:s) with two per station, and Item (i) with four levels, crossed with Station.

Participant is the facet of differentiation; Station, Rater, and Item are all facets of generalization. Rater is nested in Item, and all others are crossed. The analysis is shown in Table C.2. As before, the largest variance component is Person (0.665). However, there are also large error variances related to Rater (i.e. a rater bias term), P × S (some

Table C.2 ANOVA table—example 2: admissions OSCE

Effect	df	SS	MS	VC
p	17	658.56	38.739	0.664
S	5	43.17	8.634	−0.225
R:S	6	227.21	37.869	0.468
L	3	12.97	4.325	0.016
pS	85	585.26	6.885	0.402
pR:S	102	370.25	3.629	0.834
pI	51	13.60	0.226	−0.005
SI	15	12.53	0.835	0.000
RI:S	18	13.98	0.776	0.026
pSI	255	83.79	0.328	0.018
pRI:S	306	89.42	0.292	0.292

Source: unpublished data

applicants do well on some stations and others on other stations), and P × R (different raters like different applicants).

We can now proceed to let the computer calculate the G coefficients. First, with R as the random facet of generalization (inter-rater reliability), the formula looks like (again, for the Relative Error coefficient):

$$G(R) = \frac{V(p) + V(pS) + V(pI) + V(pSI)}{V(p) + V(pS) + V(pI) + V(pSI) + V(pR:S) + V(RI:S) + V(pRI:S)}$$
$$= \frac{1.08}{2.23} = 0.48.$$

For Item as the facet of generalization, the coefficient looks like:

$$G(I) = \frac{V(p) + V(pS) + V(pR:S)}{V(p) + V(pS) + V(pI) + V(pSI) + V(pR:S) + V(RI:S) + V(pRI:S)}$$
$$= \frac{1.90}{2.23} = 0.85.$$

However, it may actually be more appropriate to consider the equivalent of the internal consistency, which amounts to dividing any term with i by 4. The new formula then looks like:

$$G(IAverage) = \frac{V(p) + V(pS) + V(pR:S)}{V(p) + V(pS) + \dfrac{V(pI)}{4} + \dfrac{V(pSI)}{4} + V(pR:S) + \dfrac{V(RI:S)}{4} + \dfrac{V(pRI:S)}{4}}$$
$$= \frac{1.90}{1.98} = 0.96.$$

Then, for generalizing across stations (inter-station reliability), the G coefficient would be:

$$G(S) = \frac{V(p) + V(pI)}{V(p) + V(pS) + V(pI) + V(pSI) + V(pR:S) + V(RI:S) + V(pRI:S)}$$
$$= \frac{0.66}{2.23} = 0.295.$$

Finally, the overall reliability of the test is:

$$G(RSIAverage) =$$
$$\frac{V(p)}{V(p) + \dfrac{V(pS)}{6} + \dfrac{V(pI)}{4} + \dfrac{V(pSI)}{24} + \dfrac{V(pR:S)}{12} + \dfrac{V(RI:S)}{48} + \dfrac{V(pRI:S)}{48}}$$
$$= \frac{0.664}{0.807} = 0.81$$

OSCE with applicant nested in a stratification facet

It is not always the case that the facet of differentiation is crossed with all the other facets. As one example, the OSCE is often run with separate circuits or on separate days to accommodate all the candidates. Under these circumstances, Candidate would be nested in Circuit or Day and we would call Circuit or Day a stratification facet. Of course, in this case, the hope would be that there is no effect of Day since this would amount to a bias in the test, perhaps because of poor security, so that on later days, the students hear about the questions and do better. On the other hand, one might be genuinely interested in some of these variables. For example, in the admissions OSCE described earlier, do women, who have on average higher verbal ability, do better on the MMI? In these circumstances, Gender would be another grouping variable, with Candidate nested in Gender.

There may be even more explicit interest in seeing a difference between groups; for example, a test of problem-solving skill might be administered to senior and junior students, and an effect of educational level would provide a test of validity. Alternatively, the groups may result from a true experiment, such as a contrast between two strategies for teaching clinical skills. As a specific example, another study conducted with the MMI had a nine station test run over four successive days. The investigators were also interested in the effect of Gender on performance; so, this was included as an explicit between-subject factor. There was only one rater per station, and the analysis will just look at the total score per station.

The inclusion of between-subject factors results in a bit more complex specification of the design to include these factors. The resulting analysis of variance then provides a direct test of the effect of the factors. The presence of a stratification facet has a small effect on the G coefficient; the hypothesis of interest dictates whether you use the Relative (Effect assumed) or Absolute (No effect assumed) coefficient.

Setting up the program, there are four facets—Day (D; with four levels), Gender (G; with two levels), both stratification facets; Applicant (A; the facet of differentiation with varying numbers in each Day/Gender combination); and Station (S; with nine). Applicant is nested in both Day and Gender so is written A:DG. The analysis of variance is shown in Table C.3. As we can see, there is no evidence of an effect of Day or Gender on the scores, since both computed variance components are negative, equivalent to an F-ratio less than 1.

The calculation of the G coefficient is straightforward as it is actually a one-facet design, and all we can consider is generalizing across stations.

The G coefficient for a single observation, equivalent to the average correlation between any two station scores, is just (again a Relative Error coefficient omitting main effect of Station and interactions with stratification facets):

$$G(S) = \frac{V(A:DG)}{V(A:DG) + V(SA:DG)} = \frac{0.366}{2.01} = 0.18,$$

and for the nine-station test it equals:

$$G(S, Average) = \frac{V(A:DG)}{V(A:DG) + \dfrac{V(SA:DG)}{9}} = \frac{0.366}{0.548} = 0.67.$$

Table C.3 ANOVA table—example 3: admissions OSCE, applicant nested in Day and Gender

Effect	df	SS	MS	VC
D	3	6.66	2.219	−0.036
G	1	0.47	0.469	−0.019
A:GD	109	537.54	4.932	0.366
S	8	68.07	8.510	−0.007
DG	3	24.75	8.250	0.013
DS	24	155.05	6.460	0.112
GS	8	43.36	5.420	0.036
DGS	24	77.09	3.212	0.110
AS:GD	872	1430.80	1.640	1.640

Source: data from Eva, K.W. et al., An admission OSCE: The multiple mini interview, *Medical Education*, Volume 38, Issue 3, pp. 314–26, Copyright © 2004 Blackwell Publishing Ltd.

An overall reliability of 0.67 would be generally viewed as unacceptably low. If we wanted to see how many stations are required to achieve a reliability of 0.80, for example, we can simply insert various numbers into the equation until the computed G coefficient exceeds 0.80. In this case, it would take about 16 stations.

The unique aspects of this design are the combination of the between- and within-subject factors that characterize many experiments, where students are allocated to two or more groups, then take some test with multiple components. While in this case we were hoping that the nesting variables (Day, Gender) would not be significant, and they weren't, in an experiment, where subjects are nested in treatment groups, the primary effect of interest may well be these nesting variables.

There are some interesting concepts arising from this design which we alluded to earlier. If the study really does arise from an experiment or quasi-experiment, where we anticipate differences between the groups, one easy but dishonest way to inflate the G coefficients is to analyse the study ignoring the grouping factor (e.g. educational level). The consequence is that whatever variance is attributable to this grouping factor—the experimental intervention or intact differences between cohorts—would be treated as subject variance. The correct approach is to analyse the data as we have, with Subjects nested in Groups.

Moreover, herein lies the paradox identified by Cronbach (1957), in his classic paper, 'The Two Disciplines of Scientific Psychology'. In an experiment, we really do not want the subject variance to be large, since this will eventually become the denominator of the statistical test. In the present example, the effect of Gender would be determined by an F-test equal to $0.469/4.931 = 0.095$, where the denominator is the variance due to Applicant, which appears in the numerator of the G coefficient. Therefore, strangely, we could argue that, when we are using the design to examine treatment differences, we might want to actually show low reliability.

However, it is not quite so paradoxical if we examine the variances more carefully. Low reliability can arise from small between-subject variance or large error variance (relatively). In an experiment, we want both of these sources of variance to be small; in a psychometric study, we want the subject variance to be large and error variance small. We can achieve low subject variance in an experiment by sampling from homogeneous populations (hence long lists of inclusion and exclusion criteria in most drug trials); error variance is reduced in both circumstances by precise measurement.

Student rating of teachers

Frequently, universities build teacher ratings into a course. In this case, the Rater is nested in Teacher, since we will assume that every teacher has a different class with different students (we'll ignore the possibility that some students may be in more than one class in our study). Further, it is plausible that every class is a different size. Just to complicate things slightly, let us assume that the teacher evaluation questionnaire has five items, so Item is another facet, crossed with Teacher and Rater (all students fill out the same items on all teachers).

There are three facets in the design—Teacher, Rater (student), and Item. Suppose we have a study involving six teachers. The class sizes are, respectively, 25, 30, 35, 15, 40, and 55, so Rater:Teacher has these numbers of observations nested in each teacher.

Some attention must be paid to the layout of the data. It is likely reasonable to consider one line on the spreadsheet for each student rater, so each line will have five observations. urGENOVA and G_String do not use indexes; the entire data array is specified simply by the order in which data are encountered. So, we would need to have the successive lines carefully arranged so all the Teacher 1 ratings occur together (the first 25 records), then Teacher 2 (records 26–55) and so on. The design must mirror this layout, so there are two additional facets beyond Teacher: Rater (nested in Teacher) and Item (crossed with Teacher).

The ANOVA would look like Table C.4. There is a large variance due to teachers, suggesting reasonably high reliability, and a relatively large variance associated with raters—different students like different teachers. Perhaps not surprisingly, the variance components related to items are very small, suggesting a 'halo' effect.

Now, in thinking about the G coefficients, in this example it is necessary to rethink our restriction to the Relative Error coefficients. The problem is that the main effect of Rater, when it is nested, is actually equivalent to the sum of the Rater variance and

Table C.4 ANOVA table—example 4: student rating of teachers

Effect	df	SS	MS	VC
T	5	2,968.19	593.64	3.59
R:T	194	2,367.19	12.20	2.39
I	4	1.20	0.30	0.0002
TI	20	5.19	0.26	0.0002
RI:T	776	196.32	0.25	0.253

Rater × Teacher variance, and the latter is the major source of error. So we will carry the main effect of Rater in the calculations.

Computing G coefficients, the G coefficient for generalizing across raters is:

$$G(R) = \frac{V(T) + V(TI) + V(I)}{V(T) + V(TI) + V(R:T) + V(I) + V(RI:T)} = \frac{3.59}{6.23} = 0.58.$$

The average correlation between items is:

$$G(I) = \frac{V(T) + V(R:T)}{V(T) + V(TI) + V(R:T) + V(I) + V(RI:T)} = \frac{5.98}{6.23} = 0.96,$$

which shows that the items are really not independent. We should expect that this would result in a very high internal consistency (coefficient α):

$$\alpha = \frac{V(T) + V(R:T)}{V(T) + \dfrac{V(TI)}{5} + V(R:T) + \dfrac{V(I)}{5} + \dfrac{V(RI:T)}{5}} = \frac{5.98}{6.03} = 0.99.$$

Finally, we can compute the overall generalizability. However, to do so, we must overcome yet another conceptual hurdle. With unbalanced designs, we have to compute the harmonic mean of the number of raters. In this case it is 6/(1/25 + 1/30 + ⋯ +1/55) = 28.3. (The arithmetic mean would be 33.3.) The formula is then:

$$G(R,I) = \frac{V(T)}{V(T) + \dfrac{V(TI)}{5} + \dfrac{V(R:T)}{28.3} + \dfrac{V(I)}{5} + \dfrac{V(RI:T)}{141.5}} = \frac{3.59}{3.67} = 0.98.$$

The extremely high value is a consequence of two characteristics unique to this design. While there are relatively few items, the inter-item correlation (internal consistency) is very high so this contributes little to error variance; conversely, while the inter-rater reliability is relatively low, each Teacher is evaluated by a large number of raters, effectively reducing the contribution of this error variance.

Econometric versus psychometric approaches to rating of health states

As we discussed in Chapter 4, one goal of health utility assessment is to attach a utility—a number from 0 to 100 (or 1.0)—to objective health states, so that rational policy decisions can be made regarding resource allocation to one programme or another. This might be viewed as an 'econometric' perspective. On the other hand, getting patients to rate their own health state can be useful in treatment decisions at the individual patient level, and since the goal is to obtain reliable measurement on an individual, we will refer to this as a 'psychometric' perspective.

Previously, we briefly noted that some of the early studies of the Standard Gamble appeared to show high inter- and intra-rater reliability, as a result of an incorrect analytical approach, and more recent studies have shown much poorer results. The contrast between the approaches used in earlier and later methods is an instructive application of G theory.

If we return to the econometric versus psychometric approaches, and distinguish them in G theory terminology, in the first case, the 'facet of differentiation' is the described health state, and the patient is a rater of the state; in the second, the facet of differentiation is the patient.

In a typical study using the econometric approach (e.g. Torrance 1976), a group of patients (or healthy people) is assembled and asked to rate a number of health states described on paper. They may also be asked to do the ratings a second time a week or two later in order to examine the reproducibility of the ratings. Imagine a study with a total of ten health states, 50 patient raters, and two occasions. This is a three-facet completely crossed study. The facets are State (10 levels), Patient (50 levels), and Time (2 levels). The most likely way to organize the data would be to treat the ten states as items on a test, so that the database would consist of 50 rows (patients), with 20 observations (10 states × 2 levels) on each row.

Note that if we did lay the data out this way, we would treat Patient as the default facet of differentiation. We will eventually override this, and examine the consequences of using State as the facet of differentiation; however, it is precisely this substitution of Patient for State that led to misleading conclusions of the studies cited earlier.

The ANOVA table would look like Table C.5. While these data are fictitious, the resulting coefficients are realistic (e.g. Schunemann et al. 2007). Most of the variance is related to Patient, with variance due to State about ⅓ as large, and variance due to Time very small.

If we consider first the psychometric perspective, we are asking the somewhat obtuse question 'To what extent do ratings of standard health states differentiate among patient raters?' The facet of differentiation will be Patient, and we might examine

Table C.5 ANOVA table—example 5: patient rating of health states

Effect	df	SS	MS	VC
p	49	129,360	2,640	115.0
S	9	55,710	6,190	45.0
pS	441	48,510	110	35.0
T	1	2,270	2,270	1.0
pT	49	9,310	190	15.0
ST	9	13,860	1,540	30.0
pST	441	17,640	40	40.0

generalization across State—a measure of internal consistency, treating States as items on a test, and generalization across Time (test–retest) reliability. The test–retest reliability for a single rating would look like:

$$G(T) = \frac{V(p) + V(pS)}{V(p) + V(pS) + V(pT) + V(pST)} = \frac{150}{205} = 0.73,$$

which shows reasonable consistency of a patient's ratings of an individual state over two occasions. If we were to use this as a ten-item test of patient ratings of health states, we would divide the S variances by 10, as in:

$$G(T) = \frac{V(p) + \dfrac{V(pS)}{10}}{V(p) + \dfrac{V(pS)}{10} + V(pT) + \dfrac{V(pST)}{10}} = \frac{118.5}{137.5} = 0.86$$

showing very good test–retest reliability of the ten-item test. We can also compute the internal consistency in a similar manner:

$$G(T, Average) = \frac{V(p) + V(pT)}{V(p) + \dfrac{V(pS)}{10} + V(pT) + \dfrac{V(pST)}{10}} = \frac{130}{137.5} = 0.95.$$

To finish it off, the overall reliability of the ten-item test averaged across two occasions would be:

$$G(T, Average) = \frac{V(p)}{V(p) + \dfrac{V(pS)}{10} + \dfrac{V(pT)}{2} + \dfrac{V(pST)}{20}} = \frac{115}{126} = 0.90.$$

Thus the test shows very good reliability *in differentiating among patients*. These are the analyses reported in Torrance (1976), who used CTT, one factor at a time. Consequently, he used total scores for each patient across health states to look at test–retest reliability, and Time 1 data to examine internal consistency. The difficulty is that his goal was to examine the use of the instrument to differentiate among health states. Similar analyses were also reported in Feeny (2004), except that, to deal with a single factor at a time, he examined reliability *within* each health state, again examining the ability to tell patients, not health states, apart.

However, from an econometric perspective, patients are not the facet of differentiation; they are raters of health states and it is the health state that is the facet of differentiation. Moreover, it might be well to consider the Absolute agreement, as it is evident from the ANOVA table that there are large systematic differences between patients. This means that we have to include the main effect of patient and time and the Patient × Time interaction in the denominator.

The test–retest reliability now looks like:

$$G(T) = \frac{V(S)+V(pS)}{V(S)+V(p)+V(pS)+V(T)+V(ST)+V(pT)+V(pST)} = \frac{80}{281} = 0.28,$$

so states are not rated consistently over time. The critical test, however, is the generalizability across raters, which has the formula:

$$G(p) = \frac{V(S)+V(ST)}{V(S)+V(p)+V(pS)+V(T)+V(ST)+V(pT)+V(pST)} = \frac{75}{281} = 0.27.$$

Thus, there is very poor between-patient agreement about the utility of different health states. (As we pointed out earlier, the data, while fictitious, are realistic. Actual values of test–retest reliability are reported as 0.67, and for inter-rater 0.26–0.46; Schunemann et al. 2007). Of course, if one uses this method, the actual utility of the state will be an average over the patient raters in the study, so in this case, the generalizability, with 50 patients, is:

$$G(p) = \frac{V(S)+V(ST)}{V(S)+\dfrac{V(p)}{50}+\dfrac{V(pS)}{50}+V(T)+V(ST)+\dfrac{V(pT)}{50}+\dfrac{V(pST)}{50}} = \frac{75}{80.1} = 0.87,$$

which is acceptable.

Author Index

Subject Index

For the benefit of digital users, indexed terms that span two pages (e.g., 52–53) may, on occasion, appear on only one of those pages.

Tables and figures are indicated by *t* and *f* following the page number